AF614954

PHARMACOCHEMISTRY LIBRARY – VOLUME 4

# STRATEGY IN DRUG RESEARCH

Proceedings of the second IUPAC-IUPHAR Symposium held in Noordwijkerhout (The Netherlands), August 25–28, 1981

PHARMACOCHEMISTRY LIBRARY, edited by W.Th. Nauta and R.F. Rekker

Volume 1 The Hydrophobic Fragmental Constant. Its Derivation and Application. A Means of Characterizing Membrane Systems
*by* R.F. Rekker

Volume 2 Biological Activity and Chemical Structure. Proceedings of the IUPAC-IUPHAR Symposium held in Noordwijkerhout (The Netherlands), August 30–September 2, 1977
*edited by* J.A. Keverling Buisman

Volume 3 Pharmacochemistry of 1,3-Indandiones
*edited by* W.Th. Nauta and R.F. Rekker

Volume 4 Strategy in Drug Research. Proceedings of the second IUPAC-IUPHAR Symposium held in Noordwijkerhout (The Netherlands), August 25–28, 1981
*edited by* J.A. Keverling Buisman

PHARMACOCHEMISTRY LIBRARY
Editors: W.Th. Nauta and R.F. Rekker

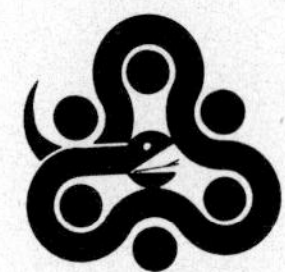

Volume 4

# STRATEGY IN DRUG RESEARCH

Proceedings of the second IUPAC-IUPHAR Symposium held in Noordwijkerhout (The Netherlands), August 25–28, 1981

Edited by

J. A. KEVERLING BUISMAN

*c/o Duphar BV, Weesp, The Netherlands*

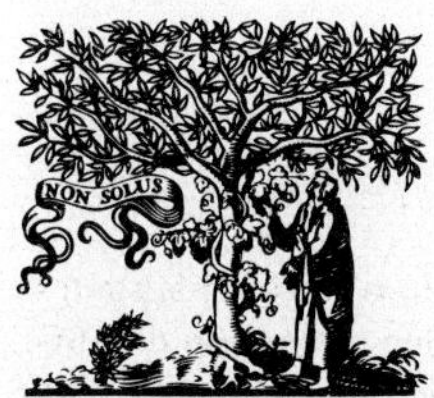


ELSEVIER SCIENTIFIC PUBLISHING COMPANY
Amsterdam – Oxford – New York 1982

ELSEVIER SCIENTIFIC PUBLISHING COMPANY
Molenwerf 1
P.O. Box 211, 1000 AE Amsterdam, The Netherlands

*Distributors for the United States and Canada:*

ELSEVIER SCIENCE PUBLISHING COMPANY INC.
52, Vanderbilt Avenue
New York, NY 10017

Cover design by Dr. C. van der Stelt

**Library of Congress Cataloging in Publication Data**
Main entry under title:

Strategy in drug research.

(Pharmacochemistry library ; v. 4)
Organized by the Medicinal Chemistry Division of the Royal Netherlands Chemical Society under the sponsorship of the International Union of Pure and Applied Chemistry, Commission on Medicinal Chemistry, and others.
Includes index.
1. Pharmaceutical research--Congresses. 2. Structure-activity relationship (Pharmacology) I. Keverling Buisman, J. A. (Jan Anne) II. International Union of Pure and Applied Chemistry. Commission on Medicinal Chemistry. III. International Union of Pharmacology. IV. Series. [DNLM: 1. Pharmacology--Congresses. 2. Research--Methods--Congresses. W1 PH272L v.4 / QV 20.5 I92 1981s]
RS122.S77 615'.1'072 81-19476
ISBN 0-444-42053-3 (v. 4) AACR2

ISBN 0-444-42053-3 (Vol. 4)
ISBN 0-444-41564-5 (Series)



Printed in The Netherlands

CONTENTS

## Preface

The second Noordwijkerhout IUPAC-IUPHAR Symposium "Strategy in Drug Research" was organized by the Medicinal Chemistry Division of the Royal Netherlands Chemical Society under the sponsorship of the International Union of Pure and Applied Chemistry (IUPAC) (Commission on Medicinal Chemistry), the International Union of Pharmacology (IUPHAR), the European Federation for Medicinal Chemistry (EFMC), the Fédération Internationale Pharmaceutique (FIP) and the Royal Netherlands Association for the Advancement of Pharmacy (KNMP).

As for the first symposium in this new series it was the aim of the organizers of the meeting to intensify the dialogue between the two major groups of scientists active in the field of medicinal chemistry, the chemists and the pharmacologists.

The symposium was held during the period of August 25-28, 1981 in Congress Centre Leeuwenhorst in Noordwijkerhout, the Netherlands; 275 participants from 25 countries came to Noordwijkerhout.

The topic "Strategy in Drug Research" was chosen because such strategies can be based upon both chemical and biological findings. Within the subjects : Receptor Studies and Research Strategy; Lessons from Enzyme Chemistry; Toxicological Parameters as a Lead; Pharmacokinetics as a Starting Point; Biological Measurements, Methods and Data Handling; 14 lectures had been chosen as examples for the respective fields which gave together with ± 45 posters a good overview of the actual state of affairs. Interesting results of the designing of 'better' molecules, being the central aspect in the broad field of medicinal chemistry, on basis of receptor studies, theoretical considerations in enzyme mechanisms, toxicological and pharmacokinetic studies as well as on molecular pharmacological investigations were presented. Much emphasis was put on the need for reliable biological parameters in all studies aiming at the design of new molecules.

In the opening lecture special attention was called to drug research strategy for tropical diseases. According to professor Ariëns, in his concluding remarks the pharmacologists and the chemists meet at the receptor level - the receptor being defined broadly -; they should therefore also discuss at this meetingpoint, he said. It is clear that in modern medicinal chemistry, results can only be expected when this discussion takes place in a language understandable for all participants to it. In this respect the symposium "Strategy in Drug Research" contributed in a very positive way.

The proceedings include the full texts of all lectures presented, as well of the four presented during the satellite symposium "The value of predictions in Structure-Activity Analysis", during which symposium the predictive merits of QSAR studies have been amplified.

H. Timmerman
Chairman Organizing Committee

J.A. Keverling Buisman (Editor), *Strategy in Drug Research* 


# DRUGS FOR DEVELOPING COUNTRIES

ADETOKUNBO O. LUCAS, M.D., Director
UNDP/WORLD BANK/WHO Special Programme for
Research and Training in Tropical Diseases

## ABSTRACT

Tropical parasitic infections remain major public health problems in many developing countries. Efforts to control some of these diseases have been hampered by a number of factors both medical and managerial. One specific constraint is the lack of drugs which can be suitably applied in largescale control programmes in the endemic countries. Such drugs should be highly effective, safe, and simple to apply in the field.

This problem has been tackled by the World Health Organization in collaboration with scientists and institutions all over the world, including the pharmaceutical industry. A Special Programme for Research and Training in Tropical Diseases, co-sponsored by the United Nations Development Programme (UNDP), the World Bank, and the World Health Organization (WHO), is seeking new and improved tools for the control of six major tropical diseases - malaria, schistosomiasis, filariasis (including onchocerciasis), trypanosomiasis (both African and the American form called Chagas' disease), leishmaniasis and leprosy. The scientific programme is planned and executed by multidisciplinary groups of scientists. The research programme ranges from metabolic studies of the parasite and the screening of candidate compounds, to clinical evaluation and field trials. Existing drugs are being re-examined and innovative drug delivery systems are being sought.

The issue of drugs for developing countries resolves itself into two separate problems. The first concerns the availability to the people of developing countries, especially to the most needy, of those drugs which are already in general use. This issue is being tackled by the Essential Drug Programme of the World Health Organization which, in collaboration with governments, is examining the various problems associated with the manufacture, purchase and distribution of a basic list of drugs required by the health services of each country.

The second issue concerns the need for new and improved drugs required to deal with diseases which are common in, and mostly peculiar to, the developing countries in the tropics. In dealing with this question, it is important to understand the basis for the geographical distribution of these diseases which are highly endemic in the tropics. Some diseases acquired this distribution in historical times, being cosmopolitan with no special predilection for the tropics until relatively recently. Through the inevitable pressures of development, and in particular, the improvement in environmental sanitation and personal hygiene, these diseases have retreated from the developed countries and are now found mostly in developing countries. Thus epidemics of cholera, for example, no longer occur in developed countries, while they remain a persistent menace in developing countries. The distribution of cholera is now mainly tropical, but its global distribution in earlier times shows that the tropical environment was not a prerequisite for its occurrence. Many such examples can be cited - plague, tuberculosis, and so on. These diseases can be seen as being tropical in the historical perspective.

There is another group of diseases for which the tropical climate plays a significant role in their occurrence and distribution. Some, of these, like African trypanosomiasis, onchocerciasis and other filariases, are clearly diseases of warm climates with no possibility of sustained transmission in colder climates. In other cases, such as malaria, minimal transmission did occur in some countries with temperate climate, but because of the biological requirements of the parasite and its vector, the infection had a tenuous hold in these areas. The intensity of transmission graduates from this low level in cold, hypoendemic areas to the wet tropics where the disease is hyperendemic to holoendemic. In parts of tropical Africa, for example, the transmission of malaria is intense, occurring at a rate which is several thousand fold the critical level required to sustain transmission.

In this paper, I will specifically examine the second question - the search for new and improved drugs for the control of tropical parasitic and infectious diseases.

What is the role of drugs in the control of these diseases? In the treatment of infected persons, drugs may prove life-saving in severe cases or, in less seriously ill patients, they may relieve symptoms, arrest and reverse pathological processes. In the public health context, drugs may have an impact on transmission by reducing or eliminating the reservoir of infection in man or, when used prophylactically, by protection of the susceptible persons in the population. The limitations of drugs in the control of these diseases are well recognized; they have been emphasized almost to the point of exaggerating the limitations and underestimating the value of the rational use of drugs in the control of tropical and parasitic diseases. What must be emphasized is that drugs must be used in association with other measures - environmental sanitation and modification of human behaviour - to enhance the impact of chemotherapy and perhaps render the gains more permanent. Without doubt, drugs are useful, even essential, elements in the armamentarium of weapons against tropical diseases.

In response to the call for intensification of research and development in this area, there has been much debate and discussion, and the authorities in this field are apparently divided into two dissenting camps. Some point to the wide variety of anti-parasitic and other anti-infective agents which have been introduced into the pharmacoepia in recent years: piperazine, tetramisole and mebendazole for the treatment of intestinal helminths; niridazole, metrifonate, oxamniquine, and praziquantel for schistosomiasis, and so on.

Whilst welcoming the discovery and duly acknowledging the value of these new drugs, the other camp draws attention to areas of need. For some of the tropical diseases there is a clear need for safe and effective remedies; the available drugs are judged inadequate to meet the needs of programmes for the control of these diseases in endemic areas of the tropics. Authorities differ, not so much on fundamental issues, but rather on emphasis. The first group favours a pragmatic approach, emphasizing the need to apply vigorously the available drugs in association with other measures in the control of these diseases. The second group, no less practical, draws attention to the limitations of some of these drugs, especially in situations where such limitations constitute a significant constraint on control programmes. In such cases, there is a clear indication for research aimed at the development of new drugs or new formulations of existing ones.

The specifications of the ideal drugs for controlling these diseases are dictated by a number of important features of the diseases and the environment in which they occur. Often a high proportion of the community is affected or at risk and therefore control measures must be suitable for large-scale application in the field rather than in hospitals. In view of the shortage of highly trained personnel in most of the affected areas, the ideal drug would be safe enough to permit its administration without supervision by highly trained personnel. It should be effective in producing clinical improvement of disease in the affected individual; and in the context of control, it should also be capable of making a significant impact on transmission. Since these diseases most commonly affect the poor rather than the affluent, the ideal drug must be reasonably cheap so that the governments and the people in most need of it can afford it. In summary, the ideal drug for dealing with each of these tropical diseases should be highly effective, safe, simple to apply and cheap. These specifications are highly demanding, but should be retained as the ultimate goal, and as the yardstick for monitoring progress.

One major effort aimed at intensifying the search for such drugs was initiated by the World Health Organization and co-sponsored by the United Nations Development Programme (UNDP) and the World Bank.

The Special Programme has two interdependent objectives.

1) Development of new and improved tools to control tropical diseases - to develop new preventive, diagnostic, therapeutic and vector control methods specifically suited to prevent, treat and control selected tropical diseases in the countries most affected by them. The new methods must be susceptible to implementation:

- at a cost that can be borne by developing countries;
- requiring minimal skills or specialized supervision; and

- in a manner which allows their integration into the health services, especially the primary health care systems of developing countries.

2) The second objective is the strengthening of biomedical research capability in the countries most affected by tropical diseases, through training in biomedical sciences and various forms of institutional support. Biomedical research capability in tropical countries must be strengthened because major activities in the specification, development and testing of new tools must occur in the tropical countries where the diseases are endemic, to ensure that these tools are effective in controlling the target diseases in these countries.

The six diseases initially included in the scope of the Special Programme are: malaria, schistosomiasis, filariasis, trypanosomiasis (both African sleeping sickness and the American form called Chagas' disease), leishmaniasis and leprosy.

Criteria for selection of the diseases included:

- impact of the disease as a public health problem;
- the absence of satisfactory methods for control of the disease in prevailing circumstances of the tropical countries;
- the presence of research opportunities leading to improved control methods.

The activities of the Programme are directed towards development of any practical tool needed to solve the problems of the selected diseases. Development is focused on drugs, vaccines, methods for biological control of vectors, and diagnostic tests which are simple to perform.

The research and development component of the Programme is therefore concentrated on:

- chemotherapy and chemoprophylaxis,
- immunotherapy and immunoprophylaxis,
- biological control of vectors,
- diagnostic aspects, especially immunodiagnosis

The research is focused upon specific objectives and involves investigators from all relevant areas of the biomedical, physical and social sciences.

Since several major problems requiring research apply to most or all of the six diseases, in addition to disease components, the Programme includes components on epidemiology and operational research, vector control, socio-economic and biomedical research.

Epidemiology and operational research serve to provide the basis for the specifications of the required tools and to assess their effectiveness. The research therefore ranges from the most sophisticated laboratory investigations to the use of simple diagnostic tests in the field. The research and development interlinks with related sectors such as nutrition, economics and education.

Each component is developed under the guidance and with the participation of multidisciplinary groups of scientists organized into a number of Scientific Working Groups, each with clearly defined research goals.

These Scientific Working Groups (SWGs) are the modus operandi of the Programme's research and development activities. An SWG comprises all the scientists who plan and/or carry out research on a specific aspect of the Programme. Members of the Group define the research objectives, devise a strategic plan to achieve them, carry out the research according to the plan, and review the plan and the research as the work progresses. The Steering Committee of a Scientific Working Group manages and guides the Group's activities towards the objectives.

Individual Scientific Working Groups are formed according to needs identified by the Programme's Scientific and Technical Advisory Committee (STAC).

The SWG mechanism for research implies clear goals and precise steps to achieve them, assembled into a time-related strategic plan of action. To develop such a plan and operate an SWG, the scientists must describe:

(1) the detailed objective(s) of the SWG, e.g. the specifications for a malaria vaccine applicable and effective in rural areas;

(2) the current state of the art in relation to the objective(s);

(3) the problems which remain to be solved, i.e. the gaps in knowledge;

(4) the possible research approaches and disciplines which may solve these problems, as well as the feasibility, sequence and cost of the activities, or projects, in each line of research;

(5) a clear strategic plan including each research approach and its line(s) of research, leading towards the final objectives.

One of the major objectives of the Special Programme is to develop and apply appropriate and effective tools for control of the tropical diseases in the affected countries. This goal predicates that the research and development operations cover the entire spectrum of activities required to fill the gaps in knowledge between the current stage of development of these tools and their actual application in the field. These activities will vary, for example, from research into the molecular structure and functions of parasite cell membranes as an early step in vaccine development, to clinical and operational research involving the application of a new or modified chemotherapeutic agent in a rural tropical setting.

Experience over the past four years of the operation of the Programme has confirmed the value of the SWG mechanism. The SWGs involve the participation of scientists from a wide variety of disciplines including:

| | | | |
|---|---|---|---|
| 1. | Immunology | 5. | Pharmacology |
| 2. | Biochemstry | 6. | Epidemiology |
| 3. | Molecular Biology | 7. | Behavioural Sciences |
| 4. | Genetics | 8. | Vector Ecology |

Together with experts in parasitology, tropical medicine and tropical public health, these scientists plan, implement and evaluate the scientific programme. For some of the scientists, this activity represents their first involvement with tropical parasitic diseases. They bring to bear on these age-old problems fresh minds, new perspectives and innovative approaches to their solution.

The chemotherapy section of the working group on each disease is using the same basic strategy: re-examination of the existing drugs, with research aimed at improving their performance in control programmes, and a search for new drugs.

There is reason to hope that the usefulness of the existing drugs can be enhanced by suitable modifications of formulations and dosage. One obvious improvement would be the production of long-acting formulations which would make single-dose applications feasible. Another area of improvement would be revision of dosages to optimize efficacy and minimize toxicity. For some of these drugs, the dosage schedules had been determined by trial and error without the guidance through pharmaco-kinetic studies. Such studies are now being undertaken, and it is hoped that these would provide useful clues for improving the performance of the existing drugs.

The development of new drugs is being tackled using the traditional approach of screening compounds that are identified on the basis of various leads and taking the promising agents through the standard phased testing in man. In addition, aspects of the biology of the parasite are being studied in the hope of identifying metabolic pathways which have features peculiar to the parasite. Such metabolic quirks are possible targets for custom-made chemotherapeutic approaches. The possibility of obtaining more precise targetting of drugs is also being explored by the use of liposomes, lysosomotropic agents and antibody-drug complexes

Some concrete examples will illustrate the approaches that are being made.

## Malaria

The emergence of strains of *Plasmodium falciparum* which are resistant to 4-aminoquinolines, and some other drugs in common use, is a most challenging problem. In order to define the dimensions and the dynamics of the problem, the programme has sponsored projects on the detection and monitoring of drug resistance. Kits for testing the sensitivity of *P. falciparum* *in vitro* are being supplied to scientists and institutions in endemic areas. *In vivo* tests are also being conducted parallel with the *in vitro* assessment. Alternative drug regimes are being tested in areas where the parasite is proving resistant to standard treatment schemes. Studies aimed at the elucidation of the mechanisms of the action of chloroquine suggest that selective binding of the drug to products of haemoglobin digestion may be an important factor in its schizonticidal activity. It has been suggested that the process of selective binding differs in the sensitive strains as compared with those resistant to chloroquine.

Mefloquine, a new drug which was discovered by the Walter Reed Army Institute of Research (WRAIR) is in process of development in collaboration with industry. Phases I and II clinical trials have been completed and more extensive supervised field trials are now planned for the near future.

The Scientific Working Group on the Chemotherapy of Malaria is actively pursuing other approaches in the search for better anti-malarial drugs. In collaboration with Chinese scientists, the group has promoted research on Qing Hao Su, a traditional remedy derived from the plant *Artemesia annua*. The active principle of this plant is a novel compound in anti-malarial chemotherapy. Chinese scientists have tested the parent compound and a number of chemical derivatives have shown to be more potent in their anti-malarial action.

Anti-malarial drugs with long-lasting action could greatly simplify the logistics of drug distribution in mass campaigns. The Group are approaching this question from two main directions. Using the existing technology for producing longacting formulations of drugs, they have been investigating this approach using existing anti-malarial drugs. For example, more effective and less toxic formulations of primaquine are being developed by covalently linking the drug to the hepatotropic carrier, asialofetuin or by using some of its aminoacyl derivatives. In addition, the Group funded research which led to the design of a biological screen specifically designed to identify compounds which have long-acting anti-malarial action.

Metabolic studies on *Plasmodium falciparum* have been greatly facilitated by the landmark discovery by Dr. William Trager of a method for the continuous *in vitro* culture of the parasite. Intensive effort is now being applied in the study of the energy metabolism of the parasite, its lipid metabolism with particular reference to its membranes, its nitrogen metabolism in relation to the digestion of host haemoglobin and so on. In all these studies, there is a search for metabolic pathways and requirements, which differ significantly from those of the mammalian host, as possible targets for drug action.

## Filariasis

Of the various forms of filariasis, river blindness, the disease caused by infection with *Onchocerca volvulus*, has the most serious effect on the population. Furthermore, the existing drugs for the treatment of this infection are inadequate. The highest priority has been accorded to the development of a new drug, especially one which is capable of killing the adult worms of *Onchocerca volvulus* in man. The only macrofilaricide in use against this infection is suramin - a drug which tends to provoke dangerous side effects; furthermore, it has to be administered intravenously over a six-week period.

Whilst the search for a new drug continues, the Group are concerned about improving the use of existing filaricides. They are anxious to determine the safest and the most practical schedules for the immediate treatment of patients who are at risk of blindness from ocular onchocerciasis. They are looking for methods of reducing the damage resulting from the inflammatory response to the dying worms.

The Onchocerciasis Control Programme (OCP) has carried out field trials which indicated that a smaller dose than is normally prescribed remains effective, but is better tolerated than the standard course. Pharmacological studies of suramin are being carried out so as to further refine its use and to provide leads for the development of new drugs related to the parent compound. Similar studies are being done on diethylcarbamazine (DEC); the drug is microfilaricidal in this infection, i.e. it has no significant effect on the adult worms. Furthermore, it provokes unpleasant side effects. Evidence has been produced suggesting that the excretion of DEC is significantly affected by the pH of the urine. Further study of this phenomenon may guide the use of the drug in future.

With regard to the search for a new macrofilaricidal drug, the activities of a network of screening laboratories is being coordinated by the Programme. The biological screens extend from small animal models which serve as the primary and secondary screens, to the cattle screen (*O.gibsoni*, *O. gutturosa*) which so far is the most valid screen for predicting macrofilaricidal activity in man. This screen has indicated that mebendazole in combination with l-tetramisole has embryostatic action, and these findings are now being confirmed in man. Meanwhile, the search continues for truly macrofilaricidal compounds.

The other diseases within the Programme are being tackled in a similar manner. Steps are being taken in each case to re-examine the currently available drugs and seeks ways of optimizing their use in the field. New drug development is being undertaken in collaboration with other agencies, including the pharmaceutical industry. In those cases where industry has undertaken initiatives to develop new drugs, the Programme has collaborated by assisting in the clinical and field evaluation of the new compounds. Where there is little evidence of such interest, the Programme has taken the initiative to promote relevant activity. In these endeavours, the Programme also seeks the collaboration of the pharmaceutical sector.

## Conclusion

The Special Programme represents a new front in the battle against tropical parasitic and infectious diseases. This initiative of the 154 Member States of the World Health Organization represents international collaboration on a global scale involving both north and south, east and west, academia and industry. It complements other efforts such as the Expanded Programme for Immunization, the Water Decade, the Malaria Action Programme and other thrusts against these crippling and killing diseases. It is cast in the context of the drive towards the goal of Health for All by the Year 2000.

...........

Note: This paper is based on the information contained in the Fourth Annual Report of the UNDP/WORLD BANK/WHO Special Programme for Research and Training in Tropical Diseases.

J.A. Keverling Buisman (Editor), *Strategy in Drug Research*



# THE BENZODIAZEPINE RECEPTOR AND ITS LIGANDS

H. Möhler

Pharmaceutical Research Department, F. Hoffmann-La Roche & Co., Ltd., CH-4002 Basle, Switzerland

ABSTRACT

The main central actions of benzodiazepines are due to the enhancement of GABAergic synaptic transmission. This effect is based on the interaction of the benzodiazepines with specific membrane proteins, the benzodiazepine receptors, which are localized in GABAergic synapses and may be part of the postsynaptic GABA receptor unit. Activation of the benzodiazepine receptor by agonists may modulate the GABA-dependent regulation of the chloride channel. Recently, selective benzodiazepine antagonists have been found. Their main representative, Ro 15-1788, is per se pharmacologically inactive at doses which are adequate to block all major central benzodiazepine actions.

## NEURONAL INHIBITION

The nervous system consists of many different populations of nerve cells which can be distinguished by the type of neurotransmitter they use for communication with their respective target (effector) cells. Basically, a neurotransmitter, irrespective of its chemical structure, triggers either an inhibitory or an excitatory response in the effector cell. This signal transfer occurs in specialized contact zones, the synapses. The neurotransmitter is released from its neuron, diffused across a narrow gap to the target cell and is recognised there by specific surface receptors.

Inhibitory signals play a very important role in brain function. They keep the excitatory processes "in check", e.g. by preventing overstimulation of a cell. In addition, they are involved in filtering processes which ensure that "important" information gets priority in brain processing as compared to "less important" information. The excitatory signals have to make their way through arrays of inhibitory mechanisms.

In the brain the most abundant inhibitory neurons are those which use γ-aminobutyric acid (GABA) as neurotransmitter. When GABA interacts with the GABA receptor on the target cell, the associated chloride channel is opened and chloride ions are

*References p. 20*

free to flow through the membrane in the direction dictated by the transmembrane chloride concentration gradient and the membrane potential. This increase in chloride conductance is the basis of the inhibitory action of GABA. In most cases (postsynaptic inhibition) chloride ions flow into the cell. The resulting increase in negative charges (hyperpolarization) makes the cell more resistent to excitatory signals. In case of the nerve endings of primary afferent neurones (presynaptic inhibition) GABA causes a depolarization which reduces the amplitude of the action potential. Consequently less neurotransmitter is released from the nerve ending resulting in a diminution of the excitatory signal of primary afferent neurones.

## BENZODIAZEPINE RECEPTORS

Benzodiazepines have found wide therapeutic application as anxiolytics, hypnotics, anticonvulsants and muscle relaxants. A breakthrough in the understanding of the mechanism of action of benzodiazepines came from mainly electrophysiological studies which showed that benzodiazepines enhance GABAergic synaptic inhibition in the central nervous system (ref. 1). The reinforcement of this physiological inhibitory mechanism is the basis of the main central actions of benzodiazepines.

The discovery of specific high-affinity binding sites for benzodiazepines (ref. 2, 3) opened the way for the biochemical investigation of benzodiazepine actions on the molecular level. The present day view (Fig. 1) stems mainly from four findings.

1) Benzodiazepine actions in the central nervous system are mediated via specific target structures, the benzodiazepine receptors, to which benzodiazepines bind with high affinity. The presence of stereospecific benzodiazepine binding sites in the brain could be demonstrated in in vitro equilibrium binding studies using $^{3}$H-diazepam as labeled ligand. The potency of various benzodiazepines in displacing $^{3}$H-diazepam from these sites corresponded to their potency in exerting their main central actions (Figs. 2,3). The excellent correlation between the binding affinities of a large number of benzodiazepines and their pharmacological potencies provided evidence that the benzodiazepine binding sites were part of brain structures which were involved in triggering the pharmacological response of benzodiazepines. The macromolecules carrying the benzodiazepine binding sites were therefore termed benzodiazepine receptors (refs. 2,3).

2) Using $^{3}$H-flunitrazepam as a photoaffinity probe, the benzodiazepine receptor was shown to be a membrane protein consisting mainly of a protein of molecular weight 50 000 (ref. 4). There are indications that a benzodiazepine receptor may contain more than one benzodiazepine binding site (ref. 4).

3) The benzodiazepine receptor could be visualized autoradiographically on the electronmicroscopic level. The receptors were found to be localized exclusively in synapses (ref. 4). At least some of these synapses could be identified as GABAergic

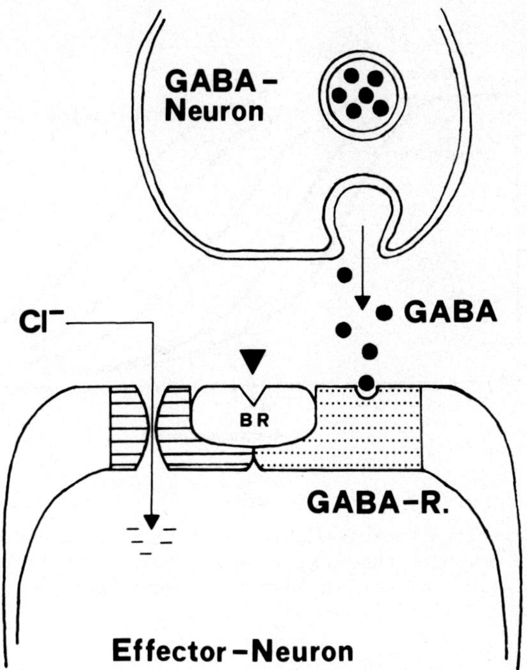


Fig. 1. Simplified working hypothesis of the molecular events in benzodiazepine actions. BR = benzodiazepine receptor ; a benzodiazepine molecule is depicted as triangle ; GABA-R. = GABA-receptor ; $Cl^-$ = chloride, which enters the cell through the chloride channel. For explanation see text.

by immunohistochemical techniques (ref. 5).

4) Although a presynaptic localization of benzodiazepine receptors cannot be excluded, biochemical evidence (refs. 6-8) indicates that the benzodiazepine receptor may be a constituent of the postsynaptic membrane. It may be part of a supramolecular complex, the GABA receptor unit, consisting of the GABA receptor, its associated chloride channel, the benzodiazepine receptor and other proteins. These components are operative in the generation of the postsynaptic potential. The activation of the GABA receptor by the neurotransmitter GABA triggers the opening of the chloride channel. Various protein components, including the benzodiazepine receptor, may be involved in the allosteric interaction between the GABA receptor and the chloride channel. In the presence of benzodiazepines the dynamics of the protein-protein interaction in the GABA receptor unit may be modulated in such a way that the GABA-ergic synaptic transmission is enhanced.

*References p. 20*

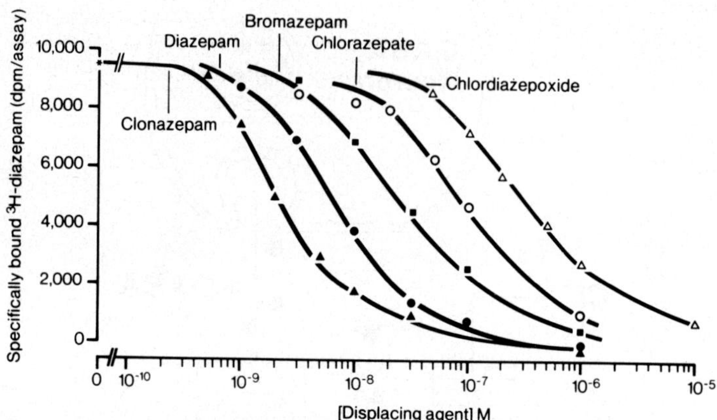


Fig. 2. Potency of various benzodiazepines in displacing specifically bound $^3$H-diazepam. Homogenates of human cerebral cortex were incubated with 1.5 nM $^3$H-diazepam and increasing concentrations of various benzodiazepines (ref. 26).

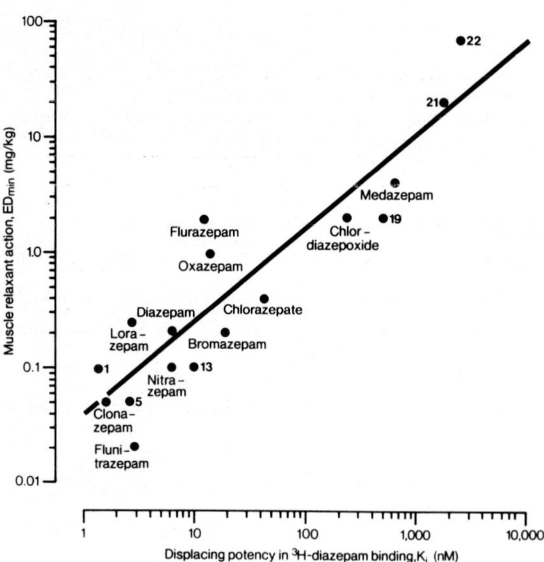


Fig. 3. Correlation between the inhibitory potency (Ki) of various benzodiazepines in $^3$H-diazepam binding in vitro with their pharmacological potency (cat muscle relaxant action, minimum effective oral dose, EDmin) (ref. 3).

## HETEROGENEITY OF BENZODIAZEPINE RECEPTORS

Benzodiazepine receptors in various brain areas cannot be differentiated on the basis of ligand affinity when tested with classical 1,4-benzodiazepines such as diazepam, clonazepam or flunitrazepam (refs. 2,3). However, the triazolopyridazine CL 218 872, which showed moderate affinity to the benzodiazepine receptors in rat cerebral cortex, had a considerably higher affinity to the benzodiazepine receptors in cerebellum (ref. 10). This finding gave rise to the concept of benzodiazepine receptor heterogeneity. Furthermore, photoaffinity labeling of benzodiazepine receptors with $^3$H-flunitrazepam (ref. 4) showed regional differences in the protein pattern. In addition to the main receptor protein (MW 50 000) found in all brain regions, one to three additional proteins were photolabeled (MW 55 000 to 59 000) in hippocampus and several other brain areas while e.g. the cerebellum showed none of the additional photolabeled proteins (ref. 11).

It remains to be seen whether the heterogeneity of benzodiazepine binding sites demonstrated in vitro, is of pharmacological significance. For instance, CL 218 872 seems to maintain only the anti-conflict and anti-metrazol activities while having weak sedative and muscle relaxant components (ref. 10). However, at present, it is not clear whether the pharmacological profile of this compound is indeed due to its regionally different affinity to benzodiazepine receptors or due to so far unknown interactions of the drug with other neuronal systems. Nevertheless, the concept of benzodiazepine receptor heterogeneity may be useful for drug development.

## BENZODIAZEPINE RECEPTOR AGONISTS

The benzodiazepine receptor is highly selective for compounds of the benzodiazepine- and benzazepine - series. They include the classical 1,4-benzodiazepines e.g. chlordiazepoxide or diazepam, the 1,2-anellated benzo- resp. thieno-1,4-diazepines, e.g. triazolam or midazolam resp. Ro 11-7800, the 1,5-benzodiazepinones such as clobazam and the 1- or 2-benzazepines (Fig. 4). In addition, some compounds chemically unrelated to benzodiazepines have been found to bind to benzodiazepine receptors with moderate affinity such as zopiclone (ref. 9), some triazolopyridazines e.g. CL 218 872 (ref. 10) and the phenyl-chinoline derivative PK 8165 (ref. 12) (Fig. 5). These compounds show at least some benzodiazepine-like pharmacological activity.

Other CNS depressants, like barbiturates, meprobamate, ethanol, methaqualone, haloperidol, muscimol do not interact with the benzodiazepine binding sites.

## SELECTIVE BENZODIAZEPINE ANTAGONISTS

Selective antagonists are very valuable tools for the investigation of drug- and neurotransmitter-receptor mediated events.

*References p. 20*

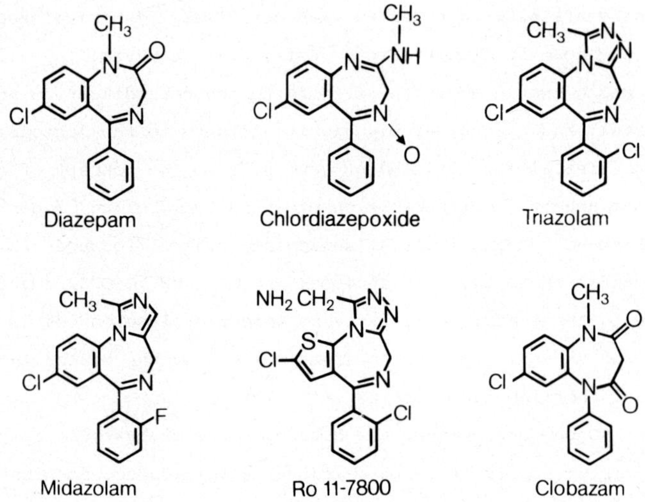

Diazepam Chlordiazepoxide Triazolam

Midazolam Ro 11-7800 Clobazam

Fig. 4. Structural formula of some benzodiazepine receptor agonists.

CL 218 872 Zopiclone PK 8165

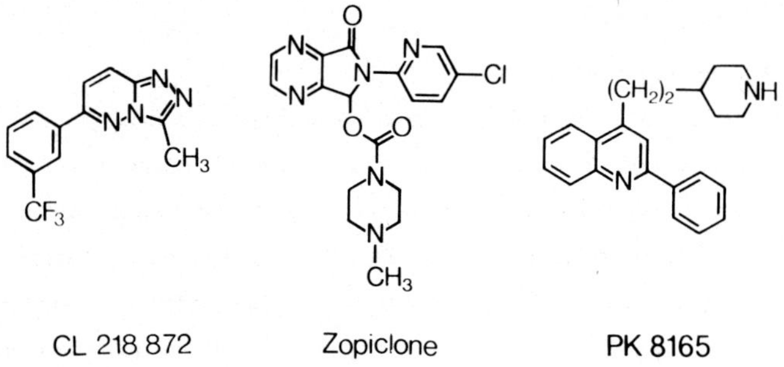

Fig. 5. Benzodiazepine receptor agonists chemically unrelated to benzodiazepines.

In the case of the benzodiazepines no compound was so far available which blocked their actions on the level of the benzodiazepine receptor.

Recently, Ro 15-1788 (Fig. 6), a representative of a series of imidazodiazepines, was found to be a very potent inhibitor of the high affinity binding of $^{3}$H-diazepam to brain synaptic membranes in vitro ($IC_{50}$ = 2 $nmol \cdot l^{-1}$) but failed to produce any of the behavioural or neurophysiological effects of benzodiazepines. Detailed analysis revealed that Ro 15-1788 selectively and potently inhibited all major central actions of benzodiazepines by competitive interaction at the level of the benzodiazepine receptor (refs. 13-15).

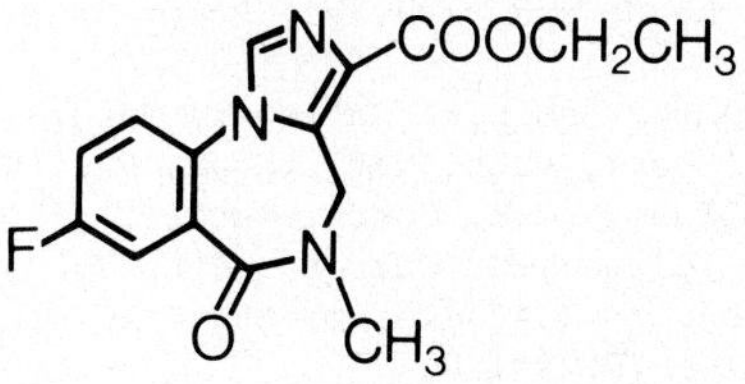

Fig. 6. Structural formula of Ro 15-1788 (ethyl-8-fluoro-5,6-dihydro-5-methyl-6-oxo-4H-imidazo[1,5][1,4]benzodiazepine-3-carboxylate.

The antagonistic action of Ro 15-1788 is restricted to pharmacologically active ligands of the central type of benzodiazepine receptor, i.e. benzodiazepines and chemically unrelated compounds such as zopiclone and CL 218 872. The effects of central depressants which do not act via the benzodiazepine receptor sites such as ethanol, phenobarbitone, methaqualone, meprobamate, haloperidol, etazolate, l-cycloserine and muscimol were not antagonized by Ro 15-1788 (refs. 13-15).

Ro 15-1788 could find therapeutic application as an antidote in cases of intoxication involving overdoses of benzodiazepines, and in anaesthesiology for abbreviating the state of sedation when a benzodiazepine is used as inducing agent. Ro 15-1788 will be used to counteract the central effects of 3-methyl-clonazepam, a benzodiazepine which is very effective in the treatment of schistosomiasis (refs. 16,17). Ro 15-1788 by itself has so far not been found to have intrinsic pharmacological effects in man (ref. 18) and does not impair the schistosomicidal action of 3-methyl-clonazepam (ref. 13).

The chemically unrelated compounds methyl- or ethyl-β-carboline-3-carboxylate (ref. 19) and CGS 8216 (ref. 20) also antagonize at least some benzodiazepine actions. These compounds however, are non-selective benzodiazepine antagonists since they are convulsants or proconvulsants or antagonize also barbiturate and meprobamate effects (refs. 20-25).

ACKNOWLEDGEMENT

I thank Dr. W. Haefely for critical reading of the manuscript.

*References p. 20*

REFERENCES

1 W. Haefely, A. Kulcsar, H. Möhler, L. Pieri, P. Polc and R. Schaffner, Advances in Biochemical Pharmacology, 14(1975)131-151.
2 R.F. Squires and C. Braestrup, Nature, 266(1977)732-734.
3 H. Möhler and T. Okada, Science, 198(1977)849-851.
4 H. Möhler, M.K. Battersby and J.G. Richards, Proc. Natl. Acad. Sci. USA, 77(1980)1666-1670.
5 H. Möhler, J.G. Richards and Y.-J. Wu, Proc. Natl. Acad. Sci. USA, 78(1981) 1935-1938.
6 J.F. Tallman, W. Thomas and D.W. Gallager, Nature, 274(1978)383-385.
7 M. Karobath and G. Sperk, Proc. Natl. Acad. Sci. USA, 76(1979)1004-1008.
8 A. Guidotti, G. Toffano and E. Costa, Nature, 275(1978)553-555.
9 J.C. Blanchard, A. Boireau, C. Garret and L. Julou, Life Sci., 24(1979)2417-2420.
10 A.S. Lippa, E.N. Coupet, C.A. Greenblatt, C.A. Klepner and B. Beer, Pharmacol. Biochem. Behav., 11(1979)99-106.
11 W. Sieghart and M. Karobath, Nature, 286(1980)285-287.
12 G. Lefur, J. Mizoule, M.C. Burgevin, O. Ferris, M. Heaulme, A. Gauthier, C. Gueremy and A. Uzan, Life Sci., 28(1981)1439-1448.
13 W. Hunkeler, H. Möhler, L. Pieri, P. Polc, E.P. Bonetti, R. Cumin, R. Schaffner and W. Haefely, Nature, 290(1981)514-516.
14 H. Möhler, W.P. Burkard, H.H. Keller, J.G. Richards and W. Haefely, J. Neurochem., 37(1981)714-722.
15 P. Polc, J.-P. Laurent, R. Scherschlicht and W. Haefely, Naunyn-Schmiedeberg's Arch. Pharmacol., 316(1981)317-325.
16 H.R. Stohler, in W. Siegenthaler and R. Lüthy (Eds.), Current Chemotherapy, American Society for Microbiology, Washington DC, 1978, pp.147-148.
17 R. Pax, J.L. Bennett and R. Fetterer, Naunyn Schmiedeberg's Arch. Pharmacol., 304(1978)309-315.
18 A. Darragh, M. Scully, R. Lambe, I. Brick, C. O'Boyle and W.W. Downie, The Lancet, July 4(1981)8-10.
19 C. Braestrup, M. Nielsen and C.E. Olsen, Proc. Natl. Acad. Sci. USA, 77(1980) 2288-2292.
20 P. Bernard, K. Bergen, R. Sobiski and R.D. Robson, Pharmacologist., 23(1981)150.
21 R. Mitchell and I. Martin, Europ. J. Pharmacol., 68(1980)513-514.
22 P.J. Cowen, A.R. Green, D.J. Nutt and I.L. Martin, Nature, 290(1981)54-55.
23 R.A. O'Brien, W. Schlosser, N.M. Spirt, S. Franco, W.D. Horst, P. Polc and E.P. Bonetti, Life Sci., 29(1981)775-782.
24 P. Polc, N. Robert and M. Wright, Brain Res., 217(1981)216-220.
25 C. Cepeda, T. Tanaka, R. Besselievre, P. Potier, R. Naquet and J. Rossier, Neuroscience Letters, 24(1981)53-57.
26 H. Möhler and T. Okada, Brit. J. Psychiatry, 133(1978)261-268.

J.A. Keverling Buisman (Editor), *Strategy in Drug Research*



# THE PROBING AND THE MODE OF ACTION OF β- AND $\alpha_2$-ADRENERGIC RECEPTORS

A. Levitzki

Department of Biological Chemistry, The Hebrew University of Jerusalem, Jerusalem (Israel)

## ABSTRACT

β-Adrenergic agonists activate adenylate cyclase only in the presence of guanyl nucleotides, where the physiological representative is GTP. The inhibition of adenylate cyclase by $\alpha_2$-adrenergic agonists also requires GTP but at concentrations higher than those required for activation. The activation of the enzyme by a β -agonist involves the facilitation of the rate of conversion of the enzyme complex from its inactive state to its active cAMP producing state. Termination of the signal elicited by the stimulatory hormone involves the hydrolysis of GTP at the GTP regulatory site. The inhibitory action of the $\alpha_2$-agonist seems to involve a low affinity GTP site which interacts directly with the catalytic unit, or which inhibits the interaction between the catalytic unit and the stimulatory GTP site.

---

## INTRODUCTION

Catecholamines interact with specific receptors, triggering a variety of cellular processes which depend on the target cell and reaching a variety of tissues on which they again act as hormones. The interaction of the catecholamine with the receptor triggers a primary biochemical reaction executed by a catalytic apparatus coupled to the catecholamine receptor. Three types of biochemical events have been recognized: 1. activation of adenylate cyclase by β-adrenergic receptor, 2. inhibition of adenylate cyclase by $\alpha_2$-adrenergic receptor, and 3. activation of phosphatidyl inositol turnover and influx of $Ca^{++}$, both of which activate C-kinase by the $\alpha_1$-adrenergic receptor. Other events that follow the binding of an agonist to the receptor have been encountered as well; for example, the change in membrane potential and the activation of phosphatidylethanolamine methylation as a result of β-receptor occupancy. The roles of the two latter events have not yet been fully delineated.

Subsequent to the triggering reactions, a cascade of biochemical reactions is further triggered, eventually yielding the final physiological response of the cell and the tissue. Here we shall exclusively analyze the current knowledge of

*References p. 35*

the $\beta$ and $\alpha_2$-adrenergic receptors and their mode of coupling to the enzyme adenylate cyclase.

## RESULTS AND DISCUSSION

<u>Biochemical signals coupled to $\beta$-adrenergic and $\alpha_2$-adrenergic receptors</u>

### A. $\beta$-Adrenergic Receptors

Of all catecholamine receptors, the $\beta$-adrenergic receptors have been given the most attention. This may be due to the fact that the primary biochemical signal elicited upon agonist binding to the surface $\beta$-receptors has been identified and found to be the activation of adenylate cyclase producing the "second messenger" cAMP from ATP within the target cell (ref. 1).

$$\text{ATP} \xrightarrow{\text{l-catecholamine}} \text{cAMP} + \text{Ppi} \qquad (1)$$

In this respect, the coupling between the $\beta$-adrenergic receptor and the enzyme adenylate cyclase is similar to the coupling between adenylate cyclase and hormone receptors to certain polypeptide hormones such as glucagon, ACTH, and secretin. In certain cells such as the liver cell and the fat cell, $\beta$-adrenergic receptors as well as receptors for polypeptide hormones are coupled to the enzyme adenylate cyclase. The second messenger cAMP produced intracellularly by the enzyme adenylate cyclase triggers a large variety of biochemical events typical to the cell, usually through the activation of protein kinase, as a first step. The activation of adenylate cyclase by $\beta$-adrenergic agonists is mediated by the nucleotide GTP which acts in a synergistic fashion with the catecholamines (for review see ref. 2). It seems that both the occupancy of the $\beta$-adrenergic receptor with agonists and the level of intracellular GTP determine the final output of cAMP by the enzyme adenylate cyclase. The role of GTP in the activation of adenylate cyclase has been extensively studied and will be examined in detail when the mechanistic aspects of the mode of coupling of the receptor with the enzyme are discussed. The other biochemical responses which are cAMP independent were claimed to be coupled to the $\beta$-receptor. One is the catecholamine-dependent $Ca^{++}$ efflux, and the other is phosphatidylethanolamine carboxymethylation.

1. <u>$\beta$-Receptor-Induced $Ca^{++}$ Efflux</u>. It was shown in both turkey (ref. 3) and human erythrocytes (ref. 4) that $^{45}Ca^{++}$ efflux is enhanced by $\beta$-agonists and blocked by $\beta$-antagonists. This effect is not mimicked by cAMP or dibutyryl cAMP and, therefore, is most probably not mediated by adenylate cyclase. It is interesting that $\beta$-receptor-dependent adenylate cyclase from turkey erythrocytes, as well as many other adenylate cyclases, is strongly inhibited by $Ca^{++}$. For the $\beta$-receptor-dependent turkey adenylate cyclase it was shown that the $Ca^{++}$ ions interact at a specific allosteric site (refs. 5, 6). These findings suggest (ref. 3) that the first effect of a $\beta$-agonist is the deinhibition of the enzyme which

is in the resting state in the inhibited $Ca^{++}$bound form, by releasing $Ca^{++}$ from the regulatory site. These findings are so far restricted to the turkey and the human erythrocyte systems (which possess a few β-receptors), and it is not clear at this point whether the interaction between $Ca^{++}$ and β-receptors is a general feature in the action of β-adrenergic receptors. Since $Ca^{++}$ seems to be the second messenger of $\alpha_1$-adrenergic response (ref. 7) and since it was found that $\alpha_2$-agonists inhibit adenylate cyclase (refs. 8-10), it is attractive to postulate that $Ca^{++}$ functions as a regulatory link between α and β-receptors. One difficulty with this finding is of course the fact that significant inhibition occurs at the 10-0.1 mM concentration range of $Ca^{++}$, when adenylate cyclase activity is assayed in membrane fragments (ref. 5). It was observed, however, that incorporating the specific $Ca^{++}$ ionophore A-23187 into the intact erythrocyte, in the absence of added free $Ca^{++}$, is sufficient to induce 63% inhibition of the β-agonist-dependent activity in the intact cell (ref. 3). This finding may be interpreted to mean that the internalization of the membrane-bound $Ca^{++}$ is sufficient to induce enzyme inhibition, most probably by creating a high local $Ca^{++}$ concentration.

2. β-Adrenergic Receptor-Dependent Phospholipid Methylation. β-Adrenergic agonists were found to stimulate the enzymatic synthesis of phosphatidyl-N-monomethylethanolamine and phosphatidylcholine from phosphatidylethanolamine reticulocyte ghosts, in the presence of S-adenosyl-L-methionine (ref. 11). The stimulation is stereospecific, dose dependent, and inhibited by the β-blocker propranolol but not by α-adrenergic blockers. This β-receptor-dependent phospholipid methylation induces the increase of membrane fluidity with the concomitant increase in the β-receptor-dependent adenylate cyclase activity. The increase in the efficiency of the adenylate cyclase system may be due to the increased membrane fluidity which was found to play a key role in determining the efficiency of the coupling of β-receptors to adenylate cyclase in turkey erythrocytes. Similar results were recently reported for the β-adrenergic receptor-dependent adenylate cyclase from HeLa cells. The β-receptor-dependent phospholipid methylation is not cAMP-dependent and it is not clear at present what role it plays in the generation of the eventual β-adrenergic response. It remains to be established whether the role of phospholipid methylation is solely to increase the efficiency of receptor-to-cyclase coupling due to the increase in membrane fluidity. Another unknown aspect of this phenomenon is the biochemical mechanism by which the receptor activates the phosphatidylethanolamine methylating enzyme(s). It was recently observed that β-agonists induce the carboxymethylation of proteins in the rat parotid gland (ref. 12). This effect is stereospecific for l-agonists, and is specifically blocked by β-blockers and not by α-adrenergic blockers. The role of β-adrenergic-dependent protein carboxymethylation in the parotid gland is not yet known. The time course of protein methylation overlaps the time course of β-

*References p. 35*

receptor-dependent $\alpha$-amylase secretion, suggesting a relationship between protein methylation and the process of exocytosis.

B. $\alpha_2$-Adrenergic Receptors

$\alpha_2$-Adrenergic receptors are coupled to adenylate cyclase in an inhibitory mode. The inhibitory effect of $\alpha_2$-agonists on the activity of adenylate cyclase requires the presence of GTP. It is not yet clear whether the $\alpha_2$-receptor-linked GTP site is identical or different from the GTP stimulatory site known to be part of the eucaryotic adenylate cyclase system. It is interesting to note that opiates and enkephalins were shown recently to induce the inhibition of $PGE_1$-dependent adenylate cyclase in neuroblastoma glioma hybrids where the inhibitory effect is GTP and $Na^+$ dependent (refs. 16-18). Similarly, the inhibition of fat cell adenylate cyclase by the high affinity inhibitory adenosine receptor requires the presence of GTP and $Na^+$ ions (ref. 19).

C. $\alpha_1$-Adrenergic Receptors

It has been demonstrated that the primary event occurring upon occupation of the $\alpha$-adrenergic receptor by an $\alpha$-agonist in the parotid glands is the influx of $Ca^{++}$ which functions as the "second messenger" (ref. 7). Furthermore, the specific $Ca^{++}$ ionophore A-23187, when incorporated into the cell membrane, can substitute for the $\alpha$-adrenergic ligand and bypass the receptor-dependent mechanism. The influx of $Ca^{++}$ as the primary event in the salivary gland (rat parotid) causes the efflux of $K^+$ ions with water (ref. 7 and references therein). The efflux of potassium has also been recognized as an $\alpha$-adrenergic response in guinea pig liver (ref. 13) and in adipose tissue (ref. 14).

The stimulation of the pineal gland with l-epinephrine via the $\alpha$-adrenergic receptor was found to be dependent on the presence of $Ca^{++}$ in the incubation medium and results in a seven-fold increase in the cGMP level (ref. 15). It seems from these studies that the influx of $Ca^{++}$ is the first event induced by the $\alpha$-agonist. The formation of cGMP seems to result from $Ca^{++}$ influx. This is not surprising, as guanylate cyclase is a $Ca^{++}$-dependent enzyme. $\alpha_1$-Adrenergic receptors are involved in a variety of physiological activities, and it remains to be seen whether in each case $Ca^{++}$ functions as the "second messenger."

Another biochemical response elicited by the activation of $\alpha_1$-adrenergic receptors is the incorporation of inorganic $^{32}Pi$ into phosphatidylinositol in slices of the parotid gland (ref. 20). This biochemical event was shown to be unrelated to the $K^+$ efflux and water secretion also induced by $\alpha$-receptor activation. Interestingly enough, the divalent cation ionophore A-23187 which introduces $Ca^{++}$ into the cell thus causing $K^+$ release (ref. 7 ), has no significant effect on the incorporation of $^{32}Pi$ into phosphatidylinositol. Conversely, the $\alpha_1$-receptor-induced phospholipid effect is maximal in the absence of $Ca^{++}$ in the medium, when there is no $K^+$ release from the cell. In summary, it can be concluded that $\alpha_1$-

receptor activation leads to two independent biochemical events in the rat parotid gland: (1) an increase in membrane permeability toward extracellular $Ca^{++}$ that enters the cell and causes $K^{+}$ release, and (2) an increased incorporation of $^{32}Pi$ into acidic phospholipids. The findings of Nishizuka and his colleagues (ref. 21) suggest that both $Ca^{++}$ and diacylglycerol (the breakdown product of phosphatidylinositol) are required to activate C-kinase together with phosphatidylserine. Activation of C-kinase enzyme induced phosphorylations are most probably the key biochemical events linked to $\alpha_1$-adrenergic receptors.

Mechanistic aspects

A. Stimulation of Adenylate Cyclase by β-Receptors

Over the past few years it has become apparent that the receptor and the catalytic moiety are not the only components of the receptor-cyclase complex. Mainly through the pioneering studies of Rodbell and colleagues (ref. 22), it became apparent that a third component, the transducer, plays a decisive role in the processing of the hormonal signal. It turns out that the binding of the hormone or of the neurotransmitter is a necessary event for the activation of adenylate cyclase but not sufficient of itself (refs. 23, 24, and refs. therein). The nucleotide GTP *must* be present so that the hormone-induced activation of adenylate cyclase will take place. The role of the GTP regulatory unit was not recognized for a long time, probably because the substrate ATP used in the cyclase assay is usually contaminated with enough GTP to saturate the GTP regulatory site that binds the nucleotide with an affinity constant in the micromolar range. Indeed, when ATP free of GTP is used in the cyclase assay, the dependence of the cyclase activity on GTP can be demonstrated.

It is now generally accepted that GTP functions as an intracellular regulator which interacts with a specific regulatory site on the receptor-cyclase system and activates the enzyme with the hormone in a synergistic manner. It was also found to be generally true that GTP analogs such as GppNHp, GTPγS, and $GppCH_2p$ (see ref. 24 and references therein) activate the hormone-dependent adenylate cyclase in a quasi-irreversible fashion and, in the presence of hormone, induce the formation of a highly active and extremely stable adenylate cyclase. Detailed kinetic analysis on the β-adrenergic receptor-dependent adenylate cyclases (refs. 23-25) reveal that the role of the agonist is to facilitate the activation of the adenylate cyclase by the guanyl nucleotide. The efficiency of the β-receptor directed ligand diminishes progressively where: l-epinephrine = l-isoproterenol = l-norepinephrine > dopamine > l-phenylephrine > l-isoterenol > metanephrine. That is, the lower the efficacy of the agonist, the less efficient is the process of ligand-induced cyclase activation (ref. 26). Pure antagonists such as l-propranolol have no effect on the rate of cyclase activation. The extent of enzyme activation by the guanyl nucleotide alone (basal activity) varies from system to

References p. 35

system, although in every case the agonist facilitates the activation process. In our elucidation below we depict the cyclase unit as E, where E includes the GTP regulatory unit. Independent evidence indicates that the E and the GTP unit are associated with each other, even in the detergent-solubilized state (ref. 27).

The activation of adenylate cyclase to its activated state requires the simultaneous binding of the agonist and of the guanyl nucleotide to their respective sites. When both sites are occupied, the enzyme is converted from its inactive E state to its activated state E'. Termination of the hormonal signal occurs concomitantly with the hydrolysis of GTP as the guanyl nucleotide regulatory site to GDP and Pi. Indeed, in turkey erythrocytes (ref. 28), the β-receptor-dependent GTPase activity can be measured directly. The hydrolysis step *per se* is independent of the continued presence of the agonist at the receptor site (refs. 23-25). The enzyme cannot, however, be reactivated until a new molecule of GTP binds to the guanyl nucleotide regulatory site, while the hormone still resides on the receptor.

In the presence of hormone and GTP, the only two species of cyclase in the system are E, the inactive form of the enzyme, and the cAMP producing form E'. Once the steady state has been reached, the system can be described by the following equation:

$$E \underset{k_{off}}{\overset{\text{GTP, agonist, } k_{on}}{\rightleftharpoons}} E' \qquad (2)$$

Thus, the total enzyme concentration in the membrane $[E_T]$ under these conditions is given by:

$$[E_T] = [E] + [E'] \qquad (3)$$

Applying the steady-state conditions:

$$k_{on}[E] = k_{off}[E'] \qquad (4)$$

Inserting (3) into (4), one obtains (ref. 23):

$$[E'] = \frac{[E_T]}{1 + \frac{k_{off}}{k_{on}}} \qquad (5)$$

Namely, only a fraction of the total cyclase pool is in its active form. The fraction $[E']/[E_T]$ can, in fact, be measured directly by determining the ratio of the maximal specific activity in the presence of GTP to that in the presence of GppNHp. In the latter situation, all of the enzyme pool is converted to the active form and thus the specific activity is given by the term "$k_{cat}[E_T]$", where $k_{cat}$ is the turnover number of the cyclase system. In the presence of GTP, however, the maximal specific activity is given by the term "$k_{cat}[E']$". It follows that the ratio between the two specific activities yields directly the ratio of $[E']/[E_T]$. According to the two state models derived here, the ratio $[E']/[E_T]$

is determined by the ratio $k_{off}/k_{on}$. The kinetic constant $k_{on}$ depends on hormone concentration and its maximal value is attained upon saturation of the agonist concentration. It is apparent from Equation 5 that the level of cyclase activity increases as $k_{on}$ increases. The first order rate constant $k_{off}$, depicting the decay of the activated state into its inactive form, represents the GTPase step at the regulatory site. For the turkey erythrocyte β-adrenergic-dependent adenylate cyclase, the values of $k_{on}$ and $k_{off}$ (refs. 25, 26, 28, 29) were measured directly. $k_{on}$ was determined by following the rate of adenylate cyclase activation upon saturating the concentrations of l-epinephrine and of GppNHp (refs. 25, 30). Under these conditions, $k_{off} = 0$, since the GppNHp cannot be hydrolyzed, and thus *all* the cyclase molecules are converted to the activated form of the enzyme, as was indeed found — namely, $[E'] = [E_T]$. This value was found to be in the range of $k_{on} = 0.4$ to $1.0\ min^{-1}$ at 37°C. The value of $k_{off}$ was also measured directly by two independent methods for the turkey erythrocyte system. One method involves the measurement of the rate constant of GTP hydrolysis at the regulatory site by the GTPase assay which was recently developed (ref. 28). The second method involves the measurement of the rate decay of the activated state E' to its inactive form by a quenching experiment (refs 25, 26) carried out as follows: The enzyme is incubated with hormone, GTP, and non-radioactive ATP; at zero time an excess of antagonist and α[$^{32}$P]ATP are added simultaneously. At this time E cannot be reconverted to E' as this conversion requires the continued presence of agonist at the receptor site and E' decays into E with the characteristic $k_{off}$. Concomitantly with this decay [$^{32}$P]cAMP continues to be produced by the vanishing activated form of the enzyme E'. The time course of [$^{32}$P]cAMP formation reflects the time course of the decay of E' to E. The characteristic rate constant of this process is $k_{off}$ and thus can be easily obtained. When an antagonist is not available, the quenching can be performed by GDPβS (ref. 31). The latter replaces GDP at the regulatory site, subsequent to its formation, and because of its tight binding, prevents the binding of GTP and therefore blocks reactivation of the enzyme. It must be emphasized that these methods can be applied to *any* adenylate cyclase system, whereas the success of the GTPase assay depends substantially upon its ability to measure the specific hormone-dependent GTPase activity over the high background non-specific nucleotide triphosphatase activity. Equation 5 can be rearranged to:

$$\frac{[E_T]}{[E']} = 1 + \frac{k_{off}}{k_{on}} \qquad (6)$$

and one can examine whether the two-state model discussed here for the cyclase system is indeed applicable. This can be done as follows: both the ratio $k_{off}/k_{on}$ and the ratio $[E_T]/[E']$ can be measured independently. The latter ratio represents the ratio of the specific activity, in the presence of GppNHp, to that in the

*References p. 35*

presence of GTP. One can then examine whether indeed the ratios $[E_T]/[E']$ and $k_{off}/n\ k_{on}$ are related by Equation 6.

Such a comparison has in fact been carried out for the turkey erythrocyte β-receptor system, and the correspondence was found to be excellent (refs. 23, 26). This finding supports the view that the two-state model for the cyclase system accounts well for the experimental data. The simple model described in Equations 2 through 5 suggests also a mechanistic approach to the study of the nature of partial agonism in the cyclase system. Partial agonists induce a smaller fraction of the cyclase to be converted into its active form E', thus yielding a lower specific activity as compared with full agonists. This may result either from a lower $k_{on}$ value or a higher $k_{off}$ value (or both). This was recently examined in detail in the case of turkey erythrocyte β-receptor-dependent adenylate cyclase. It was found that $k_{off}$ is identical for nine full and partial agonists, whereas $k_{on}$ is the parameter which is agonist dependent. Since it was also found in the latter case that $k_{off} \gg k_{on}$, it became apparent from Equations 5 or 6 that the level of cyclase activation, E', is linearly dependent on $k_{on}$. Indeed, when the steady-state level of cyclase activity is plotted against $k_{on}$ for nine different agonists, a linear relationship is obtained (ref. 26). This finding further corroborates the claim that it is sufficient to consider a two-state model for the cyclase system. Another recent finding (see also below) is that the cholera toxin induced ADP-ribosylation of the GTP binding protein is the origin of the increase in the activity of adenylate cyclase (E' according to our notation). It can be shown (ref. 32) that this covalent modification results in the decrease of the GTPase step ($k_{off}$), hence yielding an increase in the steady-state level of active cyclase in the presence of GTP. These data lend further support to the model of cyclase activation discussed above.

B. The GTP Binding Protein

The hypothesis that the guanyl nucleotide regulatory site represents a separate regulatory unit was recently verified directly. By exposing Lubrol-PX-solubilized pigeon erythrocyte membranes to a GTP-sepharose matrix, GTP binding proteins can be separated from the cyclase catalytic unit (refs. 27, 33). These proteins can then be dissociated from the GTP-matrix by GppNHp or GTP and, upon their addition to the cyclase which was deprived of the guanyl nucleotide binding proteins (G-protein), reconstitution occurs and adenylate cyclase activity is regenerated in the presence of GppNHp (refs. 33, 34). Furthermore, Pfeuffer has found that the guanyl nucleotide binding protein isolated from pigeon erythrocytes is also capable of activating rabbit myocardial adenylate cyclase which was previously depleted from GTP binding proteins (refs. 33, 34). This latter finding strongly indicates that this regulatory protein is a *universal* unit of the adenylate cyclase system and, therefore, can couple with a catalytic unit from many species. Affinity labeling experiments (ref. 33), using a GTP derivative, indicate that probably only one of the GTP binding proteins — possessing a molecular weight of approximately 42,000 — which binds to the GTP matrix, is the guanyl nucleotide regulatory unit that is strongly attached to cyclase. More recently (see below) it was found that it is the same 42,000 GTP binding subunit that is ADP ribosylated when the pigeon erythrocyte membrane is exposed to cholera toxin (refs. 35, 36). It remains to be established whether the GTP binding protein responsible for cyclase activation possesses the GTPase activity. The fact that ADP ribosylation inhibits the β-receptor-dependent GTPase activity in turkey erythrocytes supports this assumption.

The presence of the GTP binding protein is essential also for the reconstitution of fluoride activity (see ref. 37 and references therein). That is, the ability of NaF to stimulate adenylate cyclase requires the association of the catalytic moiety with the GTP binding protein. For this reason the GTP binding protein has also been termed the G/F protein. Membranes from mutant S49 cells possessing β-adrenergic receptors but lacking hormone-dependent cyclase activity ($AC^-$) were shown to regain hormone responsiveness upon addition of the G/F protein extracted from the wild type cells (ref. 37). Thus it seems that the stable association of the GTP binding protein with the adenylate cyclase moiety does not require penetration of the protein into the membrane. More recently, the G/F protein (or the N protein as it is sometimes designated) has been purified from rabbit liver (ref. 38) and from turkey erythrocytes (ref. 39). Upon solubilization of the β-receptor-dependent adenylate cyclase, the receptor (R) separates easily from the cyclase (C) (ref. 39), whereas the GTP regulatory unit (G) tends to associate with the catalytic unit C (ref. 33). In fact, these findings are not in contradiction with the assumption that the receptor does not form a stable complex with the cyclase complex altogether. There is, however, evidence that the receptor can associate with the GTP binding protein (ref. 40). The mechanistic significance of this finding is not as yet clear.

C. The Dynamics of the Topographical Interrelationship Between Cyclase and the β-Receptor

Although it is well established that the three basic components of the adenylate cyclase system: the receptor, the G-protein (the GTP binding protein) and the catalytic unit represent separate macromolecules, little is known about their organization within the membrane, their stoichiometry, and the mode of coupling between them. Certain theoretical arguments (ref. 41) favor the assumption that the stoichiometry is close to 1:1:1 or near to that ratio, although no direct proof is yet available as none of these components has been purified to homogeneity. However, more has been learned recently about the mechanism of coupling between these components in one experimental system, namely the turkey erythrocyte β-adrenergic system. It is already established that the guanyl nucleotide regulatory unit is

*References p. 35*

tightly attached to the catalytic unit and can only be separated from the latter upon solubilization in non-ionic detergents as well as the bio-specific absorption of the guanyl nucleotide protein onto a GTP-sepharose matrix. The β-receptor usually separates rather easily from the cyclase. The separation of the cyclase from the β-receptor upon membrane solubilization has been demonstrated in a number of cell types. In each case the solubilized cyclase could respond to GppNHp and to NaF, which indicates that the catalytic moiety and the GTP regulatory protein remain associated, even subsequent to solubilization. Thus, the $C_1G_m$ complex ($C_1$ = 1 enzyme units, $G_m$ = m GTP regulatory units) is a stable structure with an as yet unknown stoichiometry. Since the structural work on hormone-activated cyclases is progressing rather slowly, the approach taken to study the mode of coupling between receptors and denylate cyclases has been mainly a kinetic one. First, we shall consider the various theoretical models which have been formulated and, secondly, the experiments designed to explore the validity of these models.

## D. Possible Modes of Receptor to Enzyme Coupling

In this section we shall consider the mode of coupling of β-adrenergic receptors to adenylate cyclase. When referring to the "enzyme", we mean the whole complex between the catalytic moiety and the GTP regulatory protein. The theoretical considerations are usually applicable to other receptor cyclase systems and other receptor signal systems where the signal is not cyclase. Such a signal can be transported via an ionophore coupled to the receptor. The experimental data discussed below will be confined to the β-receptor-dependent adenylate cyclase system, not only because it is the subject of this review, but also because detailed experimen aimed at the delineation of receptor to signal coupling have so far been performed only on that system. In principle, four possible modes of coupling can occur (ref. 25):

1. The precoupled model where the enzyme unit and the receptor regulatory unit are permanently attached to one another, as in the regulatory enzyme aspartate transcarbamylase. In this case the process of enzyme activation can be described by a simple scheme. The model predicts non-cooperative agonist and antagonist binding. This model also predicts that the time course of enzyme activation to its permanently active state ($k_{off}$ = 0), in the presence of hormone and GppNHp, is first order.

2. The dissociation model assumes that the enzyme and the receptor are permanently attached to each other in the absence of agonist and that subsequent to hormone binding, the two units separate concomitantly with enzyme activation. This model predicts negatively cooperative ligand binding as well as non-first-order kinetics of enzyme activation when exposed to agonist in the presence of GppNHp.

3. The floating receptor model assumes that the hormone, the receptor, and the enzyme are in equilibrium and, thus, the fraction of enzyme attached to the recepto

can vary with the amount of agonist in the system. This model, like model 2, predicts negatively cooperative hormone binding and complex kinetics of enzyme activation.

4. The collision coupling model predicts first-order kinetics of enzyme activation by hormone and GppNHp, and non-cooperative ligand binding, as model 1.

In one system, the turkey erythrocyte β-receptor-dependent cyclase, experiments were performed to explore the nature of the coupling between the receptor and the enzyme. Binding experiments of β-antagonists and β-agonists reveal that the mode of binding is *always* non-cooperative in the turkey erythrocyte system (refs. 25, 42). Furthermore, the kinetics of enzyme activation in the presence of GppNHp are first order (refs. 25, 30). These two observations, even taken separately, constitute a firm basis for the rejection of models 2 and 3 for the turkey erythrocyte system. Both the binding experiments of β-ligands and the kinetic experiments can be accounted for equally well by either model 1 or its diametrically opposed model 4. A closer look (ref. 25) at these two models reveals that model 1 predicts that in the presence of GppNHp ($k_{off} = 0$), the rate constant of enzyme activation ($k_{on}$) is *independent* of receptor concentration and that the maximal number of activatable catalytic units is *directly proportional* to the concentration of receptor. In contrast, the collision coupling model (model 4) predicts the opposite: the rate constant of enzyme activation is *directly proportional* to the concentration of intact receptor, whereas the maximal number of catalytic units which can be activated is *independent* of receptor concentration. Using an irreversible β-adrenergic blocker (ref. 25), it was possible to demonstrate that the turkey erythrocyte β-adrenergic receptors are *not* permanently attached to the cyclase but activate the enzyme by the collision coupling mechanism. Using an identical approach to investigate the mode of coupling between the adenosine receptor and the cyclase in the turkey erythrocyte system, the opposite situation was found (ref. 43): the progressive inactivation of the adenosine receptor by an irreversible blocker results in a proportional decrease in the maximal number of activatable catalytic units in the presence of GppNHp, but *no change* in the rate constant characterizing the activation process ($k_{on}$) is effected. The fact that the adenosine receptor and the β-receptor are coupled differently to the adenylate cyclase was, in fact, predicted on kinetic grounds (see ref. 44 and references therein).

The conclusion that the adenosine receptor is permanently attached to the cyclase while the β-receptor is not, is corroborated by an entirely different experimental approach. The progressive increase in membrane fluidity by the insertion of *cis*-vaccenic acid causes a dramatic increase in the rate constant ($k_{on}$) of cyclase activation by the β-agonist bound β-receptor but no change in the rate constant characterizing the activation of cyclase by adenosine (ref. 45). These findings corroborate the assertion that the process of adenylate cyclase activation by β-receptors is bimolecular, whereas the activation by adenosine is monomolecular.

E. The Effect of GTP on β-Receptors

A number of reports have shown that besides the role of GTP in the activation of adenylate cyclase, guanyl nucleotides also affect the interaction of the receptor with the agonists. Thus, GTP and its analogs were found to reduce the affinity of glucagon to its receptors (ref. 46). The GTP-induced reduction in the affinity of the glucagon receptor toward the hormone is retained subsequent to its solubilization with Triton X-100 (ref. 47). Similarly, GTP was shown in two cell types to reduce the affinity of β-adrenergic receptors toward β-agonists but not toward β-blockers (ref. 48). These effects of guanyl nucleotides are usually attributed to a receptor-linked nucleotide site which is different from the nucleotide site coupled to cyclase. The evidence for the existence of such a site, however, is so far indirect and further experimentation is necessary in order to confirm this assertion.

F. The Role of the Lipid Matrix

Numerous studies reveal that the lipid matrix plays a role in the coupling between hormone receptors and adenylate cyclase. The treatment of membranes with phospholipases is known to damage the coupling between the hormone receptors and the cyclases. These observations may be taken as an indication that specific phospholipids are essential for the interaction between the hormone receptor and the cyclase and/or the G-protein. In the absence of more direct studies on this question, one cannot at the present time identify specific lipids essential for the function of adenylate cyclase. Similarly, the introduction of the membrane perturbing agent filipin (ref. 49) uncouples the β-adrenergic receptors from the cyclase and eliminates the ability of β-agonists to stimulate the cyclase, without affecting the binding of β-adrenergic ligands or the ability of NaF to activate the catalytic moiety of the cyclase. On the other hand, certain membrane fluidizing agents such as unsaturated fatty acids (ref. 50, 51) induce an increase in the efficiency of coupling between the β-adrenergic receptor and the cyclase in the turkey erythrocyte system. Similar findings were recently observed in cultured Chang liver cells (ref. 52). Fluidization of cell membrane may also lead to the reversible cryptization (ref. 53) of receptors at higher temperatures, with a concomitant decrease in hormone-dependent adenylate cyclase activity. This effect is independent of the effect of fluidization on the efficiency of coupling and can be separated from it.

The overall scheme for cyclase activation by hormone and GTP is summarized in Fig. 1.

The inhibition of adenylate cyclase by $\alpha_2$-adrenergic receptors

$\alpha_2$-Adrenergic agonists inhibit adenylate cyclase in a number of systems (refs.

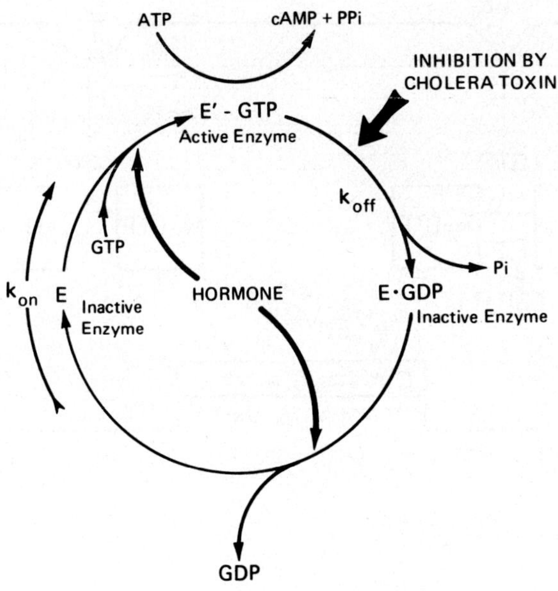


Fig. 1. The role of GTP and hormone in adenylate cyclase activation, E'. GTP is the active species of the enzyme. $k_{off}$ is the GTPase step, whereas $k_{on}$ is the rate constant characterizing the transition of the inactive enzyme E . GTP to the active state. Activation involves the removal of GDP from the regulatory site, which by itself is not rate limiting. This figure was drawn from the model developed by Levitzki (ref. 23), and Cassel and Selinger (ref. 32).

8-10). The mechanism of this inhibition is currently the subject of investigation in a number of laboratories. In our laboratory, we have studied the kinetic features of the $\alpha_2$-adrenergic inhibition of both basal and $PGE_1$-dependent adenylate cyclase in human platelets. We found that $\alpha_2$-adrenergic agonists do not affect the value of $k_{on}$ and $k_{off}$ (Equations 5 and 6). Also, direct measurements of $PGE_1$-dependent GTPase in purified human platelet membranes reveal that $\alpha_2$-agents do not influence the turnover of this enzyme (refs. 54, 55). We have therefore concluded that $\alpha_2$-inhibition is not directly mediated by the same GTP binding protein which mediates enzyme activation. We have suggested that $\alpha_2$-adrenergic inhibition is mediated through a different GTP regulatory site which, like the stimulatory GTP site, interacts directly with the catalytic unit and attenuates its activity. Alternatively, we have suggested that the inhibitory GTP site uncouples the interaction between the stimulatory GTP site and the catalytic unit. Both mechanisms can account for the absence of an inhibitory effect of $\alpha_2$-adrenergic agonists on the intrinsic parameters $k_{on}$ and $k_{off}$, or on the $PGE_1$-dependent GTPase reaction. Both possibilities are summarized in Fig. 2. Other investigators, however, reported that the inhibitory neurotransmitter enkephalin, which inhibits adenylate cyclase in

*References p. 35*

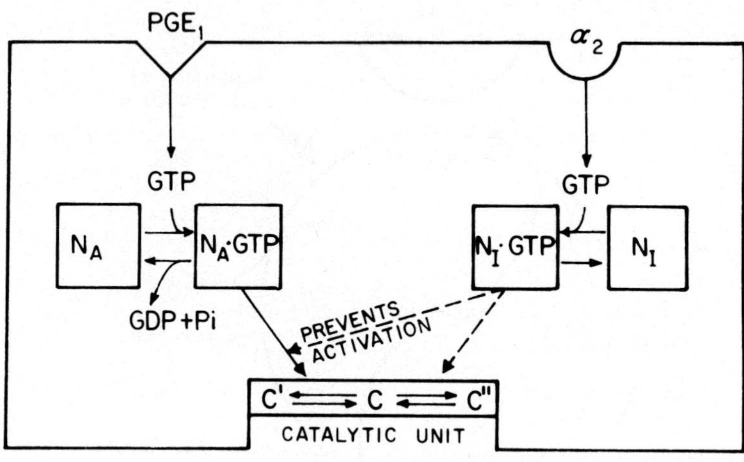


Fig. 2. Possible mechanisms by which adenylate cyclase is inhibited by GTP and $\alpha_2$-agonists. The activatory GTP binding protein ($N_A$) is associated with the stimulato receptor ($PGE_1$), while the inhibitory GTP site ($N_I$) is associated with the $\alpha_2$-receptor. Both nucleotide sites can exist in their free and GTP-liganded states, and the equilibria between these states is regulated by hormone occupancy of the receptor. Reversion of $N_A$·BTP to $N_A$ is regulated by a $PGE_1$-stimulated GTPase. The mechanism by which the reversion of $N_I$·GTP to $N_I$ has not been defined. The catalytic unit (C) can be activated to its cAMP producing state (C') by $N_A$·GTP. Inhibition, mediated by $N_I$·GTP, results from one of two possible events: either $N_I$·GTP converts C into state C' which has a lower catalytic rate, or $N_I$·GTP interferes with the conversion of C to C' by $N_A$·GTP without altering the cycle of $N_A$ + GTP → $N_A$·GTP → $N_A$ + GDP + P

neuroblastoma glioma NG-108-15 cells, stimulates a low $K_m$ GTPase in the same system (ref. 56). In the latter system the adenylate cyclase was shown to be inhibited by enkephalin only in the presence of $Na^+$. Indeed, $Na^+$ was found to *inhibit* the low $K_m$ GTPase (ref. 56) and to *stimulate* cyclase (Koski and Klee, unpublished results). Thus, enkephalins and morphine *reverse* the effect of $Na^+$ in this system. Such $Na^+$ effects are not found in the purified platelet system which we have studied.

Abbreviations used:

ADP = adenosine-5'-diphosphate
ATP = adenosine-5'-triphosphate
cAMP = adenosine-3',5'-phosphate
GDP = guanosine 5'-diphosphate
$GppCH_2p$ = guanylyl-methylene diphosphate
GppNHp = guanylyl-imido diphosphate
GTP = guanosine-5'-triphosphate
GTP$\gamma$S = guanosine-triphosphate-$\gamma$-SH
Pi = inorganic phosphate
Ppi = pyrophosphate

## REFERENCES


1 E.W. Sutherland, I. Øye and R.W. Butcher, Recent Prog. Horm. Res. 21(1965)623-646.
2 A. Levitzki, Biochem. Pharmacol. 27(1979)2081-2088.
3 M.L. Steer and A. Levitzki, Arch. Biochem. Biophys 167(1975)371-375.
4 H. Rassmussen, W. Lake and J.E. Allen, Biochim. Biophys. Acta 411(1975)63-73.
5 M.L. Steer and A. Levitzki, J. Biol. Chem. 250(1975)2080-2084.
6 E. Hanski, N. Sevilla and A. Levitzki, Eur. J. Biochem. 76(1977)512-520.
7 M. Schramm and Z. Selinger, J. Cycl. Nucl. Res. 1(1975)181-192.
8 K. Aktories, G. Schultz and K.H. Jakobs, FEBS Lett. 107(1979)100-104.
9 S.L. Sabol and M. Nirenberg, J. Biol. Chem. 254(1979)1913-1920.
10 M.L. Steer and A. Wood, J. Biol. Chem. 254(1978)10791-10797.
11 F. Hirata, J. Strittmatter and J. Axelrod, Proc. Natl. Acad. Sci. USA 76(1979) 368-372.
12 W.J. Strittmatter, C. Gagnon and J. Axelrod, J. Pharmacol. Exp. Ther. 207(1979) 419-423.
13 D.G. Haylett and D.J. Jenkinson, J. Physiol (London) 255(1972)752-770.
14 L. Girardier, J. Seydoux and T. Clausen, J. Gen. Physiol. 52(1968)925-940.
15 R.E. O'Dea and M. Zatz, Proc. Natl. Acad. Sci. USA 73(1976)3398-3402.
16 S.K. Sharma, W.A. Klee and M. Nirenberg, Proc. Natl. Acad. Sci. USA 74(1977) 3365-3369.
17 A.J. Blume, Life Sci. 22(1978)1843-1852.
18 A.J. Blume and G. Boone, Fed. Proc. 38(1979)628-633.
19 C. Londos, D.M.F. Cooper, W. Schlegel and M. Rodbell, Proc. Natl. Acad. Sci. USA 75(1978)5562-5566.
20 Y. Oron, M. Lowe, and Z. Selinger, Mol. Pharmacol. 11(1975)79-86.
21 A. Kishimoto, Y. Takai, T. Mori, U. Kikkawa and Y. Nishizuka, J. Biol. Chem. 254(1980)3692-3695 and references therein.
22 M. Rodbell, M.C. Lin, Y. Salomon, C. Londos, J.P. Harwood, B.P. Martin, M. Rendell and M. Berman, Adv. Cyclic Nucl. Res. 5(1975)3-29.
23 A. Levitzki, Biochem. Biophys. Res. Commun. 74(1977)1154-1159.
24 A. Levitzki and E.J.M. Helmreich, FEBS Lett. 101(1979)213-219.
25 A.M. Tolkovsky and A. Levitzki, Biochemistry 2(1978)3795-3810.
26 H. Arad and A. Levitzki, Mol. Pharmacol. 16(1979)743-756.
27 T. Pfeuffer and E.J.M. Helmreich, J. Biol. Chem. 250(1975)867-876.
28 D. Cassel and Z. Selinger, Biochim. Biophys. Acta 452(1976)538-551.
29 D. Cassel, H. Levkovitz and Z. Selinger, J. Cyclic Nucl. Res. 3(1977)393-406.
30 N. Sevilla, M.L. Steer and A. Levitzki, Biochemistry 15(1976)3493-3499.
31 D. Cassel, F. Eckstein, M. Lowe and Z. Selinger, J. Biol. Chem. 254(1979) 9835-9838.
32 D. Cassel and Z. Selinger, Proc. Natl. Acad. Sci. USA 74(1977)3307-3311.
33 T. Pfeuffer, J. Biol. Chem. 252(1977)7224-7234.

34 T. Pfeuffer, FEBS Lett. 101(1979)85-90.
35 D.M. Gill and R. Meren, Proc. Natl. Acad. Sci. USA 75(1978)3050-3054.
36 D. Cassel and T. Pfeuffer, Proc. Natl. Acad. Sci. USA 75(1978)2669-2673.
37 A.C. Howlett, P.C. Sternweis, B.A. Mauk, P.M. Van Arsdale and A.G. Gilman, J. Biol. Chem. 254(1979)2287-2290.
38 J.K. Northup, P.C. Sternweis, H.D. Smigel, L.S. Schleifer, E.M. Ross and A.G. Gilman, Proc. Natl. Acad. Sci. USA 77(1980)6516-6520.
39 E. Hanski, P.C. Sternweis and A.G. Gilman, J. Biol. Chem. 1981, in press.
40 A. DeLean, J.M. Stadel and R.J. Lefkowitz, J. Biol. Chem. 255(1980)7108-7118 and references therein.
41 A. Levitzki, N. Sevilla, D. Atlas and M.L. Steer, J. Mol. Biol. 37(1975)35-53.
42 E.M. Brown, S.A. Fedak, C.J. Woodard, G.D. Aurbach and D. Rodbard, J. Biol. Chem. 251(1976)1239-1246.
43 S. Braun and A. Levitzki, Biochemistry 10(1979)2134-2138.
44 A.M. Tolkovsky and A. Levitzki, Biochemistry 17(1978)3811-3817.
45 G. Rimon, E. Hanski, S. Braun and A. Levitzki, Nature (London) 276(1978)394-396.
46 M. Rodbell, H.M.J. Krans, S.L. Pohl and L. Birnbaumer, J. Biol. Chem. 246(1971) 1861-1871.
47 A.F. Welton, P.M. Lad, A.C. Newby, M. Yamamura, S. Nicosia and M. Rodbell, J. Biol. Chem. 252(1977)5947-5950.
48 M.E. Maguire, P.M. Van Arsdale and A.G. Gilman, Mol. Pharmacol. 12(1976)335-339.
49 G. Puchwein, T. Pfeuffer and E.J.M. Helmreich, J. Biol. Chem. 249(1974)3232-3244
50 E. Hanski, G. Rimon and A. Levitzki, Biochemistry 18(1979)846-853.
51 J. Orly and M. Schramm, Proc. Natl. Acad. Sci. USA 72(1975)3433-3437.
52 A. Bakardjieva, M.J. Galla and E.J.M. Helmreich, Biochemistry 18(1979)3016-3023.
53 G. Rimon, E. Hanski and A. Levitzki, Biochemistry 19(1980)4451-4460.
54 M.L. Steer, H.A. Lester, S. Braun and A. Levitzki, J. Biol. Chem. (1981) in pres
55 H.A. Lester, M.L. Steer and A. Levitzki, Proc. Natl. Acad. Sci. USA (1981) in pre
56 G. Koski and W.A. Klee, Proc. Natl. Acad. Sci. USA (1981) in press.

J.A. Keverling Buisman (Editor), *Strategy in Drug Research*



# CLONIDINE-N=C=S, AN AFFINITY LABEL FOR $\alpha_2$-ADRENERGIC RECEPTORS ON HUMAN PLATELETS AND RAT BRAIN

D. ATLAS, M.L. STEER* and Y. PLOTEK

Department of Biological Chemistry, The Hebrew University of Jerusalem, Jerusalem (Israel). *Permanent address: Department of Surgery, Beth Israel Hospital and Harvard Medical School, Boston, Mass. (U.S.A.)

## ABSTRACT

An affinity label for $\alpha_2$-adrenergic receptors, derived from clonidine, was synthesized. Its irreversible tagging of the $\alpha_2$-receptors was observed in human platelets and rat brain membranes. Exposure of intact human platelets or platelet membranes or rat brain membranes to this clonidine derivative, p-isothiocyanato clonidine+ (clonidine-N=C=S), followed by extensive washing results in the loss of the ability of [$^3$H]yohimbine binding to platelet $\alpha_2$-receptors and [$^3$H]clonidine binding to rat brain $\alpha_2$-receptors. In addition, exposure of intact platelets to clonidine-N=C=S, followed by extensive washing, results in the loss of the ability for the epinephrine-induced inhibition of adenylate cyclase activity in freeze-thawed platelets and in purified platelet membranes. This effect is time and concentration -dependent ($t_{½}$ at 30°C < 15 min; half-maximal effect with clonidine-N=C=S concentrations < 10 μM). Clonidine-N=C=S appears to interact by irreversibly blocking the platelet $\alpha_2$-receptors since (a) it abolishes $\alpha_2$-receptor effects of adenylate cyclase activity (*i.e.*, epinephrine-induced inhibition of basal and prostaglandin $E_1$-stimulated activity), while not altering other cyclase activities (basal, prostaglandin $E_1$- and NaF-stimulated), and (b) its effect on both [$^3$H]yohimbine binding and epinephrine-induced inhibition of adenylate cyclase can be specifically prevented by α-agonists ((-)epinephrine and clonidine) and α-antagonists (yohimbine and phentolamine). These observations indicate that clonidine-N=C=S is an effective affinity label for platelet $\alpha_2$-receptors as well as for rat brain $\alpha_2$-receptors, and thus can serve as a general irreversible probe for $\alpha_2$-receptors.

## INTRODUCTION

Alpha adrenergic receptors are subdivided into two distinct classes, namely,

+Abbreviations used: clonidine-N=C=S = p-isothiocyanato clonidine; $PGE_1$ = prostaglandin $E_1$; $K_d$ = dissociation constant; $B_{max}$ = maximal specific binding.

*References p. 45*

the $\alpha_1$ and $\alpha_2$ receptors (refs. 1-4). The $\alpha_1$-receptors are associated with movements of $Ca^{++}$ ions across cell membranes, whereas $\alpha_2$-receptors are coupled in an inhibitory fashion to adenylate cyclase (refs. 5-11). One of the functions attributed to the $\alpha_2$-adrenergic receptors in the central nervous system is the control of neurotransmitter release. At such receptors clonidine is a highly specific agonist, and yohimbine is a potent and specific antagonist.

The high affinity of clonidine (ref. 12) and of p-amino-clonidine (refs. 13-16) for the $\alpha_2$-receptors made them excellent probes in studies of these receptors in the central nervous system as well as in the periphery. In the present communication we describe the properties of an irreversible $\alpha_2$-ligand derived from clonidine. The new analog, p-isothiocyanato clonidine (clonidine-N=C=S), acts specifically and irreversibly at the $\alpha_2$-adrenergic site of human platelets as well as in rat brain. In addition, this ligand prevents the specific inhibition of adenylate cyclase induced by (-)epinephrine in fresh human platelets. Thus, this ligand appears to be an effective affinity label for the platelet $\alpha_2$-adrenergic receptors.

## EXPERIMENTAL

Materials. $[^3H]$Clonidine (22.2 Ci/mmole) and $[^3H]$yohimbine (83 Ci/mmole) were purchased from New England Nuclear. $[\alpha\text{-}^{32}P]$ATP and $[^3H]$cAMP were obtained from the Radiochemical Centre, Amersham (England). The following were generous gifts: phentolamine, from Ciba-Geigy (U.S.A.); clonidine, from Boehringer-Ingelheim (Germany); p-amino clonidine, from Makor Chemicals (Jerusalem, Israel); and prostaglandin $E_1$, from Upjohn (U.S.A.). (-)Epinephrine, (-)norepinephrine and yohimbine were purchased from Sigma, and (+)epinephrine from K & K Company (U.S.A.). All other chemicals were of reagent grade and all experiments were performed using double distilled water.

Synthesis of clonidine-N=C=S. The synthesis of clonidine-N=C=S will be published elsewhere (Fig. 1).

Membrane preparation. Human platelet membranes and rat brain membrane preparations were carried out according to established procedures (refs. 9 and 16, respectively).

Binding studies. Studies of binding to $\alpha_2$-adrenergic receptors in rat brain membranes and in human platelets were carried out with tritiated clonidine and with tritiated yohimbine respectively (ref. 16).

Adenylate cyclase assay. Studies characterizing the (-)epinephrine-induced inhibition of adenylate cyclase activity in freshly prepared human platelet membranes were carried out essentially as previously described(ref. 17).

## RESULTS

Effects of clonidine-N=C=S on $[^3H]$yohimbine and $[^3H]$clonidine binding in human platelets. Exposure of human platelet membranes to 30 μM clonidine-N=C=S, followed by extensive washings, reduced the binding capacity ($B_{max}$) for [$^{3}$H]yohimbine by 80% without altering the $K_d$. Incubation of platelet membranes with 30 μM clonidine-N=C=S together with 100 μM clonidine reduced $B_{max}$ by only 65%, thus indicating a partial protection of the irreversible effect (Fig. 2). Under identical conditions, reversible ligands (100 μM clonidine, 100 μM p-amino-clonidine or 100 μM (-)epinephrine), followed by extensive washings, exhibit essentially the same binding capacity as untreated membranes.

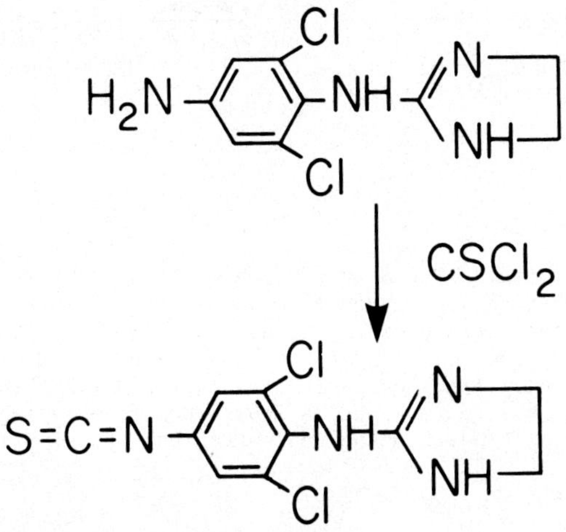

Fig. 1. Outline of synthesis of clonidine-N=C=S from p-amino clonidine.

Effects of clonidine-N=C=S on [$^{3}$H]clonidine binding in rat brain membranes. About 70% loss of [$^{3}$H]clonidine sites in rat brain membranes were observed after treatment with 70 μM clonidine-N=C=S, while 4 μM caused only about 45% loss of specific binding sites (Fig. 3).

Effects of clonidine-N=C=S on inhibition of adenylate cyclase by epinephrine in freeze-thawed platelets. Platelet adenylate cyclase, in both its basal and $PGE_1$-stimulated states, is inhibited by (-)epinephrine (refs. 7, 9). This process is specifically blocked by α-antagonists and is believed to be mediated via $\alpha_2$-adrenergic receptors. Preincubation of intact platelets with clonidine-N=C=S, followed by extensive washings and cell disruption by freeze-thawing, reduces the extent of epinephrine-induced cyclase inhibition. This phenomenon is dependent upon the concentration of clonidine-N=C=S used (Table I, Fig. 4) and the duration

*References p. 45*

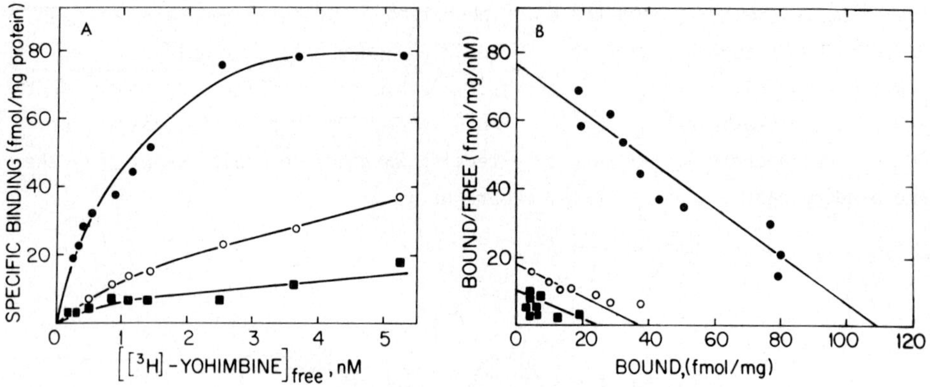


Fig. 2. Effect of clonidine-N=C=S on [$^3$H]yohimbine binding to platelet membranes. Purified platelet membranes prepared from outdated platelets were incubated for 30 minutes at 30°C in the absence of clonidine-N=C=S (●-●), in the presence of 30 μM clonidine-N=C=S alone (■-■), and in the presence of 30 μM clonidine-N=C=S and 100 μM clonidine (o-o). After extensive washing, [$^3$H]yohimbine binding was measured as described in the text. Panel A shows specific binding of [$^3$H]yohimbine as a function of the free [$^3$H]yohimbine concentration. Panel B is a Scatchard analysis of the data.

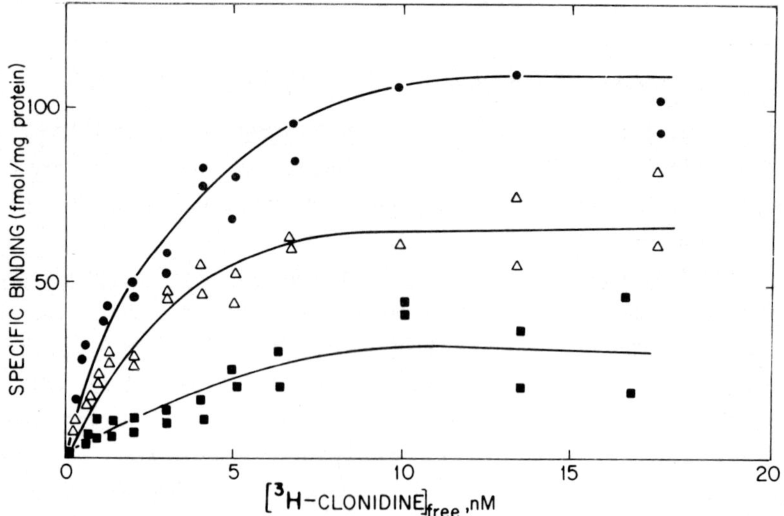


Fig. 3, A (see next page).

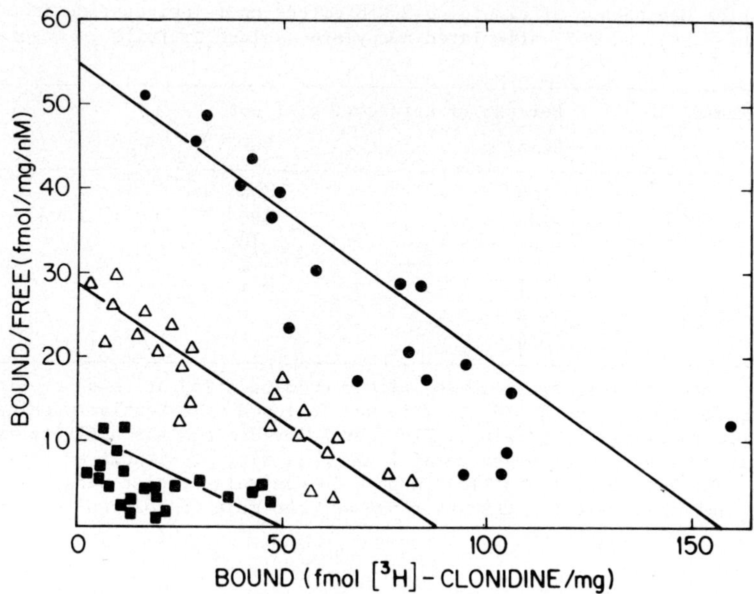


Fig. 3, B. Effect of clonidine-N=C=S on [$^3$H]clonidine binding to rat brain membrane preparations. Rat brain membranes were incubated for 30 min at 30°C in the absence (●-●) or presence (Δ-Δ) of 4 μM clonidine-N=C=S or 70 μM clonidine-N=C=S (■-■), followed by extensive washing and assayed as specific binding of [$^3$H]clonidine, as presented in Panel A. Panel B represents the Scatchard analysis of the data.

of pre-incubation with clonidine-N=C=S (Fig. 4). Half-maximal loss of epinephrine inhibition occurs with the concentrations of clonidine-N=C=S below 10 μM, and a complete loss of the (-)epinephrine effect is observed after exposure to 50 μM clonidine-N=C=S for 30 minutes at 30°C. The $t_{½}$ for loss of epinephrine inhibition is less than 15 minutes in the presence of 30 μM clonidine-N=C=S. The presence of 100 μM clonidine during the incubation time with clonidine-N=C=S partially prevents the loss of epinephrine inhibition (Fig. 5). 30 μM Phentolamine and 100 μM epinephrine effectively protected the $\alpha_2$-site (Table II). The effects of clonidine-N=C=S on platelet adenylate cyclase are selective for the inhibitory effects of (-)epinephrine; basal, $PGE_1$- and NaF-stimulated activities of adenylate cyclase are not altered significantly by treatment of intact platelets with clonidine-N=C=S (Fig. 6).

## DISCUSSION

In the present communication we report on the first successful development of an affinity label for the $\alpha_2$-adrenergic receptor. p-Isothiocyanato clonidine, a

TABLE I

Concentration dependence of clonidine-N=C=S effect on (-)epinephrine induced inhibition of basal and $PGE_1$-stimulated adenylate cyclase activity in freeze-thawed platelets

| Affinity label (μM) | Percent of epinephrine effect | |
|---|---|---|
| | Basal | $PGE_1$ |
| 0 | 100 | 100 |
| 3 | 100 | 100 |
| 10 | 14 | 10 |
| 30 | 5 | 1 |
| 50 | 1 | 1 |
| 80 | 0 | 0 |
| 100 | 0 | - |

Intact platelets were preincubated with clonidine-N=C=S at concentrations as indicated, for 30 minutes at 30°C. This was followed by extensive washing and cell disruption by freeze-thawing. Platelet adenylate cyclase activity was measured in the absence or presence of 1 μM $PGE_1$, with or without 10 μM (-)epinephrine. The extent of inhibition induced in control platelet samples is defined as 100% epinephrine effect. Results represent the mean of quadruplicate determinations.

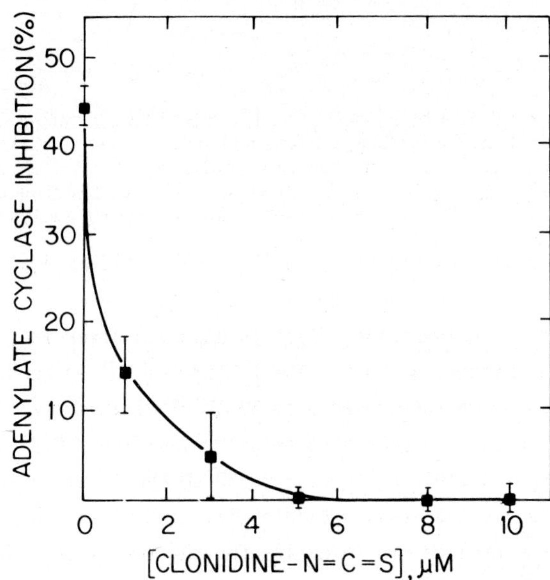


Fig. 4. Effect of clonidine-N=C=S on epinephrine-induced inhibition of adenylate cyclase in freeze-thawed platelets. Freshly prepared intact platelets were incubat for 30 minutes at 30°C with various concentrations of clonidine-N=C=S. After extensive washing and cell disruption by freeze-thawing, adenylate cyclase activity was measured in the presence and absence of 10 μM (-)epinephrine as described in the te Results represent the percent inhibition of basal activity induced by epinephrine a are the means of triplicate measurements. Vertical bars represent SE of triplicate measurements.

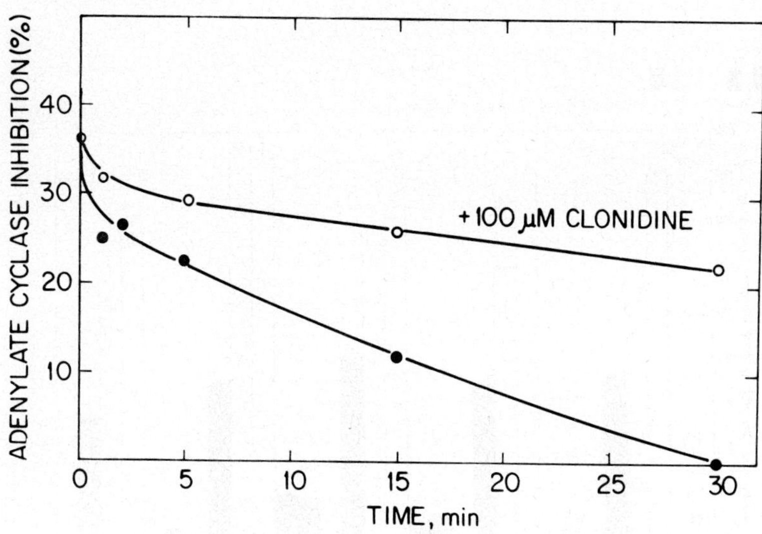


Fig. 5. Time dependence of clonidine-N=C=S effect. Freshly prepared intact platelets were incubated for various periods of time, as indicated, at 30°C in the presence of 30 μM clonidine-N=C=S alone (o-o) or combined with 100 μM clonidine (●-●). After extensive washings and cell disruption by freeze-thawing, adenylate cyclase activity was measured in the absence and presence of 10 μM (-)epinephrine, as described in the text. The percent inhibition induced by epinephrine is demonstrated, representing the mean of triplicate determinations.

TABLE II

Protection by α - ligands against loss of (-)epinephrine-induced inhibition by clonidine-N=C=S in freeze-thawed platelets

| Additions | % Inhibition by (-)epinephrine | |
|---|---|---|
| | Basal | $PGE_1$ |
| None | 47 | 21 |
| 30 μM clonidine-N=C=S | 0 | 0 |
| 30 μM clonidine-N=C=S + 100 μM clonidine | 42 | 19 |
| 30 μM clonidine-N=C=S + 30 μM phentolamine | 28 | 15 |
| 30 μM clonidine-N=C=S + 100 μM (-)epinephrine | 23 | 23 |

Intact platelets were incubated with or without clonidine-N=C=S in the absence or presence of clonidine, phentolamine, or epinephrine for 30 minutes at 30°C. After extensive washings and cell disruption by freeze-thawing, adenylate cyclase was measured in the absence (basal) or presence of $PGE_1$ (1 μM), without or with epinephrine (10 μM), and the percent inhibition induced by epinephrine was calculated. Results represent the mean of quadruplicate determinations.

*References p. 45*

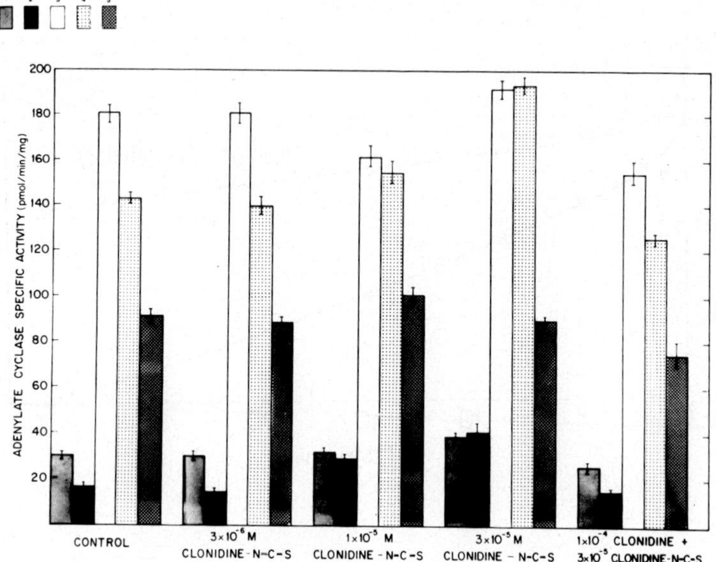


Fig. 6. Effect of clonidine-N=C=S on adenylate cyclase activity. Freshly prepared intact platelets were preincubated for 30 minutes at 30°C in the absence or presence of 30 μM clonidine-N=C=S plus 100 μM clonidine. After extensive washings followed by cell disruption through freeze-thawing, adenylate cyclase was measured as described in the text. For each preincubation condition, adenylate cyclase activity was determined under 5 different conditions which are represented by the columns, from left to right, in each group as follows: basal, 10 μM (-)epinephrine, 1 μM $PGE_1$, 1 μM $PGE_1$ plus 10 μM epinephrine and 10 mM NaF (see key for the symbols on figure).

derivative of clonidine, binds irreversibly to human platelet $\alpha_2$-receptors and rat brain membrane preparations, unlike clonidine which interacts in a reversible manner with the $\alpha_2$-receptors. The isothiocyanate group has been successfully applied in labeling transport proteins in erythrocyte membranes (refs. 18, 19).

Binding of either [$^3$H]yohimbine or [$^3$H]clonidine to whole platelet $\alpha_2$-receptors or to platelet membrane $\alpha_2$-receptors or to rat brain membranes was impaired by pre-treatment with the irreversible ligand. Studies of inhibition of platelet adenylate cyclase by epinephrine showed that pre-treatment with clonidine-N=C=S leads to a complete loss of the (-)epinephrine effect. The clonidine-N=C=S effect is specific for the $\alpha_2$-receptors, since the basal, $PGE_1$- and NaF-stimulated adenylate cyclase activities were not altered. Moreover, the specific irreversible binding to the $\alpha_2$-site is protected by $\alpha_2$-agonists (clonidine and, to a lesser extent, (-)epinephrine) as well as by $\alpha_2$-antagonists (yohimbine and phentolamine).

These observations indicate that clonidine-N=C=S is an effective $\alpha_2$-blocker for the central or peripheral $\alpha_2$-receptors. As such, clonidine-N=C=S may prove to be a potent tool for studies directed at achieving a better understanding of the molecular properties of the $\alpha_2$-receptor. Progressive inactivation of $\alpha_2$-receptors could be accomplished using this ligand and, thus, permit an evaluation of the stoichiometric relationship between $\alpha$-receptor occupancy and adenylate cyclase inhibition. In its radioactive form, clonidine-N=C=S could be used for labeling $\alpha_2$-receptors, thereby permitting their isolation and purification.

REFERENCES

1 W.Z. Langer, Biochem. Pharmacol. 23(1974)1793-1800.
2 K. Starke, Rev. Physiol. Biochem. Pharmacol. 77(1977)1-124.
3 S. Berthelsen and W.A. Pettinger, Life Sci. 21(1977) 595-606.
4 C.L. Wood, C.D. Arnett, W.R. Clarke, B.S. Tsai and R.J. Lefkowitz, Biochem. Pharmacol. 28(1979)1277.
5 L. Triner, Y. Vulliecmox, M. Verusky and G.G. Nahas, Life Sci. 9(1970)707-712.
6 J. Moskowitz, H.P. Harwood, W.D. Reid and G. Krishna, Biochim. Biophys. Acta 230(1971)279-285.
7 K.H. Jakobs, W. Saur and G. Schultz, J. Cycl. Nucl. Res. 2(1976)381-392.
8 K.D. Newman, L.T. Williams, N.H. Bishopric and R.J. Lefkowitz, J. Clin. Invest. 61(1978)395-402.
9 M.L. Steer and A. Wood, J. Biol. Chem. 254(1979)10791-10797.
10 B.S. Tsai and R.J. Lefkowitz, Mol. Pharmacol. 14(1978)540-548.
11 S.L. Sabol and M. Nirenberg, J. Biol. Chem. 254(1979)1913-1920.
12 D.C. U'Prichard, D.A. Greenberg and S.H. Snyder, Mol. Pharmacol. 13(1977)454--473.
13 B. Rouot and G. Leclerc, Eur, J. Med. Chem. Chimica Therapeutica 6(1978)521--526.
14 B. Rouot, G. Leclerc, H. Birth, C.A. Wemouth and J. Schwartz, C.R. Acad. Sci. Series D. 280(1978)909-910.
15 B. Rouot and S.H. Snyder, Life Sci. 25(1979)769-774.
16 D. Atlas and S.L. Sabol, Eur. J. Biochem. 113(1981)521-529.
17 M.L. Steer, J. Khorana and B. Galgoci, Mol. Pharmacol. 16(1979)719-728.
18 Z.I. Cabantchik and A. Rothstein, Membr. Biol. 10(1972)311-330.
19 R.E. Mullins and R.G. Langdon, Biochemistry 19(1980)1199-1205.

J.A. Keverling Buisman (Editor), *Strategy in Drug Research*



# THE STRATEGY OF THE DEVELOPMENT OF PEPTIDE DRUGS

F.J. ZEELEN

Organon Scientific Development Group, 5340 BH Oss, The Netherlands

## INTRODUCTION

There always is a tendency in research to continue working in areas where major successes were booked in the past. Plenty of know-how is available in such areas and the past successes can be used to persuade management or granting agencies to invest money in this direction of research.

Drug research is no exception. If one studies the 1980/1981 edition of Burger's Medicinal Chemistry [1] many chapters, although describing recent pharmacological results and series of new compounds, prove to be similar to those in the 1970 edition of this handbook. The 1980 volume of the Annual Reports in Medicinal Chemistry is still divided in the same 6 sections as was the first edition in 1965 [2]. This attitude has the inherent danger that while new drugs have been developed, which are somewhat more selective and more potent than the old ones, there are no novel drugs. This point is often mentioned by critics of the pharmaceutical industry.

A good strategy for any group involved in drug research would be to use part of their capacity for the exploration of novel fields. Isolation, structure elucidation and biological evaluation of natural compounds which may have a regulatory function in the human or animal organism, has proven to be a stimulating approach. New chapters in the recent edition of Burger's Medicinal Chemistry [1] describe the prostaglandins (61 pages) and cyclic nucleotides (21 pages). The chapter on peptides grew from 13 pages in 1970 to 129 pages in 1980, illustrating the rapid advancement in the peptide field.

Can we perceive a strategy for the development of peptide drugs?

*References p. 62*

---

Strategy = a preconceived plan to reach a defined goal

---

To answer this question we have to define our final goal first. This goal is to produce, in sufficient quantities at a reasonable cost price, a useful and selective drug in a form suitable for human use.
When we start from a new natural compound, structure elucidation is the first step followed by the development of a suitable method for synthesis to provide sufficient material to determine the compound's biological activities.

Analogues are then synthesized to explore whether or not compounds more selective than the parent in their activity may be found. For peptides, the usual approach for analogue synthesis is first to ascertain whether the complete peptide is necessary for activity or only part of the structure is sufficient. The next step is to discover the importance of the side chains. This can be done by stepwise replacement of the amino acids by alanine, the shortest chiral amino acid or by stepwise replacement of the amino acids by the D-enantiomer.

After this first exploratory phase a more precise definition of the goal is possible. When only one biological activity is found it may be possible to base a marketable product on the natural compound. Otherwise it may be preferred to aim at finding a more selective, more potent, more stable or less expensive compound. One then has to study the relationship between structure and biological activity. In recent years a number of techniques have been developed for this purpose.

Two peptides, ACTH and LHRH will serve to illustrate this approach.

ACTH

The adrenocorticotropic hormone ACTH is one of the pituitary hormones. Its main action is to induce the release and synthesis of the corticoids by the adrenal cortex. ACTH can be used in the clinic as a diagnostic tool to test for adrenal function and it may be used in therapy to treat rheumatic disorders and dermatological diseases. It is a peptide consisting of 39 amino acids [+].

---

[+] Standard abbreviations are used for amino acids and peptides (82)

Ser-Tyr-Ser-Met-Glu-His-Phe-Arg-Trp-Gly-Lys-Pro-Val-Gly-Lys-Lys-Arg-Arg-
1 4 10 15 18

Pro-Val-Lys-Val-Tyr-Pro-Asn-Gly-Ala-Glu-Asp-Glu-Ser-Ala-Glu-Ala-Phe-Pro-
25 26 31 33

Leu-Glu-Phe
39

Fig. 1. Structure of human-ACTH.

The structure elucidation and synthesis of the ACTH's have proved difficult due to the presence of the -Aspartyl-Glycyl- sequence (25-26) which easily leads to desamidation and rearrangement of the molecule.

The structure of human-ACTH was finally established in 1971 [3, 4].

Porcine ACTH differs from human ACTH at position 31 with leucine instead of serine. Its structure was established in 1972 [4]. Ovine and bovine ACTH are identical and differ from the human hormone only in position 33, which is glutamic acid in human-ACTH but glutamine in ovine- and bovine-ACTH [5]. A Swiss and a Hungarian group were in 1972 the first to publish a synthesis of human-ACTH using a fragment condensation approach [6, 7]. A first synthesis on a polymeric support was published in the following year [8].

It had not taken that long however for ACTH preparations of synthetic origin to reach the market. In the course of the structure elucidation of porcine-ACTH, Bell et al. [9] had prepared the 1-31, 1-30 and 1-28 fragments of porcine-ACTH by pepsin digestion followed by isolation in a homogeneous state. In the adrenal ascorbic acid depletion assay of Sayers (intravenous administration) these fragments proved as active as the parent molecule. In the clinic the 1-28 fragment proved as active as the parent-ACTH against rheumatoid arthritis. Although it was not isolated in a pure state evidence was presented that the 1-24 fragment might also have the full activity. These data indicate that only part of the ACTH molecule is essential for activity.

The above also illustrates that for the larger peptides the study of the relationship between chemical structure and biological activity starts at the same time that the structure elucidation is carried out.

The expected high activity of the 1-24 fragment of ACTH was confirmed when it was synthesized by Schwyzer and Kappeler [10, 11] and proved to be as potent as the parent molecule in the Sayers test (intravenous administration). This product was developed jointly by Ciba and Organon. For therapeutic use a suitable long acting depot preparation had to be developed. For this a formulation with a complex of tetracosactide and zinc hydroxide in a suitable buffer proved to be the answer to the problem. It was introduced in 1969 a few years before the definitive establishment of the structure of human-ACTH.

## STRUCTURE AND ACTIVITY

These data show that the carboxyl terminal region of the ACTH molecule is not essential for steroidogenesis. Shorter fragments ACTH-(1-23) [12] and ACTH-(1-20)-amide [13] also retained full activity after intravenous administration. These were however much less potent than the parent molecule after subcutaneous administration, indicating that the carboxyl terminal region is important in protecting the molecule against proteolytic attack.

The segment essential for activity seems to be the 4-10 fragment. Schwyzer et al. [14] found in vitro with isolated rat adrenal cells that this fragment could induce the same rate of steroidogenesis as the parent hormone. For this however a $10^6$ times higher molar concentration was necessary. This indicates that other segments contribute strongly to binding to the receptor. The basic sequence -Lys-Lys-Arg-Arg- (15-18) is of major importance [15]. ACTH-(1-16) which lacks part of this sequence was nearly inactive in the Sayers test even after intravenous administration [16]. The N-terminal free amino group is also important for binding.

## ACTION OF ACTH ON THE CENTRAL NERVOUS SYSTEM

A new research field was opened with the discovery of De Wied [17] that ACTH and related peptides influence the extinction of conditioned avoidance behaviour in rats. ACTH-(1-10) proved on a weight basis equipotent with the parent. As was discussed above these shorter peptides show practically no stimulation of steroidogenesis. Thus dissociation with behavioural effects proved possible. By systematic shortening of the ACTH-(1-10) from the N-terminal side, ACTH-(4-10) was found to be the shortest peptide which affected the avoidance response as potently as the parent decapeptide [18]. This peptide sequence is also found in three other pituitary

Table 1. ACTH analogues in use for diagnostic and/or therapeutic purposes.

| |
|---|
| ACTH-(1-24)<br>Tetracosactide (Synacthen, Ciba, Cortrosyn, Organon) |
| [$Gly^1$]ACTH-(1-18)-amide<br>Giractide (Acthormone, Shionogi) |
| $\alpha_h$-[$Asp^{25}$, $Ala^{26}$, $Gly^{27}$]ACTH<br>Seractide (Isactide, Ferring) |
| $\alpha_h$-ACTH-(1-28)<br>Octacosactide (Actid, Ferring) |

hormones: α-MSH (α-melanocyte stimulating hormone), β-MSH and β-LPH (β-lipotropic hormone). Both α-MSH and β-MSH affected the avoidance response in the same manner [17].

Met-Glu-His-Phe-Arg-Trp-Gly
4 5 6 7 8 9 10

Fig. 2. Structure of ACTH-(4-10)

The structure activity relationship for this small peptide was then investigated systematically. Shortening of the peptide step by step from the carboxyl end revealed that the 4-7 fragment contains the essential information for behavioural effect [19]. On a weight basis it is equipotent with the decapeptide, on a molar basis it is less active. This demonstrated that dissociation from MSH activity is also possible, since the presence both of arginine at position 8 and of tryptophan at position 9 is essential for MSH activity. This was confirmed when it was shown that in the 4-9 fragment the arginine at position 8, essential for MSH activity, could be replaced by lysine without loss of behavioural activity.

The stepwise replacement of L-amino acids in a peptide by the corresponding D-enantiomers has proven to be a fruitful approach in structure-activity studies. It gives an indication of the specific importance of the side chain for activity.

$[Lys^8]$ACTH-(4-9) which is selective in its action and sufficiently potent was used for this study [20]. It was of interest to note that the 7-D-Phe isomer facilitated instead of delayed extinction of the avoidance response in the shuttle box. This reversal of action had also been observed earlier with $[D\text{-}Phe^7]$ACTH-(1-10) [21]. The biological significance of this result needs further exploration.

Strong potentiation of the effect of the parent hexapeptide was observed for the D-$Lys^8$ isomer and somewhat smaller potentiation for the D-$His^6$ isomer. The D-$Met^4$, D-$Glu^5$ and D-$Trp^9$ isomers were at least as potent as the parent hexapeptide suggesting that many sidechain variations will be allowed for activity. To explore this further, amino acid residues were exchanged for other ones which could be expected to enhance selectivity or to lead to a reduction in the cost price of the active peptide. This is illustrated by two examples which proved successful:

a. Tryptophan, with its high reactivity for electrophilic substitution, is often the cause of side reactions in the deprotection steps of peptide synthesis. It could be replaced by phenylalanine without loss of behavioural activity [20].
b. Oxydation of the methionine sulphur to the sulphoxide level, known to decrease adrenocorticotrophic activity in ACTH and melanocyte-stimulating activity in $\alpha$-MSH, proved to enhance behavioural activity in ACTH-(4-10) and related peptides [20]. Since sulphoxides are chiral, oxydation of methionine leads to a mixture of sulphoxides, which poses a synthetic problem. For that reason methionine sulphone was introduced and proved equipotent. With the resulting ORG-2766 a potency 1000 times that of ACTH-(4-10) (subcutaneous administration) had been achieved [22]. The compound showed oral activity owing to its high potency.

Met($O_2$)-Glu-His-Phe-D-Lys-Phe

Fig. 3. Structure of ORG 2766

The compound was then selected for further pharmacological and clinical evaluation.

A number of pilot studies with oral subchronic administration of ORG-2766 suggest that this peptide has a positive and consistent effect on mood in man [24].

## INTERMEZZO

The reader may have noticed that it was assumed in the above discussion of the relationship between structure and activity that for the ACTH peptides the effect of a variation of amino acids at a given position is independent of the groups present at other positions.

For example when a variation at position a enhances potency 2-times and other variation at position c 3-times, it is assumed that a peptide combining these two variations is 6-times more potent.

$$\text{Potency} = \text{group contribution}_a \times \text{group contribution}_b \times \ldots$$

$$\log\ \text{potency} = \text{group contribution}'_a + \text{group contribution}'_b + \ldots$$

To check the validity of this assumption a Fujita-Ban analysis [25] of 55 ACTH-analogues was made, based on the potency in the pole-jumping test for conditioned avoidance behaviour [26]. Only 3 outliers were found. The potencies of 52 analogues could be described quantitatively with a multiple regression coefficient of 0,984. This justifies the initial assumption.

## A NEW CHALLENGE

The discussion on ACTH started with the simple concept of a hormone. It is produced by the pituitary and released to stimulate the target organ, the adrenal gland. Then came the pioneering studies of DE WIED and associates showing that it also has direct effects on the central nervous system [17]. The study of the synthesis of ACTH in the body recently led to another surprising discovery. It is not synthesized directly but originates from a polypeptide pro-opiocortin, which also is the precursor of β-lipotrophin [27]. Why does the body produce these two "hormones" together? To answer these questions one has to analyse the function of β-lipotropin. It is then found that β-lipotrophin can serve as precursor for an entire series of smaller peptides with interesting activities such as those of the analgesic peptide β-endorphin [28]. We would lose sight of the topic of this paper if we tried to discuss this rapidly developing field, but it illustrates the challenge and importance of this type of research.

*References p. 62*

LHRH

We now focus our attention on luteinizing hormone releasing hormone (LHRH). It is the hypothalamic hormone, which stimulates the release both of the luteinizing hormone (LH) and of the follicle stimulating hormone (FSH) by the hypophysis. Early studies suggested that LHRH's of human, sheep, pig and cow are identical [29]. In 1971 Schally and coworkers [30, 31] determined the structure of porcine LHRH. Independantly Guillemin and coworkers [32] solved the structure of ovine LHRH. Both structures proved to be identical. The first synthesis of the decapeptide were published in that same year [33, 34].

pGlu-His-Trp-Ser-Tyr-Gly-Leu-Arg-Pro-Gly-$NH_2$

1 2 3 4 5 6 7 8 9 10

Fig. 4. Structure of LHRH

Study of the relationship between chemical structure and biological activity followed the pattern indicated earlier in this paper. Shorter analogues were synthesized and tested to find the active core. Shortening from the N-terminal side ([des-$pGlu^1$]-LHRH or [des-$pGlu^1$, des-$His^2$]LHRH [35]) or from the C-terminal side ([des--$GlyNH_2^{10}$]LHRH [36]) led to significantly decreased activity. Thus the complete peptide is the active hormone and it is not a pro-drug for a shorter peptide.

Metabolism of LHRH is rapid. In the human the half-life for the first phase is 5.3 minutes [37]. Hydrolysis is possible at several positions (Fig. 5). None of the fragments showed significant activity.

This short half-life may be essential for the action of LHRH. There is evidence for pulsatile release of LHRH in the rhesus monkey [45]. Chronic stimulation by LHRH or its long acting analogues seems to lead to "down regulation" of ovarian or pituitary receptors [46]. For the treatment of infertility in hypothalamic amenorrhea a computerized portable pump has been developed by Ferring, which makes it possible to deliver an i.v. infusion every 90 minutes (15 or 20 μg LHRH in 1 minute). The first reported clinical results are promising [47].

```
  1,6    1,3   1    1   3,4    2,4     5
   ↓      ↓    ↓    ↓    ↓      ↓      ↓
pGlu——His——Trp-Ser-Tyr——Gly——Leu-Arg-Pro-Gly-NH2
```

1. kidney homogenate [38]
2. hypothalamic extract [39]
3. pituitary endopeptidase [40]
4. liver homogenate [41, 42]
5. postproline cleaving enzyme (brain, pituitary) [43]
6. pyroglutaminate aminopeptidase (brain, pituitary) [44]

Fig. 5. Degradation of LHRH

## RELATION BETWEEN STRUCTURE AND ACTIVITY

The investigators at the Salk Institute were the first to explore the functions of the side-chains of the amino acids through replacement of these amino acids by glycine, L-alanine or D-alanine. This led to two important discoveries. Replacement of histidine at position 2 by glycine yielded a partial agonist, indicating that antagonists to LHRH may be found [48]. The replacement of glycine at position 6 by D-alanine yielded a much more potent analogue with agonist activity [49].

We will come back to the antagonists later and discuss the superagonists first. Since [D-Ala$^6$]LHRH was 4 times as potent as the parent both in vitro (rat pituitary cell culture) and in vivo (i.v. administration to an estrogen primed ovariectomized rat), the authors concluded that the high potency is not due to decreased metabolism. They suggested that it might be due to a conformational effect. $^1$H- and $^{13}$C-NMR studies [50, 51] have shown that LHRH is flexible in $D_2O$ solution, occurring mainly in random coil conformations. It was then assumed that LHRH binds to its receptor in a conformation with a β-II type bend between the amino acids 5-8. Substitution of the glycine at the 6 position by D-alanine should make this a preferred conformation. This model was refined by molecular mechanics type calculations by Momamy [52]. A group at Merck then synthesized a conformationally constrained analogue (Fig. 6) to mimic this model [53].

```
                        CH2-CH2
                       /       \
pGlu-His-Trp-Ser-Tyr-NH-CH       N-CH-CO-Arg-Pro-Gly-NH2
                         \     /   |
                           C       CH2
                           ||      |
                           O       CH(CH3)2
```

Fig. 6. Conformationally constrained analogue of LHRH

References p. 62

This analogue is more potent than LHRH both in vitro and in vivo, which supports the proposed model.

Seprodi et al [54] synthesized and tested cyclic[$\beta$-Ala$^1$, D-Ala$^6$, Gly$^{10}$]LHRH and cyclic[6-Aminohexanoic acid$^1$, D-Ala$^6$, Gly$^{10}$]LHRH. These examples of conformationally constrained analogues showed only 1.2% and 0.65% of the potency of LHRH. Since these cyclic analogues are much more potent than the corresponding linear analogues this may also support the proposed bent model for the active conformation of LHRH.

These examples show the strength of an approach based on the calculation of preferred conformations. It stimulates the synthesis of unusual structures, which otherwise probably never would have been considered for synthesis.

The examples also point out weaknesses. In view of the cost of the calculations and syntheses, one may tend to produce so few examples that a statistically significant answer is impossible.

For that reason, simpler methods are necessary in the first stages of the investigations.

An analysis of the Chou and Fasman $f_j$ values [55], indicators for the tendency of the amino acids to promote $\beta$-turns shows that all amino acids in the sequence Tyr$^5$-Arg$^8$ with the exception of Leu$^7$ have $f_j > 0.070$ indicating that they promote $\beta$-turn formation (Fig. 7).

-- Tyr$^5$ - Gly$^6$ - Leu$^7$ - Arg$^8$ --

0.136 0.090 0.032 0.101

Fig. 7. Chou and Fasman $f_j$ values for the sequence 5-8 of LHRH

The low value for leucine makes the $p_t$ value ($p_t = \Pi f_j = f_i \cdot f_{i+1} \cdot f_{i+2} \cdot f_{i+3}$) too low to expect a $\beta$-turn in LHRH itself, in accordance with its NMR spectrum. One thus expects that the replacement of Leu$^7$ by amino acids like serine ($f_j = 0.095$) or better by glycine ($f_j = 0.158$), which promote $\beta$-turn conformation, will lead to more potent analogues if the model is correct. However [Ser$^7$]LHRH [56] had only 1/10 the potency of LHRH whereas [Gly$^7$]LHRH [66] was even less active. This contrasts with [Ile$^7$]LHRH [57] which still shows some 40% of the potency of LHRH

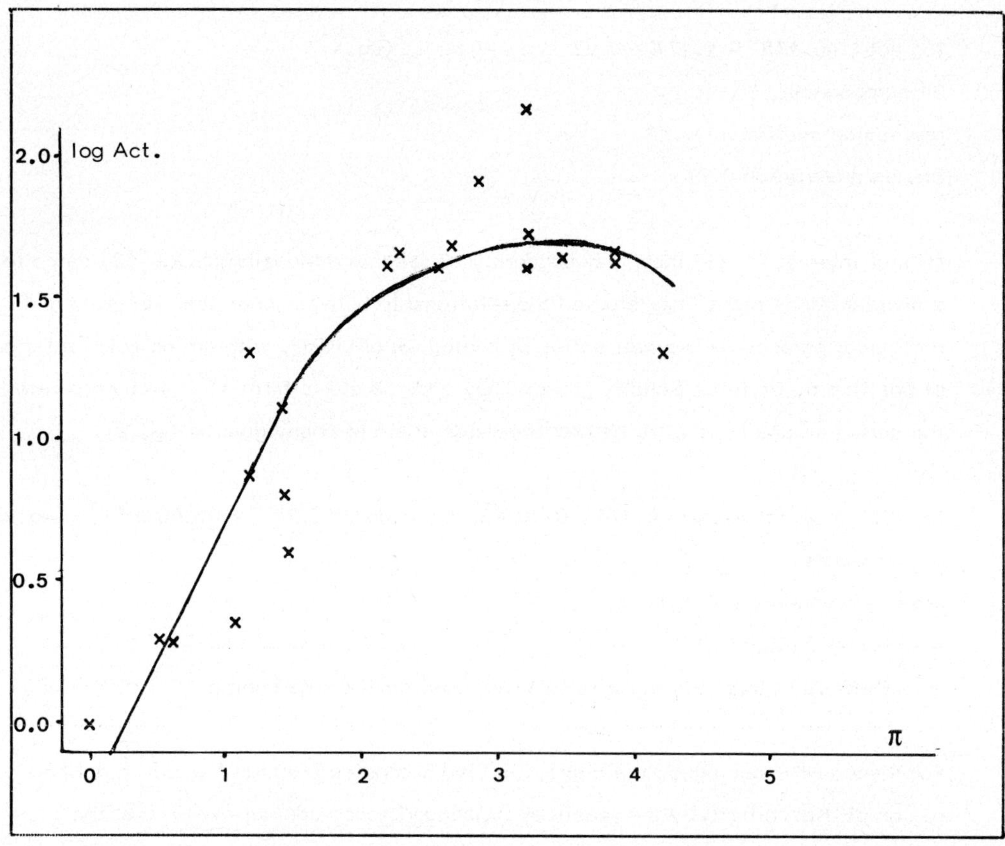


Fig. 8. Relationship between ovulation induction potency and lipophilicity

although isoleucine ($f_j$ = 0.017) is as bad at promoting β-turn conformations as leucine. These data suggest that the conformational effect may not be such a major effect in determining potency as was suggested earlier. This makes the suggestion of Fujino et al [57] that lipophilicity could be an important factor of interest.

To analyse this further we have plotted in Fig. 8 the potencies to induce ovulation against the calculated lipophilicities $\pi$ [59-61] relative to LHRH for a series of 21 analogues of [des-Gly$NH_2^{10}$]LHRH-ethylamide, with amino acid variations with a $CH_2R$ side chain at positions 6 and/or 7 (König et al. [58]).
With the exception of one outlier, [D-Cys(tBu)$^6$, Ala$^7$, des-Gly$NH_2^{10}$]LHRH-ethyl amide, the data can be fitted to a parabolic function (eq.1). The optimum $\pi$ is 3.4 relative to LHRH.

$$\log \text{act} = -0.17\pi^2 + 1.17\pi - 0.27 \qquad \text{(eq.1)}$$

21 compounds

regression coefficient 0.91

standard deviation 0.24

It is of interest to note that, independently Nadasdi and Medzihradszky [62] came to a similar conclusion. They studied the relationship between chemical structure and biological potency for a small series of analogues of LHRH, with amino acid variations at position 6, from the Schally group. They added a steric term $Y'_{\gamma,c}$ to incorporate in the series an analogue with the branched side chain of phenylglycine (eq.2).

$$\log \text{biological response} = 2.174 + 0.4078\Sigma R_f - 0.04150(\Sigma R_f)^2 - 0.3660Y'_{\gamma,c} \qquad \text{(eq.2)}$$

8 compounds

regression coefficient 0.99

standard deviation 0.071

$R_f$ = Rekkers hydrophobic fragment values [63] for the side chains.

For these LHRH analogues the highest in vivo potencies are thus found in a defined region of lipophilicity. As a practical consequence one can not expect that the variation of an amino acid at a given position and its effect on the biological activity is independent of the groups present at other positions. Thus, in contrast with the ACTH analogues, the Fujita-Ban assumption is not valid for the LHRH analogues. Many examples are reported in literature, we shall discuss two of them below.

Dutta et al, [64] studied the effect of replacement of the C-terminal glycinamide ($NHCH_2CONH_2$) by the more polar aza analogue $NHNHCONH_2$. As might be expected this replacement leads in LHRH to a somewhat less active analogue; however, in strongly lipophilic LHRH analogues it leads to enhanced potencies compared with the parent molecule. [D-Ser(tBu)$^6$, AzGly$^{10}$]LHRH (ICI 118630) is such an example. By contrast, replacement of the C-terminal glycinamide ($NHCH_2CONH_2$) by the less polar $NHC_2H_5$ yields in LHRH a 3 to 5 times more potent analogue, whereas the same replacement in the highly lipophilic [D-Nal(2)$^6$]LHRH leads to a decrease in potency [65].

The best superagonists are about 60 to 100 times more potent than LHRH.

A summary is given in Table 2. [65, 66].

Table 2. Examples of potent LHRH agonists.

| |
|---|
| [D-Trp$^6$]LHRH |
| [D-Leu$^6$, des-GlyNH$_2$$^{10}$]LHRH-ethylamide |
| [D-Ser(tBu)$^6$, des-GlyNH$_2$$^{10}$]LHRH-ethylamide |
| [D-3-(2-naphtyl)alanine$^6$]LHRH |

The LHRH case illustrates that it is important in the first phase of exploration of the relationship between chemical structure and biological activity in peptides to study the effect of variations of at least two amino acid positions at the same time. It is then possible to determine whether the Fujita-Ban assumption can be applied or not and to select the strategy for the next phase accordingly.

Free energy relationships can be derived in the next phase. This technique for the study of peptides pioneered by Kaurov and Martynov [67, 68, 69], has gained tremendously in its ease of application by the publication in recent years of parameter sets for the amino acids, see for example, refs. 59. 60, 61, 70.

If indications are obtained that conformational effects are important one may then decide to carry out molecular- mechanical or quantum-chemical calculations of low energy conformations to support the design of promising analogues.

With better knowledge of the relationships between structure and function of the peptides, the chemists will no longer stay within the limits imposed by the natural amino acids but synthesize novel structures incorporating the properties desired.

## LHRH ANTAGONISTS

The development of the LHRH antagonists, important for example as potential contraceptives, illustrates this trend. We have mentioned already the discovery of Monahan et al. [48] that [Gly$^2$]LHRH behaves as a partial agonist, indicating the possibility of developing a pure antagonist. This suggests that the N-terminal side of LHRH is not only important for binding to the receptor but is also important for the functional signal [66].

The best test to detect pure antagonists proved to be the suppression of spontaneous ovulation in the proestrus rat. In women suppression of gonadotrophin response is measured [66]. The development is summarized in Table 3.

Table 3. Summary of the development of LHRH antagonists.

| | | | Activity | |
|---|---|---|---|---|
| 1972 | [48] | [des-$His^{2}$]LHRH | | |
| 1976 | [71] | [D-$Phe^{2}$, D-$Trp^{6}$]LHRH | rat 1.5 mg | |
| | [71] | [D-$Phe^{2}$, D-$Trp^{3}$, D-$Phe^{6}$]LHRH | rat 1.0 mg | human 90 mg |
| 1978 | [72] | [Ac-$Pro^{1}$, D-$Phe^{2}$, D-$Trp^{3,6}$]LHRH | rat 0.2 mg | |
| 1979 | [73] | [Ac-D-$Phe^{1}$, D-pCl-$Phe^{2}$, D-$Trp^{3,6}$]LHRH | rat 0.03 mg | human 10 mg |
| 1981 | [74] | [Ac-$\Delta^{3}Pro^{1}$, D-pF-$Phe^{2}$, D-$Trp^{3,6}$]LHRH | rat 0.005 mg | |
| | [75] | [Ac-D-pCl-$Phe^{1,2}$, D-$Trp^{3}$, D-$Phe^{6}$, D-$Ala^{10}$]LHRH | rat 0.010 mg | |

Although the 1981 antagonists certainly do not form the end of the development of potent antagonists, they open, with an expected activity in the human in the range of 2-3 mg, the possibility for a systematic clinical exploration of the opportunities with these antagonists.

## PHARMACY

The ease of enzymatic degradation of the peptides, leading to short half lives in biological systems, makes the choice of a suitable pharmaceutical form an important step in the development of a peptide drug. Many interesting solutions have been found. The computerized pump used by Leyendecker et al. [47], which allowed programmed pulsatile intravenous administration of small amounts of LHRH was mentioned already. However, one needs strongly motivated patients for the use of such a device. With the adrenocorticotropins we briefly discussed the development of long acting depot preparations, suitable for injection, by complex formation of the peptide and a suitable carrier.

Oxytocin is used to induce and stimulate labor. It can be given as an intravenous drip but this proves rather inconvenient for the patient. Here the transbuccal route proved safe and effective. A tablet is allowed to dissolve slowly in the mouth, the onset of action is fast and can be observed easily [76, 77].

Intranasal administration was used in a clinical study with [D-Ser(tBu)$^{6}$, des-GlyNH$_2^{10}$]LHRH-ethylamide. The drug was effective but a number of users had a technical problem with the spray [78].

Vaginal administration of [D-Leu$^{6}$, des-GlyNH$_2^{10}$]LHRH-ethylamide was studied in rats. Vaginal absorption proved highly dependent on the estrous cycle of the rat. Absorption at metestrus or diestrus was 13 times higher than that obtained at proestrus or estrus [79].

However, one may be searching for too complicated methods since the high concentrations of LHRH in human- [80] and cow- [81] milk seems to suggest that the oral route is the one which evolved in nature.

## CONCLUSION

The examples given illustrate that if one can bring together a (small) team of a few good organic chemists, biochemists, endocrinologists, pharmacists and clinicians, who are willing to work closely together, peptide research can be a fruitful area for the research and development of novel drugs. The examples also illustrate how in recent years the tools have been developed to analyse systematically the relationship between chemical structure and biological activity. In the early phase when only few data are available one may then find the most important factors using the most simple models possible. These can then be tested, refined or revised when more data become available.

As soon as analogues with sufficient potency and selectivity are available a further indepth exploration of their clinical potential is necessary. Depending on the outcome, it may then be decided to enter the development phase.

## ACKNOWLEDGEMENT

Without the stimulating discussions with F. van der Vlugt, J. van Nispen and especially with H.M. Greven this paper could never have been written.

*References p. 62*

## REFERENCES


1. M.E. Wolff (Ed.), Burger's Medicinal Chemistry, 4th edition, John Wiley, New York, 1980/1981.
2. Annual Reports in Medicinal Chemistry, Academic Press, New York.
3. L. Gráf, S. Bajusz, A. Patthy, E. Barál and G. Cseh, Acta Biochim. Biophys.Acad.Sci.Hung., 6 (1971) 415.
4. B. Riniker, P. Sieber, W. Rittel and H. Zuber, Nature New Biology, 235 (1972) 114.
5. A. Jöhl, B. Riniker and L. Schenkel-Hulliger, FEBS letters, 45(1972) 172.
6. P. Sieber, W. Rittel and B. Riniker, Helv.Chim.Acta, 55 (1972) 1243.
7. L. Kisfaludy, M. Löw, T. Szirtes, I. Schön, M. Sárközi, S. Bajusz, A. Turan, A. Juhász, R. Beke, L. Gráf and K. Medsihradsky, in Chemistry and Biology of Peptides, Proceedings of the 3rd American Peptide Symposium, J. Meienhofer (Ed.), Ann Arbor Science, Ann Arbor, 1972, p.299.
8. D. Yamashimo and C.H. Li, J. Am.Chem.Soc., 95 (1973) 1310.
9. P.H. Bell, K.S. Howard, R.G. Shephard, B.M. Finn and J.H. Meisenhelder, J.Am.Chem.Soc., 78 (1956) 5059.
10. H. Kappeler and R. Schwyzer, Helv.Chim.Acta, 44 (1961) 1136.
11. R. Schwyzer and H. Kappeler, Helv.Chim.Acta, 46 (1963) 1550.
12. K. Hofmann, H. Yajima, T. Liu and N. Yanaihara, J. Am.Chem.Soc., 84 (1962) 4475.
13. K. Hofmann, H. Yajima, T. Liu, N. Yanaihara, C. Yanaihara and J.L. Humes, J. Am.Chem.Soc., 84 (1962) 4481.
14. R. Schwyzer, P. Schiller, S. Seilig and G. Sayers, FEBS Letters, 19 (1971) 229.
15. Review: J. Ramachandran in Hormonal Proteins and Peptides, C.H. Li (Ed.), Academic Press, New York Vol.II, 1973, p.1.
16. K. Hofmann, N. Yanaihara, S. Lande and H. Yajima, J.Am.Chem.Soc., 84 (1962) 4471.
17. D. de Wied, Proc.Soc.Exp. Biol., 122 (1966) 28.
18. H.M. Greven and D. de Wied, Eur.J.Pharmacol., 2 (1967) 14.
19. D. de Wied, A. Witter and H.M. Greven, Biochemical Pharmacology, 24 (1975) 1463.
20. H.M. Greven and D. de Wied, in Progress in Brain Research, E. Zimmerman, W.H. Gispen, B.H. Marks and D. de Wied (Ed.), 39 (1973) 429.
21. B. Bohus and D. de Wied, Science 153 (1966) 318.
22. H.M. Greven and D. de Wied, in Frontiers of Hormone Research, T.B. van Wimersma Greidanus (Ed.), S. Karger, Basel, Vol.4, 1977, p.140.
23. H. Rigter, R. Janssens-Elbertse and H. van Riezen, Pharmacol. Biochem. Behav., 5 (1976) suppl 1, 53.
24. R.M. Pigache and H. Rigter, in Frontiers in Hormone Research, T.B. van Wimersma Greidanus and L.H. Rees (Ed.), Karger, Basel, Vol.8, 1981, p.178
25. T. Fujita and T. Ban, J.Med.Chem., 14 (1971) 148.
26. J. Kelder and H.M. Greven, Rec.Trav. Chim. 98 (1979) 168.
27. J.L. Roberts and E. Herbert, Proc. Nat. Acad.Sci.U.S., 74 (1977) 3052.
28. J. Hope and P.J. Lowry, in Frontiers in Hormone Research, T.B. van Wimersma Greidanus and L.H. Rees (Ed.), Karger, Basel, Vol.8, 1981, p.44.
29. A.V. Schally, A. Arimura, C.Y. Bowers, I. Wakabayashi, A.J. Kastin, T.W. Redding, J.C. Mettler, R.M.G.Mc.Nair, P. Pizzolato and A.J. Segal, J. Clin.Endocrin.Metab.31 (1970) 291.

30. H. Matsuo, Y. Baba, R.M.G. Nair, A. Arima and A.V. Schally, Biochem. Biophys.Res.Commun., 43 (1972) 1334.
31. R.M.G. Nair and A.V. Schally, Int.J. Peptide Protein Res., 4 (1972) 421.
32. R. Burgus, M. Butcher, M. Amoss, N. Ling, M. Monahan, J. Rivier, R. Fellows, R. Blackwell, W. Vak and R. Guillemin, Proc.Nat.Acad.Sci.U.S., 69 (1972) 278.
33. M. Monahan, J. Rivier, R. Burgus, M. Amoss, R. Blackwell, W. Vale and R. Guillemin, C.R. Hebd.Acad.Sci.Ser.D,273 (1971) 508.
34. H. Matsui, A. Arima, R.M.G. Nair and A.V. Schally, Biochem.Biophys.Res. Commun., 45 (1971) 822.
35. A.V. Schally, A. Arimura, W.H. Carter, T.W. Redding, R. Geiger, W. König, H. Wissman, G. Jaeger, J. Sandow, N. Yanaihara, C. Yanaihara, T. Hashimoto and M. Sagakami, Biochem.Biophys.Res.Commun., 48 (1972) 366.
36. M. Fujino, S. Kobayashi, M. Obayashi, S. Shinagawa, T. Fukuda, C. Kittatada, R. Nayahama, I. Yimasaki, W.F. White and R.H. Rippel, Biochem.Biophys. Res.Commun., 49 (1972) 863.
37. S.L. Jeffcoate, R.H. Greenwood and D.T. Holland, J. Endocrinology, 60 (1974) 305.
38. M.A. Stetler-Stevenson, D.C. Yang, A. Lipkowski, L.Mc.Cartney, D. Peterson and G. Flouret, J.Med.Chem., 24 (1981) 688.
39. Y. Koch, T. Baram, P. Chobsieng and M. Friedkin, Biochem.Biophys.Res. Commun., 61 (1974) 95.
40. D. Hudson, A. Pickering, J.L.Mc. Loughlin, E. Matthews, R. Sharpe, G. Fink, I. McIntyre and M. Szelke, 5th Int. Congr. Endocrin. (1976) 18 abstract 43.
41. T.N. Akopyan, A.A. Arutunyan, A.I. Orgasiyan, A. Lajtha and A.A. Galoyan, J. Neurochem., 32 (1979) 629.
42. S. Wilk, M. Benuck, M. Orlowski and N. Marks, Neurosci. Lett., 14 (1979) 275.
43. M. Fridkin, E. Hazum, T. Baram, H.R. Lindner and Y. Koch, in Peptides, M. Goodman and J. Meienhofer (Ed.) Halsted Press, New York, 1977, p. 193.
44. K. Bauer, B. Horsthemke, H. Knitsatchek, P. Nowak and H. Keihauf, Hoppe-Seylers Z. Physiol. Chem., 360 (1979) 229.
45. P.W. Carmel, S. Araki and M. Ferin, Endocrinology, 99 (1976) 243.
46. J.P. Hanker, H.G. Bohnet, G. Leyendecker and H.P.G. Schneider, Int. J. Fertil., 25 (1980) 222.
47. G. Leyendecker, L. Wildt and M. Hansmann, J. Clin. Endocrin. Metabol., 51 (1980) 1214.
48. M.W. Monahan, J. Rivier, W. Vale, R. Guillemin and R. Burgus, Biochem. Biophys. Res. Commun., 47 (1972) 551.
49. M.W. Monahan, M.S. Amoss, H.A. Anderson and W. Vale, Biochemistry, 12 (1973) 4616.
50. P.L. Wessels, J. Feeney, H. Gregory and J.J. Gormley, J. Chem. Soc. Perkin II, (1973) 1691.
51. R. Deslauriers, G.C. Levy, W.H. McGregor, D. Sarantakis and J.C.P. Smith, Biochemistry, 14 (1975) 4335.
52. F.A. Momamy, J. Am. Chem. Soc., 98 (1976) 2990 and 2996.
53. R.M. Friedinger, D.F. Veber, D. Schwenck-Perlow, J.R. Brooks and R. Saperstein, Science, 210 (1980) 656.
54. J. Seprödi, D.H. Coy, J.A. Vilchez-Martinez, E. Pedroza, W.Y. Huang and A.V. Schally, J. Med. Chem., 21 (1978) 993.
55. P.Y. Chou and G.D. Fasman, Biochemistry, 13 (1974) 211, and 222.
56. H. Immer, V.R. Nelson, C. Revesz, K. Sestry and M. Götz, J. Med. Chem., 17 (1974) 1060.

57. M. Fujino, S. Kobayashi, M. Obayashi, T. Fukuda, S. Shinagawa, Y. Yamasak R. Nakayawa, W.F. White and R.H. Rippel, Biochem. Biophys. Res. Commun. 49 (1972) 698.
58. W. König, J. Sandow and R. Geiger, in Peptides, Chemistry, Structure, Biology R. Walter and J. Meienhofer (Ed.), Ann Arbor Science Publishers, Ann Arbor, 1975, p. 883.
59. V. Pliska and J.L. Fauchère in Peptides, Structure and Biological Function, E. Gross and J. Meienhofer (Ed.), Pierce, Rockford, 1979, p. 249.
60. J.L. Fauchère and V. Pliska in Peptides 1980, K. Brunfeldt (Ed.), Scriptor, Copenhagen, 1981, p. 637.
61. J.L. Fauchère, K.Q. Do, P.Y.C. Jow and C. Hansch, Experientia, 36 (1980) 1203.
62. L. Nadasdi and K. Medzihradszky, Biochem. Biophys. Res. Commun., 99 (198 451.
63. R.F. Rekker, The Hydrophobic Fragmental Constant, Elsevier Amsterdam, 1976.
64. A.S. Dutta, B.J.A. Furr, M.B. Giles and B. Valcaccia, J. Med. Chem., 21 (1978) 1018.
65. J.J. Nestor, T.L. Ho, R.A. Simpson, B.L. Horner, G.H. Jones, G.I. McRae and B.H. Vickery, American Peptide Symposium 1981, in press.
66. A.V. Schally, D.H. Coy and A. Arimura, Int. J. Gynaecol. Obstet., 18 (1980) 318.
67. O.A. Kaurov and V.F. Martynov, Vestn. Lening. Univ. Fiz. Khim., (1970) 137; Chem. Abstr., 74 (1971) 38743k.
68. O.A. Kaurov, V.F. Martynov, Ju. D. Mihaylov, O.A. Popernaczky and M.P. Smirnova, in Peptides 1972, H. Hanson and H.D. Jakubke (Ed.) North Holland, Amsterdam, 1973, p. 450.
69. O.A. Kaurov, Bioorg. Khim., 4 (1978) 604.
70. K.J. Schaper, Eur. J. Med. Chem., 15 (1980) 449.
71. E.J. Coy, J.A. Vilchez-Martinez and A.V. Schally, in Peptides 1976, A. Loffe (Ed.), Éditions de l'Université de Bruxelles, Brussels, 1976.
72. J. Humphries, Y.P. Wan, T. Wasiak, K. Folkers and C.Y. Bowers, Biochem. Biophys. Res. Commun., 85 (1978) 709.
73. D.H. Coy, I. Meso, E. Pedroza, M.V. Nekola, J. Vilchez, P. Piyachaturawat, A.V. Schally, J. Seprödi and I. Teplan, in Peptides, Structure and Biological Function, E. Gross and J. Meienhofer (Ed.), Pierce, Rockford, 1979, p. 775.
74. J. Rivier, C. Rivier, M. Perrin, J. Porter and W. Vale, in Peptides 1980, K. Brunfeldt (Ed.), Scriptor, Copenhagen, 1981, p. 566.
75. J. Echegyi, D.H. Coy, M.V. Nekola, E.J. Coy, A.V. Schally, I. Mezo and I. Teplan, Biochem. Biophys. Res. Commun., 100 (1981) 915.
76. J.A. Chalmers and A. Prakash, Am. J. Obstet. Gynec., (1971) 111.
77. A. Cordano and V. Kraus, Obstetrics and Gynecology, 39 (1972) 247.
78. C. Bergquist, S.J. Nillius and L. Wide, Contraception, 19 (1979) 497.
79. H. Okada, I. Yamazaki and T. Yashiki, J. Pharmacobiol. Dynamics, 4 (1981) 517.
80. A.K. Sarda and R.M.G. Nair, J. Clin. Endocrin. Metabolism, 52 (1981) 826.
81. T. Baram, Y. Koch, E. Hazum and M. Fridkin, Science, 198 (1977) 300.
82. IUPAC-IUB Commission on Chemical Nomenclature, Biochem. J., 126 (1972) 773.

J.A. Keverling Buisman (Editor), *Strategy in Drug Research* 


# ENZYMES AS TOOLS AND TARGETS IN DRUG RESEARCH

THOMAS A. KRENITSKY and GERTRUDE B. ELION

Wellcome Research Laboratories, Research Triangle Park, North Carolina USA 27709

## ABSTRACT

Enzyme inhibitors are classified here by three criteria: 1) what they structurally mimic, 2) where they bind, and 3) how they inhibit. These different classes of inhibitors vary in their relative susceptibilities to the various complex factors that can affect their activity *in vivo*. Parameters influencing both their efficacy and their selectivity are considered. Most of the examples discussed are inhibitors of enzymes involved in nucleic acid synthesis.

With these considerations as a basis, this paper will compare two general strategies for the discovery and development of enzyme inhibitors as drugs. The first, referred to as the TARGETED strategy, begins with the determination of structure-activity relationships on the isolated target enzyme. Biological tests with the most potent inhibitors follow these enzyme studies. The second strategy, referred to as the UNTARGETED strategy, depends upon biological screens to select lead inhibitors that are active *in vivo*. With this strategy, the target enzyme is not chosen, but rather revealed by investigation of the mechanism of action of the 'lead' compound. Both strategies involve a cyclical refinement process of design, synthesis, and testing on the isolated target enzyme, but the process is put into operation at different points of development. It is concluded that the TARGETED strategy is appropriate for the development of agents that act as METABOLIC REGULATORS, whereas the UNTARGETED strategy is currently the more serviceable for CHEMOTHERAPEUTIC AGENTS.

---

## INTRODUCTION

The history of pharmaceutical invention teaches that in many instances the discovery of enzyme inhibitors as therapeutic agents has involved an element of serendipity. Knowledge of the identity of the target enzyme and of its importance to the target cell have often followed, rather than preceded, the discovery of biological activity. Even when the target enzyme has been predetermined, the pitfalls *in vivo* are many. It is an unpleasant, but undeniable fact that a

*References p. 86*

high percentage of enzyme inhibitors that are potent *in vitro*, prove unsatisfactory *in vivo*. Nevertheless, enzyme studies play an important role in the modern process of pharmaceutical invention (refs. 1-3). The ultimate purpose here is to consider at what point in drug development enzyme studies are most appropriate. This paper is divided into four sections. The first is concerned with the different types of enzyme inhibitors; the second with the relative susceptibilities of each type to factors that affect efficacy *in vivo*; the third with selectivity *in vivo*; and the last, using the foregoing as a basis, with general strategies.

SCHEME I

CLASSIFICATION OF ENZYME INHIBITORS BY:

I. *What* they mimic.
   - (A) A single substrate or product
   - (B) Multi-substrate and/or product complexes
   - (C) A transition state formed during catalysis
   - (D) Allosteric regulators

II. *Where* they bind.
   - (A) Catalytic (active) site
     - (1) unoccupied
     - (2) partially occupied by co-substrate
     - (3) substrate-modified
   - (B) Non-catalytic site
     - (1) Regulatory (allosteric) site
     - (2) Non-regulatory site

III. *How* they inhibit.
   - (A) Non-covalent binding
     - (1) Non-substrate (Dead End)
     - (2) Alternate substrate
   - (B) Covalent binding (inactivating)
     - (1) Group-directed (non-substrates)
     - (2) Suicide (mechanism-based)
       - (a) Reactive-product
       - (b) Stable-intermediate

## Types of Enzyme Inhibitors

This section will classify the different types of enzyme inhibitors which will be referred to in the remainder of the paper. This is necessary because factors affecting their efficacy and selectivity are often a function of the type of inhibitor involved. Most of the examples provided involve enzymes of nucleic acid synthesis.

There are a wide variety of theoretical possibilities for interactions of inhibitors with coenzymes, apoenzymes and holoenzymes (ref. 4). For the purpose here, however, only holoenzymes will be considered. Coenzyme analogs and inhibitors that sequester coenzymes are not discussed. Although many different classifications can be devised, three major distinguishing characteristics are used here: 1) <u>what</u> the inhibitors structurally mimic, 2) <u>where</u> they bind, and 3) <u>how</u> they inhibit (Scheme I).

In the first category, an inhibitor can structurally resemble substrates, a transition state formed during catalysis, or an allosteric regulator. Mimicking a single substrate is the inhibitor oxipurinol, the major metabolite of allopurinol and a potent inhibitor of xanthine oxidase <u>in vivo</u> (ref. 5).

XANTHINE OXIDASE

XANTHINE OXIPURINOL

Inhibitors which possess the binding determinants of more than one substrate, but do not mimic the transition state, are referred to as multi-substrate inhibitors. N-(Phosphonacetyl)-L-aspartic acid [PALA], a potent inhibitor of aspartate transcarbamylase (ref. 6), is of this class.

Aspartate Transcarbamylase

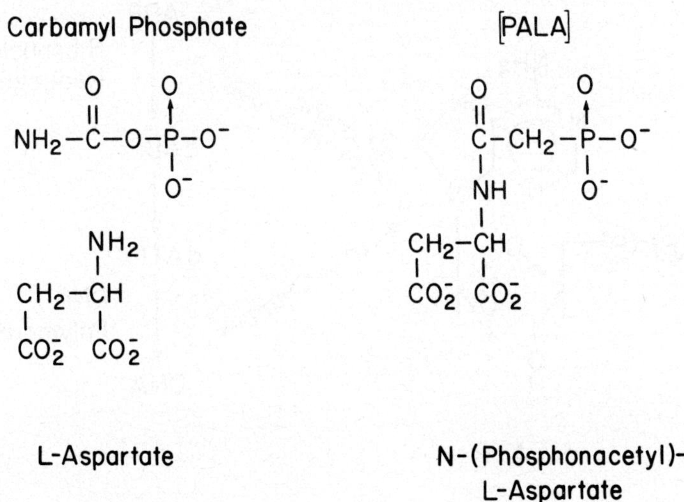


*References p. 86*

An example of an inhibitor resembling a transition state is deoxycoformycin, a potent inhibitor of adenosine deaminase _in vivo_ (ref. 7).

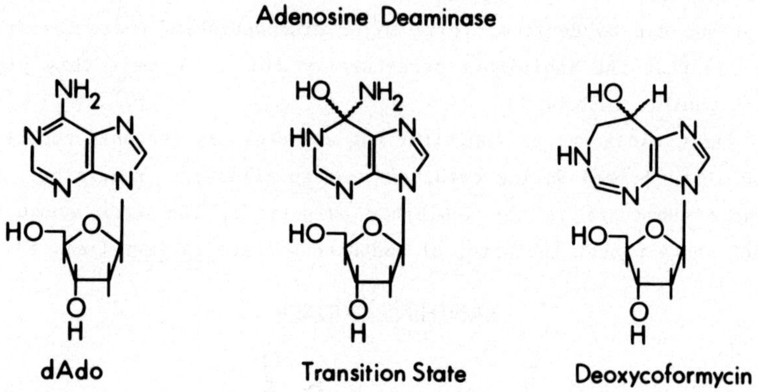

Inhibitors that bind to the target enzyme at allosteric sites might structurally resemble natural allosteric regulators of the enzyme. Such an inhibitor is the arabinosyl analogue of ATP (araATP), a metabolite of adenine arabinonucleoside. This compound competes with ATP for the allosteric activator site on ribonucleotide reductase from a human cell line (ref. 8). This results in inhibition of the purified reductase and should cause a decrease in the dATP pools _in vivo_. Since araATP also inhibits DNA polymerase in competition with dATP (ref. 9), the net result of the allosteric inhibition of ribonucleotide reductase is the self potentiation of the inhibitory effect on DNA polymerase (ref. 8).

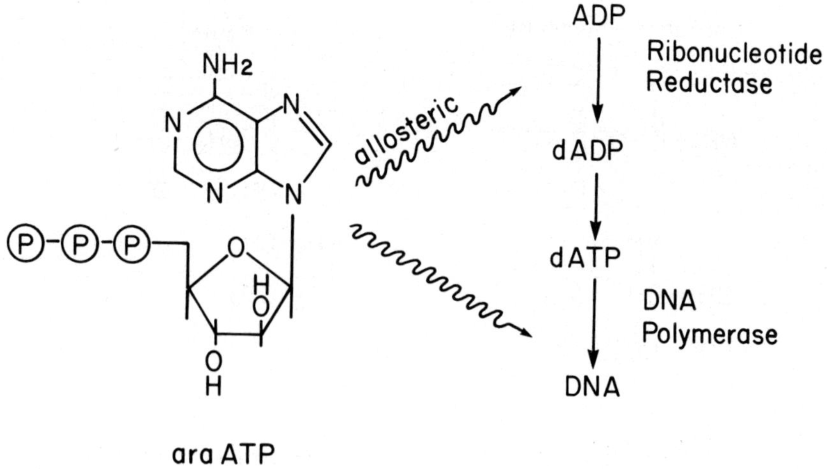

There is some redundancy between the first category in Scheme I where inhibitors are classified by what they mimic and the second category classifying them by where they bind. This is because inhibitors are most likely to bind to the same site as do the natural substrates that they structurally resemble. However, the second category is useful in that it allows for some distinctions to be made that are not possible in the first. Most commonly enzyme inhibitors bind to catalytic sites. Nevertheless, there are important inhibitors that bind to allosteric sites and some that partially bind to non-regulatory sites adjacent to the active site. For the sake of classification, therefore, in the second category two major groups of inhibitors can be distinguished: those that bind to catalytic sites and those that bind to non-catalytic sites (Scheme I).

Inhibitors that bind to the active site are further distinguished by whether they bind to a site unoccupied by substrates, to a site that has one or more - but not all - of the substrates bound, or to a site that has been modified by a substrate. This latter type occurs with enzymes that have "Ping-Pong" mechanisms. For example with oxipurinol, xanthine oxidase must be in the reduced rather than the oxidized form for the tightest binding to occur (refs. 10,11).

Among inhibitors that bind to sites other than the catalytic site, two types are distinguishable: 1) those which bind to regulatory (allosteric) sites and 2) those which bind to non-regulatory sites. Inhibitors which bind to allosteric sites can exert their effects on catalysis by their failure to induce the proper conformational changes and by competing with endogenous allosteric activators. Thusly, ATP and araATP compete for the allosteric site of ribonucleotide reductase as noted above. Another way that inhibitors can act at allosteric sites is by being more effective or by accumulating to higher levels than endogenous allosteric inhibitors.

Substrate analogs that contain large hydrophobic moieties which enhance binding might be considered to bind partly to the active site and partly to a hydrophobic region adjacent to the active site. Such hydrophobic regions do not normally have a direct regulatory function. They can, therefore, be distinguished from allosteric sites. Moreover, such sites are not necessarily hydrophobic in nature, although, it seems that in many instances, this is the case. An inhibitor that has a moiety most probably interacting with such a hydrophobic site is the adenosine deaminase inhibitor, erythro-9-(2-hydroxy-3-nonyl)adenine [EHNA] (ref. 12).

Adenosine Deaminase

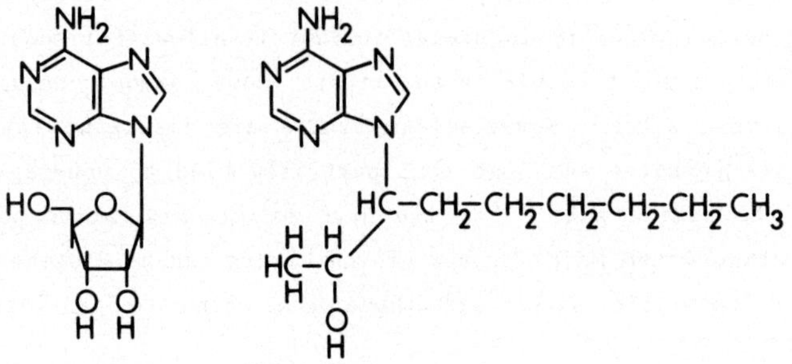

Ado EHNA

Perhaps, the most fundamental distinction among inhibitors is whether or not the interaction between the target enzyme and the inhibitor involves a covalent bond (Category III in Scheme I). This distinction has often been designated by the adjectives 'reversible' and 'irreversible'. The latter has referred to those involving a covalent bond. However, the facile reversibility of some reactions which form a covalent bond between inhibitor and target enzyme has been demonstrated (ref. 13). For this reason, the terms 'non-covalent binding' and 'covalent binding' inhibitors are used here. Within the non-covalent binding class, inhibitors can be either non-substrates or alternate substrates. The non-substrate inhibitors exert their effect simply by binding. This is the case with the dihydrofolate reductase inhibitor, trimethoprim (ref. 14).

Dihydrofolate Reductase

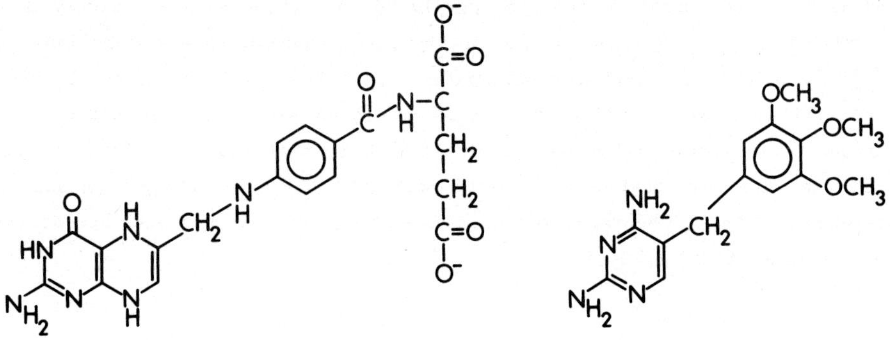

Dihydrofolate Trimethoprim

Inhibition by alternate substrates is more complex and can involve not only binding by substrates and/or products but may also depend on catalytic parameters. This is well illustrated by the alternate substrate inhibitor of xanthine oxidase (X.O.), allopurinol (ref. 15). Here the product, oxipurinol, binds much more tightly to the reduced than to the oxidized form of the enzyme. Allopurinol, therefore, serves not only to generate oxipurinol, but also to generate the reduced form of the enzyme.



Among the covalent binding inhibitors, two types can be distinguished: group-directed and suicide inhibitors. They are somewhat analogous to the non-substrate and alternate substrate types in the non-covalent binding class. The group-directed type is analogous to the non-substrate type since it need not be catalytically transformed by the enzyme to cause inhibition. The inhibitor *per se* possesses a moiety capable of reaction with a group on the target enzyme. Selectivity is achieved by the proximity between this reactive moiety and a group on the enzyme possessing complementary geometry and reactivity. This type of inhibitor has been championed by Baker (ref. 16). A group-directed inhibitor of 5'-phosphoribosyl-N-formylglycinamidine synthetase, an enzyme involved in the *de novo* synthesis of purines, is L-azaserine. This inhibitor alkylates a sulhydryl group in the active site of this enzyme (ref. 17).

## 5'-Phosphoribosyl-N-formylglycinamidine Synthetase



A similar example, that has been studied in more detail, is the inhibition of glutaminase by the homolog of L-azaserine, 6-diazo-5-oxonorleucine [DON] (ref. 18). In the normal catalytic sequence of this enzyme, a covalent thio-ester intermediate involving an active site sulfhydryl group and the γ-carbonyl of glutamine is formed. When DON serves as a substrate, an analogous intermediate is formed and diazomethane is one of the products, but inactivation of the enzyme does not occur. Alternatively, the carbon vicinal to the azo-group of DON is capable of reacting with the enzyme sulfhydryl at a rate 70 times slower than at the carbonyl position. When this unfavored reaction occurs, the enzyme is inactivated. DON is classified as a group-directed rather than as a suicide inhibitor of this enzyme because when it serves as a substrate no enzyme inactivation occurs. If it was a suicide inhibitor, the converse would apply; inactivation would occur only when it served as a substrate.

Suicide inhibitors in their native state do not contain a moiety that readily reacts with a critical group on the target enzyme. In contrast to the group-directed type, these inhibitors must undergo catalytic conversion by the target enzyme before the inactivating reaction can occur. Two sub-types of suicide inhibitors can be distinguished. With one, the catalytic conversion of the inhibitor by the target enzyme results in the formation of a reactive moiety which then reacts with a group on the enzyme in much the same way as a group-directed inhibitor does. This sub-type might be referred to as a 'reactive-product' suicide inhibitor and is exemplified by the acetylenic substrate analog of β-hydroxydecanoyl thioester dehydrase (ref. 19). Here the acetylenic form of the inhibitor must be converted by the target enzyme to the allenic isomer which then reacts with a histidine residue on the enzyme.

β–Hydroxydecanoyl Thioester Dehydrase

x = $CH_3(CH_2)_5$
y = $S(CH_2)_2NHCOCH_3$

$x{-}C{\equiv}C{-}CH_2{-}C({=}O){-}y$ (acetylene form)

⇌ Enzyme–Catalyzed

$x{-}CH{=}C{=}CH{-}C({=}O){-}y$ (allene form)

↓

$x{-}CH{=}C(\text{His–Enzyme}){-}CH_2{-}C({=}O){-}y$

The second sub-type of suicide inhibitor is found only with enzymes which form covalent intermediates with its substrates in the normal catalytic sequence. The covalent intermediate between enzyme and inhibitor is analogous to that formed with natural substrates. The essential difference is that the enzyme-inhibitor intermediate is not readily broken down to products. Consequently, the catalytic site is obstructed. For this reason, this sub-type might be referred to as a 'stable-intermediate' suicide inhibitor. A classic example is the inhibition of thymidylate synthetase by 5-fluorodeoxyuridylate (ref. 20).

Thymidylate Synthetase

O HN F O N H (P) O O H ⇌ O HN $CH_2$-$H_4$Folate F H O N S Enzyme (P) O O H

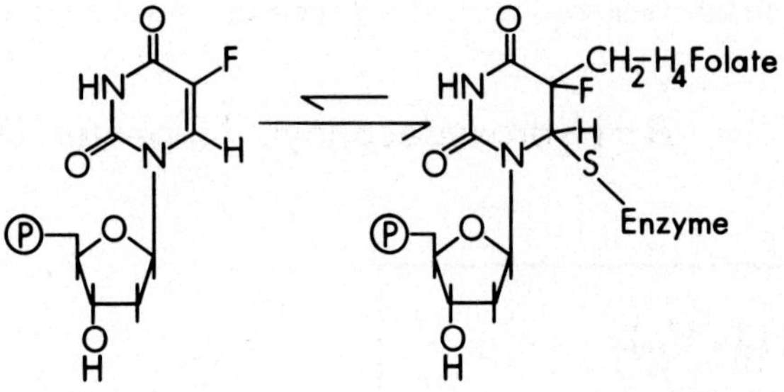

5–Fluoro–dUMP

In the normal reaction sequence, a ternary covalent intermediate between deoxyuridylate, 5,10-methylene tetrahydrofolate, and a cysteine sulhydryl on the enzyme is formed that readily undergoes conversion to products. When 5-fluorodeoxyuridylate is the substrate, the ternary intermediate formed is relatively stable, resulting in the inactivation of the enzyme by the covalent obstruction of the active site. However, the reaction involved in the formation of the ternary intermediate is slowly reversible (ref. 13). This reversibility allows for restoration of enzyme activity.

The obvious advantage of both 'reactive-product' and 'stable-intermediate' suicide inhibitors is that they have two tiers of specificity: one derived from binding and the other derived from catalysis.

One last distinction must be made before *in vivo* parameters are considered. Enzyme inhibitors can be divided into two classes on the basis of the effects that they have *in vivo*. Inhibitors which alter the metabolism of the treated subject in a beneficial manner are referred to as METABOLIC REGULATORS. Their targets are enzymes which are not foreign. The xanthine oxidase inhibitor, allopurinol, falls into this class. In the second class are inhibitors that serve as CHEMOTHERAPEUTIC AGENTS. They are specifically directed toward enzymes of foreign pathogens or aberrant cells (cancer). The relevance of this distinction will become clearer later in the discussion on general strategies.

SCHEME II

FACTORS AFFECTING EFFICACY OF ENZYME INHIBITORS IN VIVO

I. Levels and half-life of the inhibitor

II. Substrate accumulation

III. Concentration of the target enzyme

IV. Efficiency of alternate metabolic pathways

## Efficacy in vivo

Whether or not an enzyme inhibitor can exert the desired beneficial effect in vivo depends on a number of complex factors (Scheme II). For those inhibitors which are active per se (e.g., trimethoprim, deoxycoformycin, EHNA, azaserine, and PALA), the first consideration is that they reach their target enzyme in sufficient quantity for an adequate period of time. This means that they must be absorbed, distributed to the appropriate tissues, and spared from rapid catabolism and excretion. Inadequate absorption can be the result of the formulation or of the physical properties of the drug. In the latter case, the only solutions to the problem are to resort to a prodrug or a more suitable analog (ref. 21).

With inhibitors which are administered as prodrugs (e.g., adenine arabinonucleoside and acyclovir [9-(2-hydroxyethoxymethyl)guanine]), there is the added need to be transformed in vivo at adequate rates and in appropriate cells. The efficiency of this process relative to that of degradation and elimination must be favorable. These are factors whose contributions to efficacy in vivo are not easily predicted by tests performed in vitro.

The ability of the substrates of an inhibited enzyme to accumulate is particularly important with non-substrate inhibitors which simply bind to active sites. In the simplest situation with linear competitive inhibitors, the degree of inhibition is directly related to the ratio of the concentration of the inhibitor (I) divided by its inhibition constant ($K_i$) to the substrate concentration (S) divided by its Michealis-Menten constant ($K_m$) (see figure on next page). Clearly for efficacy, the extent of substrate accumulation must be overcome by the combined forces of the amount of inhibitor and the tightness of its binding relative to that of the substrate.

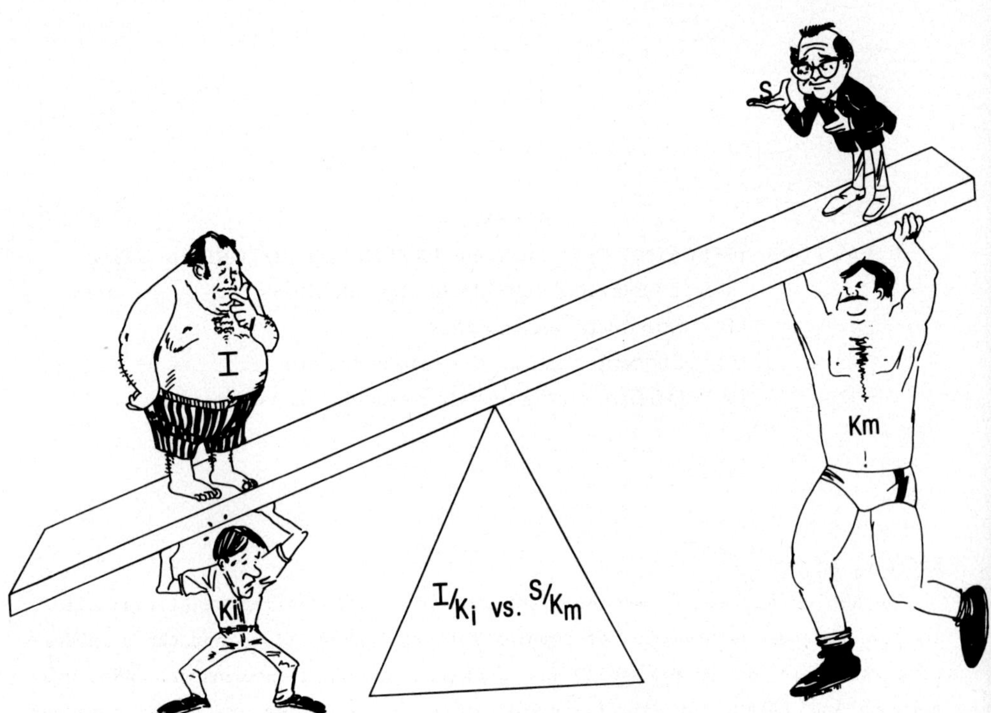


An example of where this was not achieved is with the nucleotide metabolites of allopurinol and orotidylate decarboxylase. Here substrate accumulation explains why the inhibition of this enzyme is largely overcome in vivo. These nucleotides are potent, competitive inhibitors of orotidylate decarboxylase in vitro (ref. 22). In vivo, the levels of orotidylate in rat liver were increased 73-fold just one hour after administration of the drug (ref. 23). During this time, only small transitory decreases in the pyrimidine nucleotide pools were observed (ref. 24). This illustrated the ineffectiveness of these inhibitors under substrate pressure. In this case, ineffectiveness was desirable since the target enzyme was xanthine oxidase rather than orotidylate decarboxylase. An example of the converse with another simple competitive inhibitor is trimethoprim and the bacterial dihydrofolate reductases (ref. 14). Here limited substrate accumulation, combined with adequate inhibitor levels and the high affinity of the inhibitor for the target enzyme, provides for efficacy in vivo.

With multi-substrate reactions, co-substrate accumulation can also affect inhibition even where the inhibitor directly competes with only one of the substrates. If an inhibitor competes with one substrate and the affinity of this substrate and the inhibitor are differentially affected by a co-substrate, accumulation of the co-substrate will influence the degree of inhibition (ref. 25).

**OROTIDYLATE DECARBOXYLASE**

1-Oxipurinol Nucleotide
7-Oxipurinol Nucleotide
1-Allopurinol Nucleotide

OMP → UMP + $CO_2$

Substrate accumulation also affects more complex types of inhibitors. Inhibitors which bind to allosteric sites might conceivably be influenced by the presence of substrates on the active site. This influence can be either positive or negative and could be mediated through substrate-induced conformational changes in the enzyme that affect the allosteric site. With inactivating inhibitors, substrate accumulation occurring after inactivation of only a portion of the total enzyme can help to protect the remaining active enzyme by preventing binding of the inhibitor. This has been demonstrated with 5-fluorodeoxyuridylate and thymidylate synthetase (ref. 26). The obvious general lesson here is that the most desirable situation is where substrates of an inhibited target enzyme are prevented from accumulating *in vivo* by alternative routes of metabolism or by rapid excretion.

The concentration of the target enzyme can also be of importance to the efficacy of an inhibitor *in vivo*. Certain enzymes are present at levels that appear to be in great excess over what is required for normal metabolic function. In such situations, extensive - but not complete - enzyme inhibition may have very little overall metabolic effect. Nature seems to recognize the importance of this factor since an increase in the level of the target enzyme is commonly the basis for resistance to inhibitors. The rate of synthesis of the target enzyme can be especially important with inactivating inhibitors. With both covalent and non-covalent binding inhibitors, the normal rate of enzyme degradation may be decreased by the presence of the inhibitor. This appears to be the case with orotidylate decarboxylase, where levels of the enzyme (measured after the inhibitor is removed) are higher in drug-treated than in untreated cells (refs. 22 and 27).

Another factor that can be of importance *in vivo* is the efficiency of alternate metabolic pathways. A lack of such a pathway is, of course, most desirable. But the presence of one, does not necessarily preclude efficacy *in vivo*. For example, with the inhibition of bacterial dihydrofolate reductase by trimethoprim, the critical thymidylate synthetase reaction which generates dihydrofolate from tetrahydrofolate is readily by-passed by thymidine salvage *in vitro* (ref. 28). The result is ineffectiveness of this anti-bacterial agent in any culture where the medium contains thymidine. Yet, the availability of thymidine to bacteria is so limited *in vivo* that this inhibitor is highly effective.

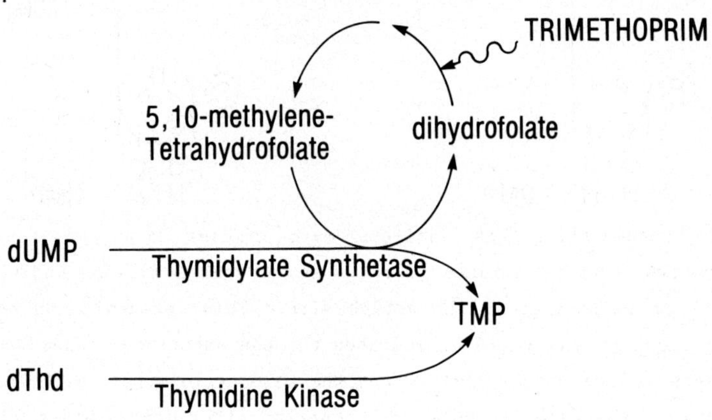


## Selectivity *in vivo*

As with efficacy, the selectivity of enzyme inhibitors *in vivo* is influenced by various complex parameters. With METABOLIC REGULATORS, the simplest and most ideal inhibitors are completely specific for the target enzyme and have no effects on other physiological processes, except indirectly through their inhibition of the target enzyme. It was noted above that with allopurinol this is so only because inhibition of orotidylate decarboxylase was overcome by substrate accumulation. This selectivity *in vivo* would have been difficult to predict solely from *in vitro* data.

With CHEMOTHERAPEUTIC AGENTS, the ideal is where the target enzyme of a pathogen has no counterpart in the host and the inhibitor is target specific. This situation is approximated with β-lactam antibiotics (ref. 2) and sulfonamides (ref. 29). On the other hand, the presence of a homologous enzyme in the host does by no means preclude selectivity, as is well demonstrated by the dihydrofolate reductase inhibitor trimethoprim (ref. 14). The $K_i$ value of this inhibitor with the bacterial enzyme is several thousand times lower than that with the host enzyme. This large difference in inhibitor specificity is likely not to be a particularly unique phenomenon. Amino acid sequencing of enzymes from diverse sources has demonstrated that genetic drift is surprisingly rapid (ref. 30). The exceptions are with amino acid residues which are directly involved in catalysis and in the binding of substrates. Here, conservation is the rule. However outside of the active site, large differences between homologous enzymes from host and pathogen are to be expected. Therefore, those inhibitors interacting with residues on the pathogen's enzyme that do not directly interact with normal substrates (non-regulatory site inhibitors, see Scheme I) are more likely to be selective. In addition, genetic drift in regions away from the active site can alter the flexibility of this site and thereby result in inhibitor specificity differences.

With prodrugs that require metabolic conversion to the ultimate inhibitor, the potential for selectivity is magnified. This situation is analogous to the double-tiered specificity of suicide inhibitors discussed above. A tier of specificity can be added by each enzyme from the pathogen involved in the selective activation of the inhibitor. The final tier is based on the difference in inhibitor specificities between the target enzyme of the pathogen and the homologous enzyme in the host. In ideal situations, not only is the target enzyme exposed to higher levels of the inhibitor, but it is also more susceptible to inhibition. An important example of such a situation is the antiviral agent, acyclovir (ref. 31).

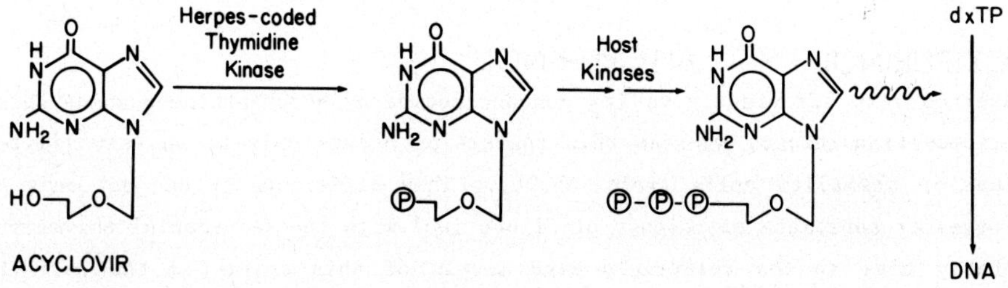

ACYCLOVIR —(Herpes-coded Thymidine Kinase)→ monophosphate —(Host Kinases)→ triphosphate —(dxTP)→ DNA

Phosphorylation of this agent is extremely low in normal mammalian cells. However in cells infected with herpes simplex virus, there is induction of a virus-coded thymidine kinase that effectively catalyzes its phosphorylation. Consequently, this drug is preferentially activated in virus-infected cells. The ultimate target enzyme appears to be the viral DNA polymerase which is inhibited by the triphosphate metabolite of acyclovir. This metabolite is probably a chain-terminating alternate substrate inhibitor (refs. 32,33). Moreover, the viral polymerase is more susceptible to inhibition than is the host enzyme. The potential opportunities for chemotherapeutically exploiting substrate specificity differences in anabolic enzymes is highlighted by this example.

Along the same lines, studies on the purine salvage enzymes of leishmania were undertaken in an attempt to understand the reasons for the toxicity of allopurinol to cultured forms of leishmania (ref. 34). Large differences between host and parasite were revealed. In the parasite, allopurinol is

MAN LEISHMANIA

RNA

OXIPURINOL ALLOPURINOL

converted very efficiently to its mononucleotide by hypoxanthine-guanine phosphoribosyltransferase, whereas this conversion occurs only to an very limited extent in mammalian cells (refs. 35,36). This difference is due not only to the greater substrate efficiency of allopurinol with the leishmanial enzyme but probably also to the relatively high levels of this enzyme in the parasite (ref. 37). In the mammal, the nucleotide of allopurinol is not further anabolized. On the other hand, in leishmania, it is converted to the corresponding adenine nucleotide analogs and incorporated into RNA (ref. 35). Enzyme studies showed that the nucleotide of allopurinol is a substrate for adenylosuccinate synthetase from leishmania, but not from mammalian tissues (ref. 38). These differences between host and parasite again demonstrate the potential of activating enzymes to endow prodrugs with selectivity.

All of the parameters discussed for efficacy _in vivo_ (Scheme II) can also influence selectivity. Permeability and metabolic parameters can result in differences in the duration and levels of an enzyme inhibitor in pathogen versus host cells. Selective delivery of inhibitors to targets is an area where imaginative approaches are being pursued. The dramatic increases in the efficacy and selectivity of the anti-leishmanial antimonials when encapsulated in liposomes (ref. 39) suggests the wider use of this approach with enzyme inhibitors. It seems especially suited for applications in diseases affecting the reticuloendothelial system. Another approach being pursued is the delivery of otherwise impermeable inhibitors to target cells by covalent attachment to appropriate carrier molecules. Interesting examples are found with amino acid analogs and their peptide derivatives (ref. 40). In many respects, bacterial transport systems for free amino acids are more specific than are those for peptides. Antibacterial peptides, like bacilysin, serve as readily transported prodrugs for amino acid analogs which are themselves poorly transported. Inside the bacterial cell, these peptides are cleaved to release the amino acid analog inhibitor, which in the case of bacilysin inhibits the enzyme glucosamine synthetase.

GLUCOSAMINE SYNTHETASE

CELL WALL

BACILYSIN

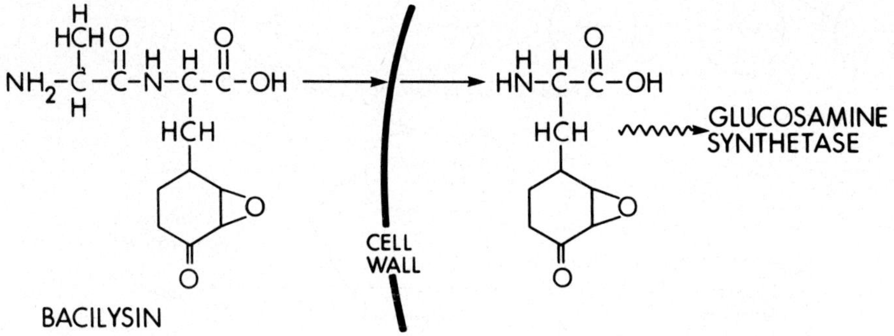

The preferential accumulation of substrates of an inhibited enzyme in the host might protect the host cells, but not the pathogen, from toxicity. A similar effect can be achieved if the natural substrate has a high $K_m$ with the pathogen target enzyme and a low $K_m$ with the homologous host enzyme.

The concentration of the target enzyme in the parasite versus that in the host can also influence selectivity. If a large excess of the target enzyme homolog were present in the host and a minimal level were present in the parasite, partial inhibition might have a profound effect on the parasite and essentially no effect on the host. With activating enzymes, the converse holds where higher levels in the pathogen would be favorable. With catabolic enzymes which can inactivate inhibitors or their precursors, normal tissues can often protect themselves from toxicity whereas tumors, generally low in catabolic enzymes, cannot.

The lack of an alternative metabolic pathway in the parasite countered by its presence in the host might also provide for a situation favorable for selective chemotherapy. This situation appears to be present in the purine salvage pathways of most pathogenic protozoa. In these pathogens, purine biosynthesis de novo is deficient or lacking (ref. 41), suggesting that they might be particularly susceptible to purine analogs. Indeed, the activities of allopurinol and its ribonucleoside against leishmania (ref. 34,42) support this view.

*References p. 86*

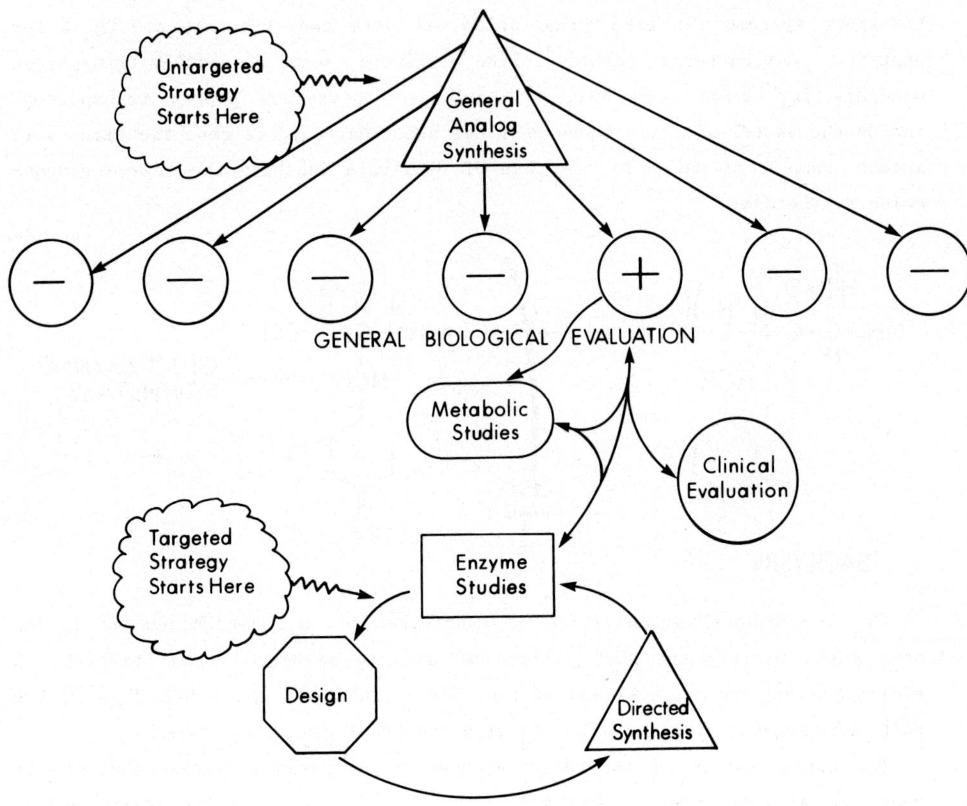


General Strategies

The foregoing considerations emphasize the multiplicity and complexity of the factors that can affect both the efficacy and the selectivity of enzyme inhibitors in vivo. These in vivo parameters may, but do not necessarily, have negative effects. Indeed, there is the potential for better performance in vivo than would have been expected from studies in vitro. Nevertheless, the majority of enzyme inhibitors which are potent in vitro are ineffective in vivo. In the face of the unknowns of the in vivo system, approaches which minimize our dependency upon chance must be fostered. The steadily growing understanding of drug metabolism, pharmacokinetics and comparative biochemistry will certainly increase the predictability of the in vivo parameters outlined above. In the meantime, many new and useful enzyme inhibitors will undoubtedly be discovered and developed. The history of drug research shows clearly that this very process will serve as a vehicle for the growth of our knowledge of in vivo parameters. Furthermore, current knowledge of genetics and comparative biochemistry emphasize that the potential for chemotherapeutic exploitation is vast. What any meaningful strategy must now face is the reality of our inability to accurately predict the effects of *in vivo* factors. Therefore, to be serviceable, strategies must attempt to minimize the impact of these unknowns.

Currently, there are two basic approaches to the discovery and development of enzyme inhibitors as drugs. The first might be called the TARGETED strategy. In somewhat idealized form, this approach initially requires the choice of the target enzyme and the type of inhibitor to be synthesized. These critical choices are difficult to make, as is emphasized by the foregoing considerations. However, having made the choices as rationally as possible, a few potential inhibitors are then synthesized and tested against the isolated enzyme for inhibitory activity. Structure-activity relationships then act as a guide to design improved inhibitors. A cyclical improvement process involving the design, synthesis, and testing of inhibitors on the isolated enzyme is pursued. When inhibitors of suitable potency are acquired, they are evaluated in biological systems. If there is insufficient activity or selectivity, the metabolism and pharmacokinetics of the inhibitor could be studied in an attempt to ascertain the basis for the inadequacy. This information might suggest the possibility that chemical modification of the inhibitor or administration as a prodrug would improve its efficacy or selectivity.

The second approach, which has been advocated by Hitchings (ref. 43), is called the UNTARGETED strategy. Analogs of naturally occurring substrates likely to cause inhibition of enzymes *in vivo* are synthesized and then tested in biological screens. The greater the variety of analogs and biological test systems, the greater the probability of uncovering useful leads. Ideally, this strategy is untargeted with respect to both molecular and biological targets. In other words, it is disease-oriented only to the extent that the variety of biological tests are limited. *In vitro* cell culture systems often serve as the primary screens. The advantages here are that a small amount of each test compound is required and a large number of compounds can be tested economically. Direct *in vivo* testing is usually relegated to the role of a secondary screen. Obviously, such biological screens can reveal drugs that act by mechanisms other than by inhibition of enzymes. However for the purpose here, let us assume that the 'lead' compound is an enzyme inhibitor. A study of the nature of the metabolites of this compound and the effects that it exerts on the pathogen or animal model should provide clues to the identity of the target enzyme. Definitive studies are then performed with isolated enzymes. From this point on, the remainder of the process is similar to that of the TARGETED strategy. The advantage is that the biological screens have eliminated those classes of compounds which might be potent inhibitors of isolated enzymes, but are not effective or selective *in vivo*. Furthermore, prodrugs can be revealed by this method of selection. Once the target enzyme is identified, specificity studies with the purified enzyme are a valuable tool in the quest for the best inhibitor of the series. The quantitative nature and rapid generation of enzyme data are ideal for guiding chemical synthesis. Here the enzymes studied can include, in addition to the target enzyme from the parasite, the homologous enzyme in the host and any relevant activating or inactivating enzymes from either parasite or host.

A fundamental difference between the TARGETED and the UNTARGETED strategies is the manner in which the target enzyme is determined. With the TARGETED strategy, a choice is made by an assessment of fact and theory and is the first step in the process. With the UNTARGETED strategy, the target enzyme is revealed by investigation of the mechanism of action of a biologically active 'lead' compound.

Each strategy confronts the pitfalls and complexities of the *in vivo* system at different points. In the TARGETED strategy, they are confronted after at least some *in vitro* enzyme specificity studies have been performed. In the UNTARGETED strategy, they are confronted directly after synthesis and before any detailed biochemical studies are begun. Both strategies have in common a cyclical process of design, synthesis, and determination of inhibitory potency with the purified target enzyme, but this process is put into action at different points.

The two strategies described above are, of course, somewhat polarized idealizations. In the real world, various combinations of both are put into practice. Xanthine oxidase inhibition by allopurinol, the METABOLIC REGULATOR used to treat hyperuricemia, was revealed by an enzyme inhibition screen (ref. 44). In this case, the target enzyme was chosen and not revealed by investigation of the mechanism of action of a 'lead' compound. Although the synthesis of allopurinol was directed only partially by enzyme data, this drug is as close to a product of a TARGETED strategy as is any of that era. An even clearer and more recent example of the execution of the TARGETED strategy is the development of another METABOLIC REGULATOR, the adenosine deaminase inhibitor EHNA (ref. 12). Here the synthesis was specifically directed by the results of the enzyme studies. The cyclical improvement process of design, synthesis, and testing was fully operative.

With enzyme inhibitors that serve as CHEMOTHERAPEUTIC AGENTS, examples of the UNTARGETED strategy are plentiful. The discovery that the 5-substituted diaminopyrimidines were antifolates (ref. 45) was unexpected and probably would have been missed if a TARGETED approach was being followed. The bacterial dihydrofolate reductase inhibitor, trimethoprim, was developed from this series. Although its synthesis predated studies with purified dihydrofolate reductase, enzyme studies did add impetus to its development by distinguishing its mode of action from that of the sulfa drugs. This distinction and their synergism ultimately led to their use in combination. Trimethoprim well illustrates the unpredictability of the effects of in vivo parameters. From a theoretical viewpoint, one would have been discouraged from pursuing this type of inhibitor for three reasons which are discussed separately above and summarized here. First, trimethoprim is a simple competitive inhibitor subject to reversal by substrate accumulation. Second, a homologous enzyme is present in the host. Third, an alternate metabolic pathway (thymidine salvage) is operative in the pathogen that was shown to be capable of bypassing inhibition in vitro. Despite these obstacles, this agent is effective and selective in vivo.

A more recent example of a product of the UNTARGETED strategy is acyclovir. It was unexpected that this CHEMOTHERAPEUTIC AGENT would be selectively activated by a virus-coded nucleoside kinase that prefers thymidine as a substrate and that its triphosphate metabolite would preferentially inhibit the viral polymerase.

On the basis of such examples, it might be concluded that the TARGETED strategy is best applied to the development of inhibitors that are useful as METABOLIC REGULATORS. Here the choice of the target enzyme is relatively uncomplicated. On the other hand, the UNTARGETED strategy is more appropriate to the development of inhibitors for use as CHEMOTHERAPEUTIC AGENTS, where initial selection of the target enzyme is more difficult. Here the in vivo parameters are complicated by the host-pathogen relationship. The utility of the TARGETED approach in the chemotherapeutic field should grow in parallel with our knowledge of comparative biochemistry and in vivo parameters.

The importance of the UNTARGETED strategy in pharmaceutical invention has been obscured by the paucity of accurate historical information. An all too understandable eagerness on the part of those involved with drug discoveries to appear brillant rather than merely lucky has undoubtedly been a factor in minimizing the role of the UNTARGETED strategy. In this paper, it has been emphasized and exemplified that the ability to predict the effects of in vivo factors on the performance of enzyme inhibitors is still limited. Clearly in many instances, it is both serviceable and rational to approach the complexities of biological systems in the empirical fashion represented by the UNTARGETED strategy.

*References p. 86*

ACKNOWLEDGEMENTS - The authors are indebted to T. Spector and E. Wise of these laboratories for their helpful discussions.

ABBREVIATIONS USED

dAdo = 2'-deoxyadenosine

ADP = adenosine -5'-diphosphate

ATP = adenosine-5'-triphosphate

dADP = 2'-deoxyadenosine-5'-diphosphate

dATP = 2'-deoxyadenosine-5'-triphosphate

OMP = orotidine-5'-monophosphate

UMP = uridine-5'-monophosphate

dUMP = 2'-deoxyuridine-5'-monophosphate

dThd = 2'-deoxythymidine

TMP = 2'-deoxythymidine-5'-monophosphate

dxTP = 2'-deoxynucleoside-5'-triphosphates

REFERENCES

1 N. Seiler, M.J. Jung and J. Koch-Weser (Eds.), Proc. Int. Symp. Substrate-Induced Irreversible Inhibition of Enzymes, Strasbourg, France, July 24-25, 1978, Elsevier, Amsterdam, 1978.
2 T.I. Kalman (Ed.), Proc. 12th Ann. Med. Chem. Symp., Amherst, New York, May 21-23, 1979, Elsevier, Amsterdam, 1979.
3 M. Sandler (Ed.), Proc. Symp. Enzyme Inhibitors as Drugs, London, April 9-10, 1979, MacMillan, London, 1980.
4 J.L. Webb, Enzyme and Metabolic Inhibitors, Vol. 1, Academic, New York, 1963, pp. 50-52.
5 G.B. Elion, S. Callahan, H. Nathan, S. Bieber, R.W. Rundles and G.W. Hitchings, Biochem. Pharmac., 12 (1963) 85-93.
6 K.D. Collins and G.R. Stark, J. Biol. Chem., 246 (1971) 6599-6605.
7 P.W.K. Woo, H.W. Dion, S.M. Lange, L.F. Dahl and L.J. Durham, J. Heterocyclic Chem., 11 (1974) 641-643.
8 C.-H. Chang and Y.-C. Cheng, Cancer Res., 40 (1980) 3555-3558.
9 R.A. Dicioccio and B.I.S. Srivastava, Eur. J. Biochem., 79 (1977) 411-418.
10 V. Massey, H. Komai, G. Palmer and G.B. Elion, J. Biol. Chem., 245 (1970) 2337-2844.
11 T. Spector and D.G. Johns, J. Biol. Chem., 245 (1970) 5079-5085.
12 H.J. Schaeffer, in E.J. Ariens (Ed.), Drug Design, Vol. II, Academic, New York, 1971, Ch. 2, pp. 129-160.
13 T.I. Kalman, see ref. #2, pp. 75-91.
14 J.J. Burchall, in J.W. Corcoran and F.E. Hahn (Eds.), Mechanism of Action of Antimicrobial and Antitumor Agents, Vol. III, Antibiotics, Springer-Verlag, Berlin, 1975, pp. 304-320.
15 T. Spector, Biochem. Pharmac., 26 (1977) 355-358.
16 B.R. Baker, Design of Active-Site-Directed Irreversible Enzyme Inhibitors, Wiley, New York, 1967, pp. 70-73.
17 T.C. French, I.B. David and J.M. Buchanan, J. Biol. Chem., 238 (1963) 2186-2193.
18 C. Walsh, Enzymatic Reaction Mechanisms, W.G. Freeman, San Francisco, 1979, pp. 133-135.
19 K. Bloch, in P.D. Boyer (Ed.), The Enzymes 3rd ed. Vol. V, Academic, New York, 1971, Ch. 15, pp. 459-461.
20 W.L. Washtien and D.V. Santi, see ref. #2, pp. 101-113.

21.S.H. Yalkowsky and W. Morozowich, in E.J. Ariens (Ed.), Drug Design, Vol. IX, Academic, New York, 1980, Ch. 3, pp. 121-185.
22 J.A. Fyfe, R.L. Miller and T.A. Krenitsky, J. Biol. Chem., 248 (1973) 3801-3809.
23 G.H. Hitchings, Arthritis and Rheumatism, 18 (1975) 863-870.
24 D.J. Nelson, C.J.L. Bugge, H.C. Krasny and G.B. Elion, Biochem. Pharmac., 22 (1973) 2003-2022.
25 T. Spector and W.W. Cleland, Biochem. Pharmac. 30 (1981) 1-7.
26 A. Lockshin and P.V. Danenberg, Biochem. Pharmac., 30 (1981) 247-257.
27 G.K. Brown, R.M. Fox and W.J. O'Sullivan, Biochem. Pharmac., 21 (1972) 2469-2477.
28 A.E. Koch and J.J. Burchall, Applied Microbiol., 22 (1971) 812-817.
29 G.H. Hitchings and J.J. Burchall, Adv. in Enzymo., 27 (1965) 417-468.
30 H. Harris, Fed. Proc., 35 (1976) 2079-2082.
31 G.B. Elion, P.A. Furman, J.A. Fyfe, P. de Miranda, L. Beauchamp and H.J. Schaeffer, Proc. Natl. Acad. Sci. USA, 74 (1977) 5716-5720.
32 P.A. Furman, M.H. St. Clair, J.A. Fyfe, J.L. Rideout, P.M. Keller and G.B. Elion, J. virol., 32 (1979) 72-77.
33 P.A. Furman, P.V. McGuirt, P.M. Keller, J.A. Fyfe and G.B. Elion, Virol. 102 (1980) 420-430.
34 M.A. Pfaller and J.J. Marr, Antimicrob. Agents Chemother., 5 (1974) 469-472.
35 D.J. Nelson, C.J. Bugge, G.B. Elion, R.L. Berens and J.J. Marr, J. Biol. Chem. 254 (1979) 3959-3964.
36 D.J. Nelson, C.J. Bugge, H.C. Krasny and G.B. Elion, Biochem. Pharmac. 22 (1973) 2003-2022.
37 J.V. Tuttle and T.A. Krenitsky, J. Biol. Chem. 255 (1980) 909-916.
38 T. Spector, T.E. Jones and G.B. Elion, J. Biol. Chem. 254 (1979) 8422-8426.
39 C.R. Alving, E.A. Steck, W.L. Chapman, Jr., V.B. Waits, L.D. Hendricks, G.M. Swartz, Jr. and W.L. Hanson, Proc. Natl. Acad. Sci. USA, 75 (1978) 2959-2963.
40 P.S. Ringrose, in J.W. Payne (Ed.), Microorganisms and Nitrogen Sources, Wiley, New York, 1980, Section 4-7, pp. 641-692.
41 W.E. Gutteridge and G.H. Coombs, Biochemistry of Parasitic Protozoa, MacMillan, London, 1977, p. 69.
42 D.J. Nelson, S.W. LaFon, J.V. Tuttle, W.H. Miller, R.L. Miller, T.A. Krenitsky and G.B. Elion, J. Biol. Chem., 254 (1979) 11544-11549.
43 G.H. Hitchings, Cancer Research, 29 (1969) 1895-1903.
44 G.B. Elion, Ann. Rheum. Dis., 25 (1966) 608-614.
45 G.H. Hitchings, G.B. Elion, H. VanderWerff and E.A. Falco, J. Biol. Chem., 174 (1948) 765-766.

J.A. Keverling Buisman (Editor), *Strategy in Drug Research* 89


# SUBSTRATE-INDUCED IRREVERSIBLE INHIBITION OF ENZYMES IN DRUG RESEARCH

P. BEY, B. METCALF, M.J. JUNG, J. FOZARD, and J. KOCH-WESER
Centre de Recherche Merrell International, Strasbourg (France)

Many drugs exert their therapeutic action by inhibiting specific enzymes. One can list more than 40 major drugs in current use whose sole or principal mechanism of action is attributable to specific inhibition of one or more of 32 different enzymes. In the majority of cases, however, the therapeutic properties of these drugs were discovered prior to the elucidation of their mechanism of action. Today, enzyme inhibition is recognized as an approach of great potential for rational discovery of new leads in pharmaceutical research. To transform this potential into fact, two requirements must be met. First, target enzymes, whose inhibition is of therapeutic usefulness have to be selected. Second, compounds must be designed and synthesized that inactivate these target enzymes _in vivo_ with sufficient completeness and specificity to cause a functionally consequential depletion of the product or accumulation of the substrate of the target enzyme.

The proper choice of enzyme targets is, of course, of critical importance for the potential "pay-off" of the research investment. Enzyme targets can be divided into two categories depending upon whether or not their inhibition has already been established to be of therapeutic consequence. Enzymes of the first category are easy to identify. Specific targets among those enzymes are usually selected on the basis of undesirable properties of the existing inhibitors such as lack of potency or selectivity and/or untoward side effects. Clinical usefulness of the inhibitors that will eventually be developed is fairly certain, but this assurance comes at the price of fierce competition. Identification of new enzyme targets of potential therapeutic interest is much more difficult and requires a multidisciplinary research effort. Success obviously relates to the current knowledge of the pathophysiology of disease processes and to our ability to identify endogenous and/or exogenous molecules whose function or dysfunction underlie disease conditions. Despite the dramatic advances during the last two decades in our understanding of the etiology of various diseases, it is fair to say that intuition still plays an important role in the selection of therapeutically interesting enzyme targets. It is in the case of infectious diseases that enzyme targets can be identified most rationally and consequently with the highest degree of certainty [1] on the basis of the rapidly expanding knowledge of biochemical differences in essential metabolic pathways between parasites and their hosts.

*References p. 104*

Once the target enzymes are defined, it devolves to chemists and biochemists to develop specific inhibitors. Among all the protein targets of potential therapeutic interest, which include hormone and transmitter receptors, contractile proteins and transport proteins, enzymes offer the greatest possibilities for inhibitor design. Not only the structures of their substrates but also those of their products can serve as starting points for molecular modification. In addition, enzymes are proteins endowed with catalytic properties. The knowledge of the molecular events which occur during enzyme catalysis has advanced more rapidly than the understanding of the factors governing ligand-protein interactions. It is, therefore, not surprising that the new approaches to specific enzyme inhibition which emerged in the last decade were based on increased understanding of the catalytic functions of enzymes. Among these approaches, substrate-induced irreversible enzyme inhibition represents a major advance in drug design. It demands that the inhibitor be a substrate of the target enzyme and incorporate a latent reactive grouping susceptible to being unmasked as the result of the normal catalytic turnover. The chemically reactive species which is then generated inside the enzyme's active site subsequently alkylates a nucleophilic residue of the active site which results in an irreversible inactivation of the enzyme. Such inhibitors, referred to as suicide substrates [2], suicide enzyme inactivators [3], Trojan Horse inhibitors [4], $k_{cat}$ inhibitors [5], mechanism-based inhibitors [6] or enzyme-activated irreversible inhibitors [7], can be expected to be extremely specific, since biotransformation of the inhibitor by the target enzyme is required before that enzyme is inactivated. Moreover, in as much as the mechanism of action of the target enzymes is established, the design of enzyme-activated inhibitors can often be approached in a rational fashion, especially when the target enzymes proceed via carbanionic intermediates.

To illustrate these points, we shall detail some aspects of our efforts aimed at the development of enzyme-activated irreversible inhibitors for ornithine decarboxylase (ODC), GABA-transaminase (GABA-T) and L-aromatic-α-amino acid decarboxylase (AADC). The presentation will be divided into three parts under the following headings: 1) Rationale underlying the choice of the target enzymes; 2) Design of the inhibitors; 3) Biochemical and pharmacological evaluation of those inhibitors.

## I) RATIONALE UNDERLYING THE CHOICE OF AADC, ODC AND GABA-T AS ENZYME TARGETS OF THERAPEUTIC INTEREST

AADC and ODC catalyze the decarboxylation of 3,4-dihydroxyphenylalanine (DOPA) and ornithine into dopamine and putrescine, respectively. GABA-T transaminates reversibly γ-amino butyric acid (GABA) with α-ketoglutarate, the products of the reaction being succinic semialdehyde and glutamic acid. In 1973 when we initiated our research program, AADC was already established as a target enzyme of therapeutic interest whereas ODC and GABA-T were not.

AADC was known to be an essential but not the rate-limiting enzyme in the biosynthesis of the biogenic amine neurotransmitters dopamine, noradrenaline, adrenaline and serotonin. As a result of the consensus of the late 1950's that compounds interfering with biogenic amine biosynthesis would be therapeutically useful, methyldopa, a competitive inhibitor of AADC, was introduced for treatment of hypertension [8]. Subsequently, inhibition of AADC proved not to be the antihypertensive mechanism of the drug [9]. Two further competitive inhibitors of AADC, carbidopa and benserazide, had been used extensively and successfully in combination with L-DOPA in the therapy of Parkinson's disease [10]. None of these inhibitors was, however, potent enough to affect endogenous levels of biogenic amines. A chemically mediated long-lasting inhibition of biogenic amine biosynthesis at the decarboxylase step thus remained to be achieved.

Ornithine was known to be the only precursor in mammals for the diamine, putrescine, and for the polyamines, spermidine and spermine. Although the precise functions of these cationic compounds had not been established, a variety of observations pointed to their fundamental role in cell growth and division [11]. Impairment of the biosynthesis of these bioamines could be expected to be useful for treating diseases characterized by abnormal cell proliferation. ODC, the rate-limiting enzyme in the biosynthetic pathways of these polyamines, appeared the logical target for inhibition.

The importance of GABA as a key inhibitory neurotransmitter substance in the CNS of mammals had become clear by the early seventies, and disturbances in its metabolism were thought to play a role in several neurological disorders in man. The central role of GABA-T in the catabolism of GABA made the inhibition of this enzyme a logical target for increasing GABA levels and perhaps modulating GABAergic neurotransmission.

In addition to these physiological and biochemical considerations, a critical factor in the selection of AADC, ODC and GABA-T as enzyme targets was their dependence on pyridoxal-phosphate (PLP) for catalytic activity. We felt confident that the design of enzyme-activated irreversible inhibitors for this class of enzyme could be approached rationally.

## II) DESIGN OF ENZYME-ACTIVATED IRREVERSIBLE INHIBITORS FOR ODC, AADC, AND GABA-T

In addition to decarboxylation of α-amino acids and transamination of ω-amino acids, PLP-dependent enzymes can catalyze a variety of other clearly distinguishable reactions on amino acids or amine substrates, such as transamination of α-amino acids, amine oxidation and α-amino acid racemization. The reasons that make enzymes of this class particularly well-suited targets for design of enzyme-activated irreversible inhibitors have been discussed in detail [12]. They can be summarized as follows:

SCHEME I

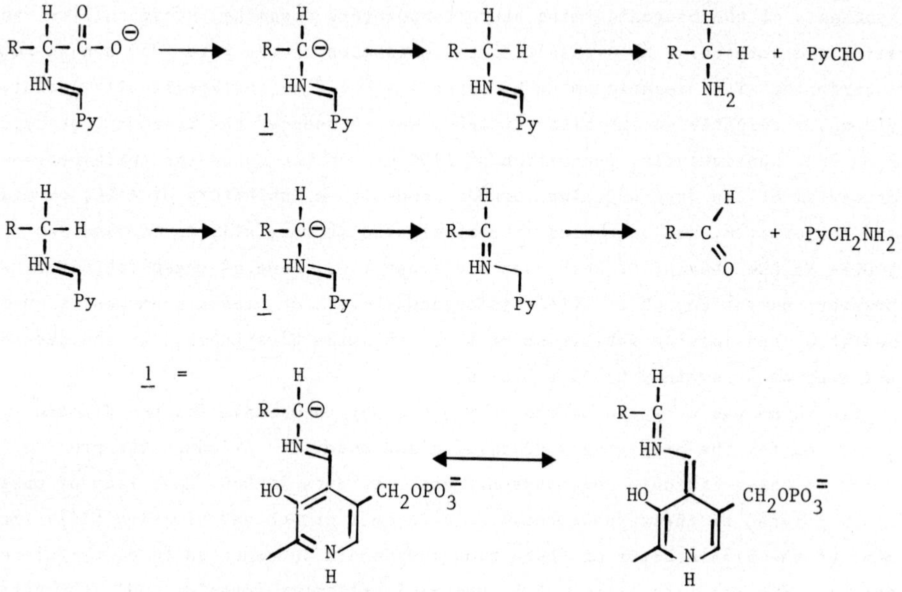

Py = pyridoxal phosphate ring system
R = side chain amino acid substrates

1) The chemical events which occur during catalysis are well established as exemplified by the mechanism of action of $\alpha$-amino acid decarboxylases and $\omega$-amino acid transaminases depicted in scheme I. The role of PLP is to labilize one of the three bonds to the carbon bearing the amino group of the substrate and then to stabilize carbanionic intermediates that can be generated at the $\alpha$, $\beta$ and/or $\gamma$ carbons to nitrogen of specific amino acid or amine substrates. This stabilization is achieved by delocalization of the extra electron density into the electron sink represented by the pyridoxal ring. In principle, the fate of these carbanionic intermediates could easily be altered by appropriately positioned groupings, such as nucleofugal, olefinic or acetylenic functions, to generate highly electrophilic Michael acceptors that would alkylate nucleophilic residues within the enzyme's active site (scheme II).

2) When performing catalysis, PLP binds covalently to the substrate via Schiff base formation between its aldehyde function and the amino group of the substrate. Such a covalent catalysis has two beneficial consequences. It prevents the reactive species that is eventually generated within the enzyme's active site from readily dissociating from the protein, thus favoring the formation of a covalent bond between the inhibitor and a nucleophilic residue of the protein. It also diminishes the risk that the reactive intermediate is released from the active site of the

SCHEME II

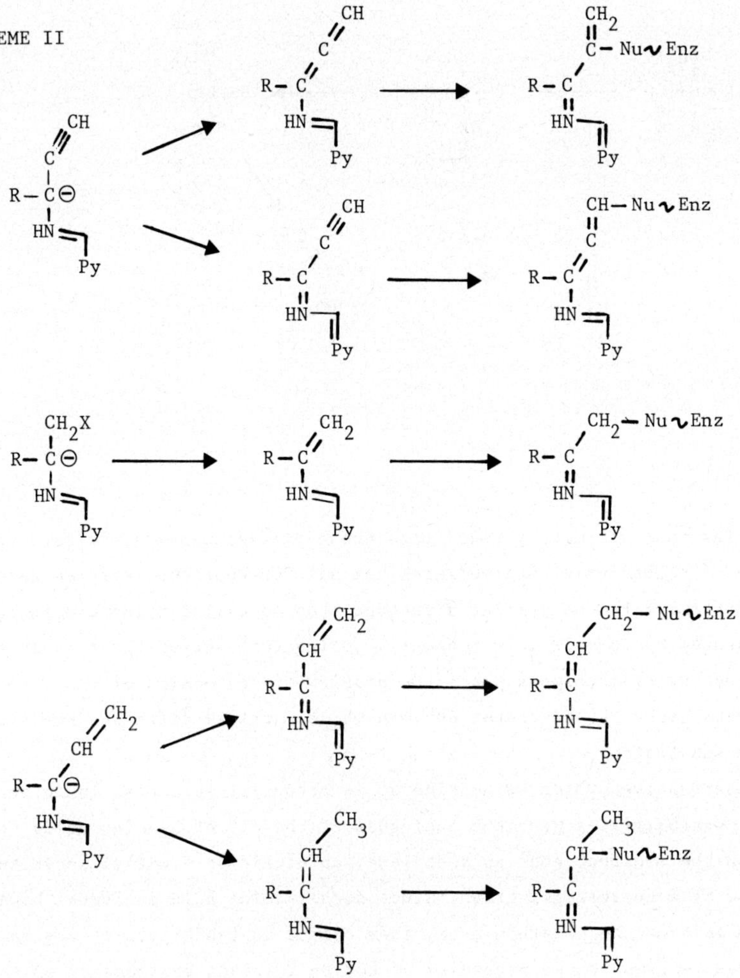

target enzyme and reacts irreversibly with nearby cellular components. This aspect is of particular importance when in vivo applications of the inhibitors are contemplated.

The difficulties of designing specific enzyme-activated irreversible inhibitors for PLP-dependent enzymes are of three types. Two of them are inherent to the concept of inhibition which demands, first, that the inhibitor be a substrate for the target enzyme and, second, that the reactive species which is eventually generated inside the enzyme's active site be positioned within bonding distance to a nucleophilic residue of the protein. These conditions impose severe limitations on the nucleofugal groups that can be used to construct the inhibitors as well as on the positioning of the latent reactive groupings along the substrate skeleton. The third difficulty is specific to PLP-dependent enzymes. The formation of the

SCHEME III

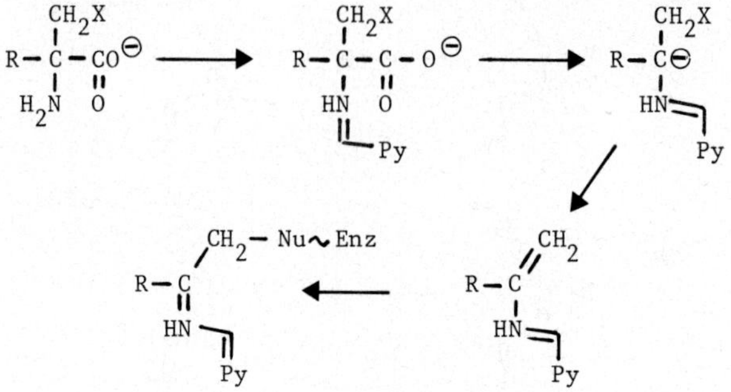

$$R-\underset{H_2N}{\overset{CH_2X}{C}}-\underset{O}{\overset{}{C}}O^{\ominus} \longrightarrow R-\underset{HN=Py}{\overset{CH_2X}{C}}-\underset{O}{C}-O^{\ominus} \longrightarrow R-\underset{HN=Py}{\overset{CH_2X}{C^{\ominus}}}$$

$$\longrightarrow R-\underset{HN=Py}{C}=CH_2 \longrightarrow R-\underset{HN-Py}{C}-CH_2-Nu\sim Enz$$

reactive species that ultimately inactivate these enzymes depends entirely upon the existence of carbanionic intermediates. As all PLP-dependent enzymes generate carbanionic intermediates of similar structure (the so-called quinonoid intermediates represented by formula 1 in scheme I) during turnover of their substrates, this common feature of catalysis poses the problem of the design of inhibitors that can discriminate among PLP-dependent enzymes which catalyze different reactions from the same substrate.

The first derivatives which we considered as potential selective inhibitors for α-amino acid decarboxylases were the analogues of the parent α-amino acids that incorporate on the α-carbon atom an acetylene, an olefin or a methyl substitutent functionalized by a nucleofugal group. Since such α-amino acid analogues have no hydrogen atom left on the α-carbon atom, they cannot be inhibitors of the majority of PLP-dependent enzymes whose mechanism of action involves abstraction of the α-hydrogen atom of the substrate. However, provided they are decarboxylated by the parent α-amino acid decarboxylases, these derivatives could still lead to the formation of highly electrophilic conjugated imines as indicated in scheme III. This assumption eventually proved to be correct.

A series of α-substituted ornithine analogues were synthesized and assayed for their inhibitory properties in vitro towards ODC [13]. The kinetic constants $K_I$ (apparent dissociation constant) and $\tau_{50}$ (half-life of ODC at infinite concentration of inhibitors) which were measured for these ornithine analogues are listed in table I. It is clear that among the α-substituted methyl ornithine analogues the

TABLE I

Inhibitory properties of α-substituted ornithine analogues towards ODC[a]

| α-Substituent | Type of Inhibition | $K_I$ (mM) | $\tau_{50}$ (min) |
|---|---|---|---|
| $CH_3$ | competitive | 0.04 | |
| $CH_2OH$ | no inhibition | | |
| $CH_2OCH_3$ | no inhibition | | |
| $CH_2CN$ | time-dependent | 8.7 | 29 |
| $CH_2Cl$ | time-dependent | no saturation kinetics[b] | |
| $CH_2F$ | time-dependent | 0.075 | 1.6 |
| $CHF_2$ | time-dependent | 0.039 | 3.1 |
| $CH=CH_2$ | time-dependent | 0.81 | 27 |
| $C\equiv CH$ | time-dependent | 0.010 | 8.4 |

[a]Partially purified from a preparation of livers of thioacetamide-treated rats. The $K_M$ of L-ornithine is 0.04 mM.

[b]At 0.1 mM, the half-life of ODC activity is 22 min.

inhibitory activity decreases with increasing bulkiness and/or decreasing nucleofugality of the leaving group. Fluorine, which is difficult to displace in $S_N2$ reactions, combines small size with good nucleofugality in alkene-forming elimination reactions. This combination of properties undoubtedly accounts for the fact that in this series the α-fluoromethyl analogues of ornithine are the most potent time-dependent inhibitors of ODC _in vitro_. α-Acetylenic ornithine displays a potency similar to that of the fluoromethyl ornithine analogues, whereas α-vinyl ornithine which has a poor affinity for the target enzyme ($K_I$ = 810 μM) is a weak inhibitor of ODC [14]. All these ornithine analogues inhibited ODC with a high degree of selectivity and met the experimental criteria for enzyme-activated irreversible inhibitors.

Similarly AADC was found to be effectively and irreversibly inactivated by the α-monofluoromethyl and α-difluoromethyl analogues of its natural substrate DOPA [15,16] (table II). α-Acetylenic and α-vinyl DOPA also inhibited AADC but the inhibition was not complete and appeared to contain both reversible and irreversible components [17]. In contrast to ODC, AADC lacks substrate specificity and is known to decarboxylate a variety of hydroxyphenylalanine derivatives [18]. Not unexpectedly, the corresponding α-monofluoromethyl and α-difluoromethyl analogues of these hydroxyphenylalanines proved also to be time-dependent inhibitors of AADC [19] as indicated in table II. There was good correlation between the substrate properties of the hydroxyphenylalanine derivatives and the inhibitory potency of the correspond-

*References p. 104*

TABLE II

AADC: Relative rates of decarboxylation of ring hydroxylated phenylalanine derivatives and inhibitory activity of corresponding α-fluoromethyl and α-difluoromethyl analogues in vitro

| Substrates | Rate[a] | Inhibitors | t1/2 (min)[b] |
|---|---|---|---|
| 3,4-dihydroxy | 100 | $-CH_2F$ | 1 to 2 at 10 μM |
| | | $-CHF_2$ | 1 at 100 μM |
| 2,3-dihydroxy | 90 | $-CH_2F$ | 1 at 10 μM |
| | | $-CHF_2$ | 1 at 100 μM |
| 2,5-dihydroxy | 83 | $-CH_2F$ | 2 to 3 at 10 μM |
| | | $-CHF_2$ | 2 at 100 μM |
| 4-hydroxy | 10 | $-CH_2F$ | 50 at 100 μM |
| | | $-CHF_2$ | no time-dependent inhibition |

[a]Value taken from ref.[18].
[b]Pseudo first order kinetics were not observed.

ing α-fluoromethyl analogues, in vitro. The α-monofluoromethyl and α-difluoromethyl analogues of 2,3-dihydroxyphenylalanine and 2,5-dihydrophenylalanine are equipotent to α-monofluoromethyl and α-difluoromethyl DOPA, respectively. Interestingly, in contrast to monofluoromethyl and difluoromethyl ornithine, which have similar inhibitory activity towards ODC, the α-monofluoromethyl analogues of the hydroxyphenylalanine derivatives are consistently more active as inhibitors of AADC than the corresponding α-difluoromethyl analogues by one or two orders of magnitude.

The important question of whether the reactive species escapes the enzyme's active site during the inhibition process was investigated using ring-$^3H$ and $^{14}C$-carboxyl α-fluoromethyl DOPA [20]. It was found that the inactivation of purified AADC from pig kidney involved a stoichiometric formation of an enzyme-inhibitor complex. Moreover, the inhibition was accompanied by release of one equivalent of radioactive $CO_2$ and fluoride ion. These results clearly demonstrated that no reactive intermediate escapes the active site of AADC during the inactivation process.

As GABA-T operates by Schiff's base-mediated formation of a carbanion on the γ carbon atom of its GABA substrate, we hypothesized that GABA analogues bearing an acetylenic or a vinyl function or a fluoromethyl group on the γ carbon might irreversibly inactivate this enzyme. These GABA analogues were synthesized and with the exception of trifluoromethyl GABA, were found to be potent substrate-induced irreversible inhibitors of purified pig brain GABA-T [21,22,23] (table III). Trifluoromethyl GABA was not even a competitive inhibitor for GABA-T. This lack of affinity of the trifluoromethyl analogue could be attributed to the large decrease

TABLE III

Kinetic constants for the inhibition of GABA-T[a] by GABA, β-alanine and δ-amino pentanoic acid derivatives

| Inhibitors | $K_I$ (mM) | $_{50}$ (min) | $t_{1/2}$ (min) at 1 mM |
|---|---|---|---|
| γ-acetylenic GABA | 0.08 | 6 | 6 |
| γ-vinyl GABA | | | 1[b] |
| γ-fluoromethyl GABA | 2.0 | 1.8 | 5 |
| γ-difluoromethyl GABA | 20 | 1.8 | 40 |
| γ-trifluoromethyl GABA | no inhibition | | |
| β-acetylenic-β-alanine | | | 15[c] |
| β-vinyl-β-alanine | | | 33[c] |
| β-fluoromethyl-β-alanine | 1.7 | 1 | 4.5 |
| β-difluoromethyl-β-alanine | 2 | 2 | 6.5 |
| δ-trifluoromethyl-δ-alanine | no inhibition | | |
| δ-fluoromethyl-δ-aminopentanoic acid | 4.7 | 2 | 11.5 |
| δ-difluoromethyl-δ-aminopentanoic acid | | | 40[b] |

[a]Purified from pig brain; The $K_M$ of GABA under the same experimental conditions as those used to study the inhibitors was 4 mM.

[b]No apparent saturation kinetics were observed.

[c]$K_I$ and $\tau_{50}$ were not determined.

in the basicity of its amine. The $pK_a$ value of the amino group decreases by more than 5 units as the number of fluorine atoms increases from 0 to 3. Like AADC, GABA-T lacks substrate specificity. It transaminates β-alanine, the lower homologue of GABA, as efficiently as GABA, and δ-aminopentanoic acid, the higher homologue of GABA, at one third the rate of GABA. As anticipated, the ω-monofluoromethyl and di-fluoromethyl analogues of β-alanine and δ-aminopentanoic as well as β-vinyl and β-acetylenic-β-alanine also proved to be substrate-induced irreversible inhibitor of GABA-T. The structure-activity relationship for GABA-T inhibition in vitro as a function of the chain length and the latent reactive grouping of the inhibition was, however, not straightforward. In the fluoromethyl series, the activity of the inhibitor decreased as the chain length increased, whereas in the vinyl and acetylenic series the opposite relationship prevailed.

Our original choice for positioning the latent reactive grouping on the GABA skeleton turned out to be fortunate. Indeed, β-methylene-β-alanine, β-methylene GABA, (E)-4-aminocrotonic acid and 4-aminotetrolic acid are β-alanine and GABA analogues in which the unsaturation occupies the same positional relationship to the amino group of β-alanine and GABA as in β-vinyl-β-alanine and γ-vinyl or γ-acetylenic GABA. Electrophilic imines could consequently be generated within GABA-T's active site from these unsaturated derivatives. Nevertheless none of them was found to inhibit GABA-T irreversibly . Surprisingly, addition of a halogen atom on the double bond of 4-aminocrotonic acid gave enzyme inhibitory activity [24].

The ω-fluoromethyl and ω-vinyl-β-alanine and GABA derivatives, as expected, proved to be highly selective inhibitors of GABA-T, at least within the class of PLP-dependent amino acid transaminases and decarboxylases [21,23]. On the other hand, β-acetylenic-β-alanine and γ-acetylenic GABA were also found to be substrate-induced irreversible inhibitors of mammalian and bacterial glutamic acid decarboxylase, the enzyme which catalyzes the decarboxylation of glutamic acid to GABA. To rationalize this unexpected finding, a mechanism relying on the principle of microscopic reversibility of enzyme catalysis was proposed [25]. Although disproved later at least in the case of inhibition of mammalian GABA-T by γ-acetylenic GABA [26], this hypothesis led to the concept that this new type of inhibition of an α-amino acid decarboxylase by an analogue of its substrate could be of a general nature. Indeed α-acetylenic derivatives of putrescine and dopamine, the products of ODC and AADC respectively, were also found to be time-dependent inhibitors of the corresponding decarboxylases [13,27]. α-Acetylenic dopamine is a relatively weak inhibitor of AADC, but the inhibitory potency of α-acetylenic putrescine towards ODC ($K_I$ = 0.002 mM, $\tau_{50}$ = 9 min) compares favorably to that of difluoromethyl ornithine (table I). Interestingly, in contrast to γ-fluoromethyl GABA analogues which do not inhibit GAD, the fluoromethyl analogues of putrescine [28] and dopamine [27] have meaningful inhibitory activity against ODC and AADC, respectively. The potency of these amine analogues is, however, less than that of the corresponding α-fluoromethyl α -amino acid derivatives.

Of the many active compounds developed, several were chosen for extensive pharmacological and biochemical evaluation. In general, in vitro and ex vivo potency and selectivity as inhibitor of the target enzymes, preliminary indication of lack of toxicity and the feasibility of synthesis of adequate amounts were the principal determinants of the compounds to be evaluated. In particular, DL-α-difluoromethyl ornithine (DFMO, RMI 71782) was chosen as an inhibitor of ODC, γ-acetylenic GABA (GAG, RMI 71645) and γ-vinyl GABA (GVG, RMI 71754) as inhibitors of GABA-T, and DL-α-difluoromethyl DOPA (DFMD, RMI 71801) and DL-α-monofluoromethyl DOPA (MFMD, RMI 71963) as inhibitors of AADC.

## III) BIOCHEMICAL AND PHARMACOLOGICAL EVALUATION OF INHIBITORS

As previously noted (section I above), the precise biological consequences likely to arise from the inhibition of ODC had not been demonstrated at the time that the first selective, irreversible inhibitor was made. Similarly, although inhibitors of GABA-T had been available before the synthesis of GAG and GVG, they were either toxic (amino-oxyacetic acid), lacking in potency (n-dipropylacetate) or penetrated poorly through the blood-brain barrier (ethanolamine O-sulphate) [22]. A thorough biochemical and pharmacological investigation of these compounds was therefore an important step towards defining those clinical conditions most likely to benefit from administration of such inhibitors. The clinical potential of new inhibitors of AADC was, on the other hand, more evident. Compounds such as carbidopa and benserazide had been used successfully to protect coadministered L-dopa from peripheral decarboxylation in the therapy of Parkinson's disease. Moreover, there remained the possibility of developing novel inhibitors of AADC sufficiently potent to render the decarboxylase step rate-limiting and, as a consequence, to deplete the endogenous monoamine transmitter stores. The primary objective of the biochemical and pharmacological analysis of the irreversible inhibitors of AADC, DFMD and MFMD, was to identify such potentially useful activity.

a) Inhibitors of ODC

Initial attempts to establish the biological significance of inhibition of ODC were made with DL-$\alpha$-methyl ornithine, a competitive inhibitor of the enzyme. The compound was used successfully to inhibit cell division in hepatoma tissue culture (HTC) cells and evidence was obtained that the effect was related directly to its ODC inhibitory properties [29,30]. It was, therefore, a logical step to test DFMO initially on HTC cells in culture. DFMO strongly decreased cell growth rate and the effect was associated with a decrease in the intracellular putrescine and spermidine concentrations [30,31]. Both the polyamine depletion and the cytostatic effect could be reversed by adding polyamines to the culture medium, establishing the functional relationship between the intracellular polyamine concentrations and the capacity of the cell for normal division [30,31]. On the basis of these data and following the establishment of suitable dose ranges and schedules to achieve inhibition of ODC in vivo [32,33,34], the effects of DFMO were investigated in two transplantable tumour models in mice, L1210 leukemia and the EMT6 mammary sarcoma. Significant slowing of the growth of both tumors was obtained concomitant with inhibition of ODC and lowering of the intracellular putrescine and spermidine concentrations [35,36]. Antitumoral effects have since been observed with DFMO in a number of animal tumour models both in vitro and in vivo. Of major significance is the fact that antitumoral effects were obtained without significant host toxicity, a reflection, presumably, of the generally low ODC activities in normal tissues [37].

Since DFMO is cytostatic, a logical extension of the development work in this area was the investigation of the effects of DFMO in combination with cytotoxic antitumoral agents. At least additive effects have been obtained when DFMO was administered together with cyclophosphamide, adriamycin or vindesine in several tumour

*References p. 104*

models with no evidence of an increase in toxicity [38] These experiments suggested that notwithstanding the antitumoral effects of DFMO _per se_, the optimal clinical benefit from the use of DFMO might be obtained in combination therapy with other antitumoral agents.

The association of an active polyamine biosynthesis with rapidly dividing or actively differentiating cell systems [11,37] suggested embryonic development as a prime target for suppression with an inhibitor of ODC. DFMO was therefore administered to mice, rats and rabbits during the period of early gestation when the maximum increase in deciduomal ODC activity occurs. Complete suppression of ODC activity and _de novo_ putrescine formation was accompanied by arrest of embryonic development [39,40]. Subsequent experiments allowed definition of a precise 12-24 hour period shortly after implantation during which administration of an inhibitor of ODC irreversibly arrests embryonic development [40]. Contragestional effects arising from inhibition of putrescine biosynthesis and manifested during early embryogenesis suggest a potentially interesting and novel approach to fertility control.

Pursuing the theme that inhibitors of ODC would be most likely to show functional effects in systems displaying rapid growth and/or where there is evidence of active polyamine biosynthesis, the capacity of DFMO to inhibit the testosterone-induced reversal of prostatic atrophy in castrated rats was studied [41]. At the doses used DFMO had little effect on the return to normal morphology of the prostatic epithelium, but markedly reduced formation of prostatic fluid . The human prostate is one of the richest natural sources of polyamines in nature [42]. Preliminary clinical studies have been performed with DFMO in chronic non-suppurating prostatis [43].

Other animal systems in which DFMO has been shown to have functional effects include ovulation in rats. Here, DFMO, given only during proestrus, abolished the gonadotrophin-dependent preovulatory rise in ODC activity and enhanced the number of eggs ovulated four days later during estrus of the following cycle [44,45]. DFMO blocked the rises in ODC associated with intestinal maturation in the new-born rat or intestinal repair following chemotherapeutic insult [46].On the other hand, no effects of prolonged treatment with DFMO on male rodent fertility or spermatogenesis were detected despite extensive depletion of putrescine and spermidine from prostate, vas deferens and testis [47].

Recent experiments have revealed that a number of parasitic infections in animals respond beneficially to administration of DFMO. These include _Eimeria tenella_ infections in chickens [48] and trypanosomiasis in mice caused both by _Trypanosoma brucei brucei_ and _Trypanosoma brucei rhodesiense_ [49].

Thus, from animal experimental studies with DFMO, a critical dependence on _de novo_ putrescine synthesis has been established in systems as diverse as early mammalian embryogenesis and the growth and multiplication of certain parasitic protozoa. Furthermore, active ODC is clearly important in the growth of both transplanted and chemically-induced animal tumours. Since inhibition of ODC per se seems not to result in toxicity, the therapeutic potential of potent selective inhibitors of this enzyme is self-evident. Clinical evaluation of DFMO is currently under way in several human malignancies as the first step towards the identification of areas in which the therapeutic promise from animal experiments can be translated into clinical usefulness.

b) Inhibitors of GABA-T

The early biochemical evaluation of GAG and GVG indicated that both compounds rapidly decreased brain GABA-T activity and concomitantly raised brain GABA concentrations up to 4 to 6 times the normal level [22,50]. GAG was approximately 10-15 times more potent than GVG, but GVG produced a longer lasting elevation in brain GABA [51].

Consistent with the role of GABA as a major inhibitory neurotransmitter in the CNS, its elevation in the brain following administration of GAG or GVG produced dose-related decreases in spontaneous motor behaviour as well as general sedation and hypothermia in both rats and mice [52]. Treated animals usually displayed a characteristic posture consisting of hunched appearance, curved spine, splayed hind paws, piloerection, lacrimation and ptosis. An interesting difference between the two inhibitors emerged during the early pharmacological evaluation. Whereas GAG could produce CNS excitation and convulsions, GVG was devoid of this effect.

Since decreases in brain GABA concentrations can be associated with convulsions in animals [53,54], GAG and GVG were tested for anti-seizure activity in a variety of animal experimental models. They produced time- and dose-related protection against audiogenic seizures in genetically susceptible mice and significant correlations were obtained between brain GABA levels and antiseizure activity for both of the inhibitors [51]. Both drugs also had anticonvulsant activity against seizures induced in mice by bicuculline, picrotoxin, metrazol, strychnine, isonazid and electroshock [52,55].

In a combined biochemical and behavioural study, the effects of increasing brain GABA concentration on the functioning of various dopamine pathways was investigated [56]. Although the response was complex, the overall effect of administration of GAG was to cause a decrease in activity in the extrapyramidal and limbic dopamine systems.

Two areas of normal behaviour in which GABA has been implicated are the regulation of feeding [57] and the control of anxiety [58]. GVG, in doses which raise brain GABA, produced a dose-related reduction in food intake in rats. The response did not show tolerance and appeared not to be mediated through either catecholaminergic or indoleaminergic mechanisms [59]. On the other hand, in a conflict model of anxiety GVG failed to produce anxiolytic effects [60].

*References p. 104*

From these experimental studies in animals, some indications of the potential clinical application of inhibitors of GABA-T have emerged. Clearly, the epilepsies represent an important field for trials of such compounds. Encouraging results were obtained in an initial clinical trial of GAG in tardive dyskinesia, a condition believed to be a consequence of dopaminergic hyperactivity [61]. More extensive trials in this condition with GVG have been initiated.

c) Inhibitors of AADC

The proven value of the existing inhibitors, carbidopa and benserazide, in combination with L-dopa in the therapy of Parkinson's disease suggested an obvious clinical utility for an inhibitor with activity against the peripheral enzyme and minimal effects in the brain. On the other hand, achievement of functional depletion of the endogenous monoamine stores would be a novel property of an inhibitor of AADC. It would require inhibitory potency greater than that displayed by any of the existing compounds in order to render the decarboxylase step in the biosynthetic pathway rate-limiting.

Following in vivo biochemical evaluation, it was clear that DFMD fell into the first category, in that its potency was adequate to prevent the peripheral decarboxylation of exogenously administered amino acids but insufficient to inhibit endogenous monoamine biosynthesis [62,63]. Moreover, DFMD appeared to act only in the periphery, there being minimal entry of the compound into the brain and negligible inhibition of central AADC [63]. The compound was therefore administered to rats alone and in combination with L-dopa and the body temperature recorded. DFMD, itself, produced no change in body temperature. The hypothermia produced by a submaximal dose of L-dopa, which reflects a central action of L-dopa was, however, enhanced dose-dependently by coadministration of DFMD [63].

Similar experiments were carried out in rats with 5-hydroxytryptophan (5-HTP) coadministered with DFMD. The functional consequence of the resultant increase in brain 5-hydroxytryptamine (5-HT) is a characteristic head and trunk movement reminiscent of a wet dog shaking itself dry. DFMD augmented "Wet Dog" shaking behaviour produced by 5-HTP and there was a significant correlation between this response and the increase in whole brain 5-HT concentration [63,64, see also fig. 1]. The qualitative similarity between DFMD and carbidopa in these experiments suggested that DFMD might have potential clinical usefulness in combination with L-dopa in the treatment of Parkinson's disease, and, perhaps, with L-5-HTP in the therapy of action myoclonus [65] and some cases of depression [66].

It soon became apparent that MFMD had properties radically different from those of DFMD. Biochemical studies in vitro showed MFMD to be much more potent than existing irreversible inhibitors of AADC. In the "Wet Dog" shake test in rats, potentiation of 5-HTP occurred, but beyond a dose of 2-5 mg/kg the effects of MFMD declined with increasing dose. At a dose of 50 mg/kg, the brain 5-HT concentration was de-

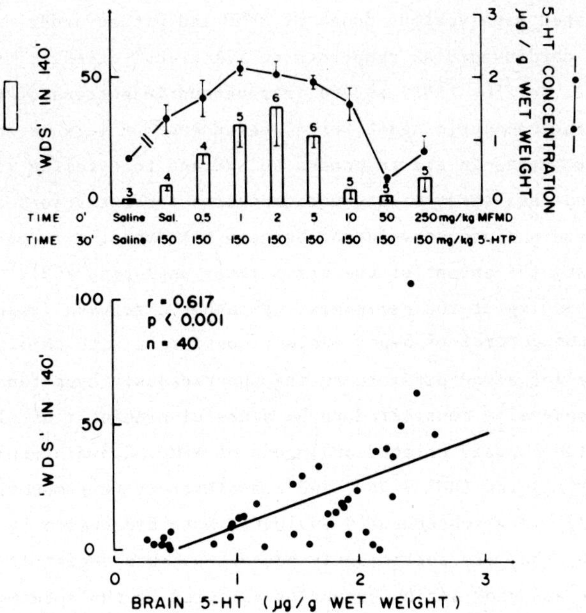


Fig. 1. Effect of DL-α-monofluoromethyldopa on "Wet-Dog" shaking behaviour (WDS) produced by 5-hydroxytryptophan (5-HTP).
<u>Upper graph</u>: WDS response ▯ ; whole brain 5-hydroxytryptamine (5-HT) concentration •——••Numbers of individual values contributing to the mean values are given above the histograms. For methodological details, see [64].
<u>Lower graph</u>: Relationship between WDS and whole brain 5-HTP concentration.

creased below the normal endogenous concentration despite the concomitant administration of 5-HTP (fig. 1). These data suggested that MFMD penetrated the CNS to prevent there the decarboxylation of exogenous 5-HTP and that in sufficient doses MFMD could inhibit endogenous 5-HT synthesis.

Biochemical analyses rapidly confirmed the exceptional potency of MFMD as an inhibitor of AADC <u>in vivo</u> and its capacity to inhibit the enzyme both in the periphery and in the CNS [67,68]. Unlike with DFMD, essentially complete inhibition of the enzyme could be obtained, resulting in depletion of the endogenous monoamine stores [67,68]. However, these studies also suggested a margin of selectivity for the periphery, and on that basis experiments were initiated to assess the relationship between depletion of the sympathetic transmitter, noradrenaline, and the functional activity of the peripheral sympathetic nervous system. In these experiments, emphasis was placed on responses of the cardiovascular system, since it is here where controlled attenuation of sympathetic function would most likely result in therapeutic benefit.

Rats were treated with various doses of MFMD and pithed under pentobarbitone anaesthesia. The cardiovascular responses to electrical stimulation of the whole spinal sympathetic outflow (SNS) and to intravenous injections of tyramine, an indirectly acting sympathomimetic agent, or of noradrenaline were measured. MFMD caused dose-dependent decreases in the responses to SNS and to tyramine without affecting those to noradrenaline. Assay of the noradrenaline concentrations of heart and portal veins showed a close correlation between the decrease in peripheral sympathetic function and the extent of the transmitter depletion [69]. Compounds which inhibit the functioning of the peripheral sympathetic nervous system have found clinical use in the control of hypertension. Consistent with this, MFMD proved effective in lowering blood pressure in the spontaneously hypertensive rat [69,70], an animal model generally considered to be a useful predictor of clinical antihypertensive action. Two closely related analogues of MFMD, 2,3-dihydroxy-DL-$\alpha$-monofluoromethylphenylalanine (RMI 72163) and 2,5-dihydroxy-DL-$\alpha$-monofluoromethylphenylalanine (RMI 72173) were subsequently evaluated both biochemically and pharmacologically. Like MFMD, they are sufficiently potent to cause depletion of the monoamine neurotransmitters and show antihypertensive activity in the spontaneously hypertensive rat [71].

In the sequence of events leading towards the development of a new chemotherapeutic agent, the conception of the compound, its chemical synthesis and its biochemical and pharmacological evaluation represent the first steps in the progress towards initial clinical evaluation. For inhibitors of the three enzymes discussed in this review, these phases have been largely completed. It remains for the future to determine whether the clinical potential indicated by the biochemical and pharmacological evaluation can be translated into therapeutic reality.

## REFERENCES


1 S.S. Cohen, Science, 205 (1979) 964-971
2 C. Walsh, Horizons Biochem. Biophys., 3 (1977) 36-55.
3 R.H. Abeles and A.L. Maycock, Acc. Chem. Res., 9 (1976) 313-319.
4 F.M. Miesowicz and K. Bloch, J. Biol. Chem., 254 (1979) 5868-74.
5 R.R. Rando, Science, 185 (1974) 320-324.
6 Drug action and design: mechanism-based enzyme inhibitors, T.I. Kalman (Ed.), Elsevier, New York, Amsterdam, Oxford, 1979.
7 Enzyme-activated irreversible inhibitors, N. Seiler, M.J. Jung, J. Koch-Weser (Eds.) Elsevier, Amsterdam, New York, Oxford, 1978.
8 A. Sjoerdsma, Brit. J. Clin. Pharmacol., in press.
9 M. Henning, in D.S. Davies, J.L. Reid (Eds.), Central action of drugs in blood pressure regulation, Tunbridge Wells: Pitman Medical (1975), 157-165.
10 The pharmacological basis of therapeutics, 6th edn. A.G. Gilman, L.S. Goodman, A. Gilman (Eds.), McMillan, New York, Toronto, London, 1980, 482.
11 H. Tabor and C.W. Tabor, Adv. Enzym., 36 (1972) 205-268.
12 P. Bey, Chem. and industry, (1981) 139-144; See also ref. 2,3,5,6 and 7.
13 B.W. Metcalf, P. Bey, C. Danzin, M.J. Jung, P. Casara and J.P. Vevert, J. Am. Chem. Soc., 100 (1978) 2551-2553.

14 C. Danzin, P. Casara, N. Claverie and B.W. Metcalf, J. Med. Chem., 24 (1981) 16-20.
15 P. Bey, in ref. 7,27-41.
16 J. Kollonitsch, A.A. Patchett, S. Marburg, A.L. Maycock, L.M. Perkins, G.A. Doldouras, D.E. Duggan, S.D. Aster, Nature (London), 274 (1978) 906-908.
17 G. Ribereau-Gayon, C. Danzin, M.G. Palfreyman, M. Aubry, J. Wagner, B.W. Metcalf and M.J. Jung, Biochem. Pharmacol., 28 (1979) 1331-1335.
18 R. Ferrini, A. Gläser, Biochem. Pharmacol., 13 (1964) 793-801.
19 P. Bey, F. Gerhart, M. Gittos, M.J. Jung, in preparation.
20 A.L. Maycock, S.D. Aster and A.A. Patchett, Biochem., 19 (1980) 707-718.
21 B. Lippert, B.W. Metcalf, M.J. Jung and P. Casara, Eur. J. Biochem., 74 (1977) 441-445.
22 M.J. Jung, B. Lippert, B.W. Metcalf, P.J. Schechter, P. Böhlen and A. Sjoerdsma, J. Neurochem., 28 (1977) 717-723.
23 P. Bey, M.J. Jung, F. Gerhart, D. Schirlin, V. Van Dorsselaer and P. Casara, J. Neurochem., in press.
24 R.D. Allan, G.A.R. Johnston and B. Twitchin, Aust. J. Chem., 33 (1980) 1115-1122.
25 M.J. Jung, B.W. Metcalf, B. Lippert and P. Casara, Biochem., 17 (1978) 2628-2632.
26 M. Bouclier, M.J. Jung and B. Lippert, Eur. J. Biochem., 98 (1979) 363-368.
27 A.L. Maycock, S.D. Aster and A.A. Patchett, in ref. 6, 115-129.
28 C. Danzin, P. Bey, D. Schirlin and N. Claverie, in preparation.
29 P.S. Mamont, P. Böhlen, P.P. McCann, P. Bey, F. Schuber and C. Tardiff, Proc. Nat. Acad. Sci., USA, 73 (1976) 1626-1630.
30 P.S. Mamont, M.C. Duchesne, A.M. Joder-Ohlenbusch and J. Grove, in ref. 7, 43-54.
31 P.S. Mamont, M.C. Duchesne, J. Grove and P. Bey, Biochem. Biophys. Res. Commun. 81 (1978) 58-66.
32 N. Seiler, C. Danzin, N.J. Prakash and J. Koch-Weser, in ref. 7, 55-71.
33 C. Danzin, M.J. Jung, B.W. Metcalf, J. Grove and P. Casara, Biochem. Pharmacol., 28 (1979) 627-631.
34 C. Danzin, M.J. Jung, J. Grove and P. Bey, Life Sci., 24 (1979) 519-524.
35 N.J. Prakash, P.J Schechter, J. Grove and J. Koch-Weser, Cancer Res., 38 (1978) 3059-3062.
36 N.J. Prakash, P.J. Schechter, P.S. Mamont, J. Grove, J. Koch-Weser and A. Sjoerdsma, Life Sci., 26 (1980) 181-194.
37 C.W. Tabor and H. Tabor, Ann. Rev. Biochem., 45 (1976) 285-306.
38 J. Bartholeyns and J. Koch-Weser, Cancer Res., in press.
39 J.R. Fozard, M.L. Part, N.J. Prakash, J. Grove, P.J. Schechter, A. Sjoerdsma and J. Koch-Weser, Science, 208 (1980) 505-508.
40 J.R. Fozard, M.L. Part, N.J. Prakash and J. Grove, Europ. J. Pharmacol., 65 (1980) 379-391.
41 C. Danzin, M.J. Jung, N. Claverie, J. Grove, A. Sjoerdsma and J. Koch-Weser, Biochem. J., 180 (1979) 507-513.
42 H.G. Williams-Ashman and D.H. Lockwood, Ann. N.Y. Acad. Sci., 171 (1970) 882-894.
43 U. Dunzendorfer, Arzneimittel-Forsch., 31 (1981) 382-385.
44 J.R. Fozard, N.J. Prakash and J. Grove, Life Sci., 27 (1980) 2277-2283.
45 J.R. Carpenter, unpublished observations.
46 G.D. Luk, L.J. Marton and S.B. Baylin, Science, 210 (1980) 195-198.
47 J.R. Fozard, unpublished observations.
48 P.P. McCann, C.J. Bacchi, W.L. Hanson, G.D. Cain, H.C. Nathan, S.H. Hutner and A. Sjoerdsma, in C.M. Calderara, V. Zappia and U. Bachrach (Ed.), Advances in Polyamine Research, Raven Press, New York, pp.97-110.
49 C.J. Bacchi, H.C. Nathan, S.H. Hutner, P.P. McCann and A. Sjoerdsma, Science, 210 (1980) 332-334.
50 P.J. Schechter, Y. Tranier, M.J. Jung and P. Böhlen, Eur. J. Pharmacol., 45 (1977) 319-328.
51 P.J. Schechter, Y. Tranier, M.J. Jung and A. Sjoerdsma, J. Pharmac. Exp. Ther., 201 (1977) 606-612.
52 P.J. Schechter and Y. Tranier, in ref. 7, 149-162.
53 B. Meldrum, in P. Krogsgaard-Larsen, J. Scheel-Krüger and H. Kofod (Ed.), GABA-Neurotransmitters, Munksgaard, Copenhagen, 1978, pp.390-405.

54 P.J. Schechter, Y. Tranier and J. Grove, in P. Mandel and F.V. Defeudis (Eds.), GABA-Biochemistry and CNS functions, Plenum, New York, 1979 pp.43-57.
55 M.G. Palfreyman, P.J. Schechter, W.R. Buckett, G.P. Tell and J. Koch-Weser, Biochem. Pharmacol. 30, (1981) 817-824.
56 M.G. Palfreyman, S. Huot, B. Lippert and P.J. Schechter, Eur. J. Pharmac., 50 (1978) 325-336.
57 J. Kelly, G.F. Alheid, A. Newberg and S. Grossman, Pharmacol. Biochem. Behav., 7 (1977) 537-541.
58 M.H. Thiébot, A. Jobert and P. Soubrié, Neurosci. Lett., 16 (1980) 213-217.
59 S. Huot and M.G. Palfreyman, Pharmac. Biochem. Behav., submitted.
60 S. Huot, M. Robin and M.G. Palfreyman, in F.V Defeudis and P. Mandel (Ed.), Amino Acid Neurotransmitters, Raven Press, New York, 1981, pp.45-52.
61 D.E. Casey, J. Gerlach, G. Majelund, T.R. Christensen, Arch. Gen. Psychiat., 37 (1980) 1376-1379.
62 M.G. Palfreyman, C. Danzin, P. Bey, M.J. Jung, G. Ribereau-Gayon, M. Aubry, J.P. Vevert and A. Sjoerdsma, J. Neurochem., 31 (1978) 927-932.
63 M.G. Palfreyman, C. Danzin, M.J. Jung, J.R. Fozard, J.K. Woodward, M. Aubry, R.C. Dage and J. Koch-Weser, in ref. 7, pp.221-233.
64 J.R. Fozard and M.G. Palfreyman, N.S. Arch. Pharmacol., 307 (1979) 135-142.
65 M.H. Van Woert, D. Rosenbaum, J. Howieson and M.B. Bowers, New England J. Med., 296 (1977) 70-75.
66 H.M. Van Praag and J. Korf, J. Nerv. Mental Dis., 158 (1974) 331-337.
67 M.J. Jung, M.G. Palfreyman, J. Wagner, P. Bey, G. Ribereau-Gayon, M. Zraïka and J. Koch-Weser, Life Sci., 24 (1979) 1037-1042.
68 P. Bey, M.J. Jung, J. Koch-Weser, M.G. Palfreyman, A. Sjoerdsma, J. Wagner and M. Zraika, Br. J. Pharmacol., 70 (1980) 571-576.
69 J.R. Fozard, M. Spedding, M.G. Palfreyman, J. Wagner, J. Möhring and J. Koch-Weser, J. Cardiovasc. Pharmacol., 2 (1980) 229-245.
70 J.R. Fozard, J. Möhring, M.G. Palfreyman and J. Koch-Weser, J. Cardiovasc. Pharmacol., 1981, in press.
71 J.R. Fozard, M.G. Palfreyman, L.E. Roebel, H.G. Cheng and D.L. Weiner, unpublished observations.

J.A. Keverling Buisman (Editor), *Strategy in Drug Research* 


# SELECTIVE INHIBITION OF B TYPE MONOAMINE OXIDASE IN THE BRAIN: A DRUG STRATEGY TO IMPROVE THE QUALITY OF LIFE IN SENESCENCE

J. KNOLL
Department of Pharmacology, Semmelweis University of Medicine, Budapest (HUNGARY)

ABSTRACT

In the aging brain, there is a loss of neurons, compensated for by a proliferation of glial cells. We might thus predict that dopaminergic and 'trace aminergic' modulation in the brain declines in senescence because of the loss of neurons and because of the increased monoamine oxidase (MAO)-B activity present in the glia. The hypothesis was forwarded that the significant increase of the incidence of depression in the elderly, the age-dependent decline in male sexual vigor and the frequent appearance of parkinsonian symptoms in the latter decades of life might be attributed to a decrease of dopamine and 'trace amines' in the brain. The possibility to counteract these biochemical lesions of aging by chronic administration of (-)deprenyl, a selective inhibitor of MAO-B, which facilitates dopaminergic and 'trace-aminergic' activity in the brain and is a safe drug in man, was analysed in details. The restitution and long term maintenance of full scale sexual activity in aged male rats continuously treated with (-)deprenyl was demonstrated as an experimental model in support of the view that the long term administration of small doses of (-)deprenyl may improve the quality of life in senescence.

Due to medical, economic and sociological factors and to a birthrate decrease which nears zero population growth, the developed countries are becoming more and more societies of older people. For example, the proportion of the elderly - that is over 65 years of age - in the United States was slightly over 4% in 1900, is at present about 11% and is projected to reach 17% by the year 2030.

According to statistics, in the developed countries elderly are now using a disproportionate amount of medical services, they are

*References p. 132*

responsible for an extremely high percentage of national health expenditure on drug prescriptions, and these trends are expected to continue.

The 9th European Symposium on Clinical Pharmacological Evaluation on Drug Control, held in November 1980, which was devoted entirely to the question of drugs for the elderly and constituted a preparatory step for the United Nations World Assembly on the Elderly 1982, concluded that many of the 'geriatric drugs' which are used in some countries as a heritage of older drugs, are probably inefficacious for most purposes, and the validity of the clinical evidence in support of most perhaps all, of the drugs which are now widely used in the elderly for relieving symptoms associated with vascular or cerebral function or both, is open to question.

But, - as the human being is mortal, life span is finite, aging is not a disease, and, as such, it is not treatable by medicaments -, is any health-strategy based on the continuous medication of old people without disease, acceptable at all?

The consideration that there is a linear decline of a number of performances beginning at about the age of 50, even in those fortunates who avoid serious acute and any type of chronic diseases and live beyond the magic age of 100, suggests an affirmative answer to this question. It seems to be an increasingly important aspect of drug research to explore new possibilities, new strategies for improving the quality of life in advanced age.

The search for such new lines of medication of the elderly might be based on the assumption that the decline of the functional capacity of the aging organism is due to the development of age-related biochemical lesions, the consequences of which can be counteracted by appropriate continuous medication. The aim of this study is to support this approach.

## The concept that the progressive decrease in brain catecholamines and 'trace amines' is an unavoidable biochemical lesion of aging

Robinson et al. (1) demonstrated in 1971 that MAO activity progressively increases in the aging brain. The age-dependent change in MAO activity was studied in detail in a number of papers (2, 3, 4, 5, 6, 7, 8, 9, 10). It seems to be firmly established by now that B-type MAO activity is increasing selectively with increased age in both human (9) and rat brain (4, 10) and the age-dependent increase in MAO-B activity is due entirely to an increased enzyme concentration in brain tissue (9).

Looking for an explanation for the selective increase of MAO-B activity with increasing age, it has to be considered that, according to Student and Edwards (11), MAO-B is predominently localized in the neuroglia and this conclusion is further supported by Strolin Benedetti and Keane (10) who found that in the rat brain the increase in MAO-B activity was restricted to the extra-synaptosomal mitochondrial fraction of the aging brain, whereas a reduction in MAO-A activity was found in the intrasynaptosomal but not in the extrasynaptosomal fraction.

All these findings seem to support our hypothesis of a progressively developing biochemical lesion in the aging brain, which leads to a decreased catecholaminergic and 'trace aminergic' modulation (12, 13).

According to this hypothesis, well established old experiences offer a good explanation for the increase of brain MAO-B activity in the latter decades of life. Cell loss is a general feature of the aging brain. A more or less constant pattern of loss of cortical neurons, up to 30% of the total neuronal pool, was found in the human brain, with increasing age (cf. 14). In an up to date study, a drop of the number of neurons from 7890/mm$^3$ at age 45 to 5800/mm$^3$ at 90, a loss of 26%, was found in the hippocampal cortex by the aid of a highly sophisticated counting arrangement (15). As the loss of neurons is always compensated by glial cells, the progressive and cumulative loss of neurons in the aging brain gives a satisfactory explanation to the selective increase of extrasynaptosomal MAO-B activity with increasing age. This seems to be an unavoidable biochemical lesion of aging.

As to the functional consequences of the change in the brain, we have to consider the possible physiological significance of extraneuronally localised MAO-B for intracellular communication in the central nervous system. Let us take dopamine as an example, which is a substrate of MAO-B. There are essentially two possibilities for dopamine in transmitting a message from one neuron to another. The dopaminergic nerve terminal might be in a synaptic contact with the target neuron. In this case the released dopamine molecules immediately reach the target cell and are rapidly eliminated by re-uptake.

On the other hand (possibly this is the usual case) dopamine is released from the nerve terminals and there is no synaptic contact. Thus the molecules have to diffuse and travel long distances to reach the target cell. Whereas in the case of synaptic contact between the neurons, the extraneuronal MAO-B activity is evidently unable to influence the chemical message delivered by dopamine, the situation is essentially different in the case of a non-synaptic interneuronal communication. In this case the chances of the slowly diffusing molecules reaching their target cell and modulating its activity might essentially depend on the concentration of the glial MAO-B in the environment. A similar control of the modulatory functions of those trace-amines in the brain which are substrates of MAO-B is also feasible. In this context β-phenylethylamine (PEA) should be mentioned first and foremost, because this is the main substrate of the B form of MAO.

The physiological role of PEA in the central nervous system (CNS) is still obscure. The possibility that it acts as an amine modulator of affective behavior was proposed by Sabelli and Giardina (16). As PEA is a potent releaser of catecholamines from the plasmatic pool of the nerve terminals, a model of how it may act as a physiological activator of catecholaminergic neurons was also suggested (17).

Collating the facts that there is an unavoidable loss of neurons, inescapably leading to increased MAO-B activity with increasing age, makes it understandable that dopaminergic and 'trace aminergic' modulation in the brain is progressively decreasing in the aging brain. It is in agreement with this trend of changes that an age-dependent decrease in the dopamine control of the basal ganglia in man was described, first by Bertler in 1961 (18), and corroborated by many others. Riederer and Wuketich (19) found that the dopamine content of the human caudate nucleus decreased by 13% per decade over age 45.

If, in addition, we also consider that the activity of tyrosine hydroxylase, the enzyme catalysing the rate-limiting step in catecholamine biosynthesis, was also found to decrease in human brain tissue with increasing age (20), weighty arguments seem to support the view that catecholaminergic tone is progressively decreasing in the aging brain.

As the described age-dependent chain of events can be deduced to well defined biochemical lesions, the chances to develop a new drug strategy for counteracting or possibly even preventing, the adverse consequences of the age-related decrease of the catecholaminergic tone in the brain, are fair.

## The concept that the high incidence of adverse changes in affective behavior, sexual performance and motor coordination in advanced age, is due to the age-related decrease of catecholaminergic tone in the brain

A survey of the medicinal literature, prefaced by the basic statement that any age-dependent change of a brain-function can be deduced to a biochemical lesion of the nerve tissue, suggests that

a/ the significant increase of the incidence of depression in the elderly,

b/ the age-dependent decline in male sexual vigor, and

c/ the frequent appearance of parkinsonian symptoms in the latter decades of life deserve common analysis.

These three aging phenomena might be attributed to age-dependent changes in brain catecholamine metabolism, as catecholaminergic modulation is known to play a leading role in the control of mood, male sexual behavior and motor coordination, and there is a progressive decline in the activity of the catecholaminergic system in the brain with increasing age.

Depression with late onset. It is an old clinical experience that elderly are more susceptible to depression than other age groups. 'Involutional depression' as a diagnostic entity was introduced by Kraepelin in 1896 (21). In spite of the fact that, this category is omitted from the 9th revision of WHO's International Classification of Diseases (1978), the conspicuous proneness of aged persons to depression is undeniable. Per 100.000 people, aged 25 to 34 years, 76.3 psychiatric abnormalities of all types have been found, against 235.1 per 100.000 people over 65 years; depression accounts for most mental disorders occurring in the elderly (22).

The seriousness of depression in old age is shown by the increase of suicide rates in the elderly. In the United States, for example, where the general suicide rate is below 11 per 100.000 of the population, suicides of white males reached 150 per 100.000 in their seventh age decade, and 25 per cent of all suicides occurred in elderly persons.

Even if we accept the view that "in old age, death ought to be considered more as the 'finishing touch' of life than as a horrifying experience against which younger people rebel" (23), the extremely high percentage of suicides is evidently the most serious sign of depressed mood, alien to healthy people of all age groups.

According to field studies of depression in old age, performed with random samples of septuagenarians and with the aim to disclose also the mild and moderate cases of depression, some kind of a depressive disorder was found in about 25 per cent in persons over age 65 (24, 25, 26). This high incidence of depression in the elderly cannot be explained, however, simply by knowing that old age is the season of losses (loss of spouse, of children, of job, of status, etc.) and the

*References p. 132*

period of a general decline of health conditions, as about 75 per cent of aged persons manage these troubles without clinical symptoms of depressed mood, sadness and reduced activity. The facts that, on the one hand, not all the aged are depressed and, on the other hand, when recognized in due time, depression of an aged person, which misdiagnosed, may lead to premature death, is usually highly responsive to treatment, speak in favour of our assumption that objective biochemical lesions in the metabolism of the aged brain tissue might play a decisive role in the proneness of the aged to depression.

Such a conclusion is in agreement with the, by now classical, amine hypothesis concerning the biological bases of mental illnesses. It is well known that the great drug-discoveries of the 1950s, lithium for mania (27), chlorpromazine for schizophrenia (28), meprobamate as an antianxiety agent (29), imipramine (30) and MAO inhibitors (31) as antidepressants, the development of benzodiazepines, the most potent antianxiety drugs (32) and the butyrophenon family of antipsychotics (33), etc., leading to highly efficient symptomatic treatment of psychoses, revolutionized psychiatric practice.

The good hopes, however, of the 1960s, to discover the genetically determined biochemical lesions which explain mental illnesses and to find the curative drugs, in spite of heroic efforts during the last decades, have not been realized. Year by year we accumulate more and more insight into the mechanisms of action of the psychopharmacological agents, without finding ultimately defined biological lesions in either schizophrenic or maniac-depressive patients which are causative to the illness.

It might well be that in a certain percentage of the population an inherited biological lesion or metabolic error determines the proneness of the individual to a mental illness, whereas the manifestation of the disease is due to the interaction of highly complex psychological, environmental and sociocultural factors. In the case of depression a functional weakness of the brain catecholaminergic, and possibly also 'trace aminergic', systems' activity, without dramatic changes in amine metabolism, detectable by the current biochemical methodology, might be one of the important causative factors in the proneness to the disease. Other factors, like a central 5-HT defect, neuroendocrinological abnormalities, etc., were also suspected to play a role in the development of a pathological depression of mood (for review see 34).

In the elderly biological lesions leading to a decreased catecholaminergic tone in the brain are biochemically detectable, making the higher incidence of depression in aged persons easier to interpret.

The sexual vigor of the male as a function of age. Sexual activity in the human male is known to be influenced by a number of factors, like good health, stable marriage, satisfactory sexual partner(s), adequate financial and social status, etc. But even in the males who meet all the requirements for retention and maintenance of sexual functioning, there is an age-related decrease in the sexual vigor, the reason of which still remains obscure (for review see 35, 36).

Martin (37) studied coital activity as a function of age, interviewing 628 members of the Baltimore Longitudinal Study of Aging. The objects were white, married, urban residents in good health of the Washington-Baltimore area, varying from 20-95 years of age. According to this study, the median coital activity was highest, 2.1 per week, between ages 30-34 and decreased progressively with increasing age, sinking to 0.2 per week in the age-group 65-69.

The data in Martin's study (37) throw light upon the enormous individual variations in sexual vigor. The mean frequency of total sexual activity in 159 males was found to be 520 sexual events per 5 years in the age group 20 to 39, including young males performing below 100 sexual events per 5 years and those with frequencies of total sexual activity over 1000 sexual events per 5 years.

In the age group 65-79, the mean frequency of total sexual activity decreased to 75 sexual events per 5 years, but even in this group subjects producing 400-700 sexual events per 5 years were registered.

To explain the age-related decrease in sexual activity we may assume that sexual vigor of the human male is primarily related to the dopaminergic activity in the brain, as dopamine progressively decreases with increasing age. Individual differences in the activity of the dopaminergic system might lead to the observed considerable variations in sexual performance between males in the same age group. The individuals at ages 20-39 with high rates of performance (over 800 sexual events per 5 years) might have a more active dopaminergic system than the poor performers (less than 200 sexual events per 5 years). Such individual differences might explain why a number of males maintain a remarkable sexual vigor in the age-group 65-79, a few are even better performers than the average in the age-group 20-39, despite of the unavoidable age-related decrease in the activity of the dopaminergic system.

We shall come back later in detail to the validity and practical consequences of this approach using the aged male rat as an experimental model.

The appearance of parkinsonian symptoms in old age. Parkinson's disease described in 1817, will certainly achieve a special place in the history of clinical sciences as it was the first and is still the only example of the successful application of a neurochemical discovery to the efficient treatment of a prevalent degenerative neurological disorder. Charcot (38) introduced in 1892 for the symptomatic treatment of the disease the Belladona alkaloids which were then replaced by synthetic anticholinergic agents (from 1946), however, the causative biochemical lesion leading to the disease remained unknown until 1960.

In 1957 Montagu (39) detected the presence of dopamine in the central nervous system and Carlsson et al. (40) demonstrated that reserpine depletes dopamine from brain tissues and that it can be replenished by dopa. In 1959 Bertler and Rosengren (41) reported that about 80% of the dopamine in the human brain is localised in the basal ganglia. One year later Ehringer and Hornykiewicz (42) published the loss of melanin-containing neurons in the pars compacta of the substantia nigra and the resulting dramatic decrease of striatal dopamine in parkinsonian patients. This was a discovery of crucial importance, leading within a few years to the highly efficient levodopa treatment of the disease.

As has been previously mentioned, Riederer and Wuketich (19) demonstrated that the dopamine content of the human caudate nucleus decreases by 13% per decade over age 45. They concluded from clinical studies that parkinsonian symptoms appear if the striatum looses more than 70% of its dopamine content. The age-related decrease in the dopamine content of the basal ganglia explains the usual appearance of Parkinson's disease in advanced age.

In answer to the question of why all of the elderly do not exhibit parkinsonian symptoms, we may refer again to the importance of individual variations in the dopaminergic activity. We assume that individuals with relatively high dopaminergic activity in their early life maintain even during their latter decades a higher dopaminergic tone and in spite of the age-related decrease in the dopamine content of the basal ganglia, the activity of the system remains above the critical threshold for exhibiting parkinsonian symptoms. However, proneness to the disease evidently increases with age and different etiological factors are then capable of manifesting the disorder. The relationship between parkinsonian symptoms, dopaminergic activity and age is supposed to be similar to the relation between depression with late onset, catecholaminergic tone and age.

Pharmacological spectrum and therapeutic aspects of (-)deprenyl, a selective inhibitor of MAO-B, which facilitates dopaminergic and 'trace-aminergic' modulation in the brain

In the aging brain, there is a loss of neurons, compensated for by a proliferation in glial cells. We might thus predict that catecholaminergic and 'trace-aminergic' modulation in the brain declines in senescence, partly because of the loss of catecholaminergic neurons and partly because of increased MAO-B activity present in the glia. This age-related biochemical lesion might be corrected by drugs which inhibit selectively B-type MAO, facilitate the activity of catecholaminergic neurons in the brain and are safe enough in humans for chronic administration. (-)Deprenyl (N-methyl-N-propargyl-(2-phenyl-1--methyl)-ethyl-ammonium.HCl, Jumex$^R$, Chinoin) seems to comply with these requirements.

(-)Deprenyl, an MAO inhibitor without the 'cheese effect'. (-)Deprenyl, a highly potent, irreversible inhibitor of MAO, was developed in 1964 as a new spectrum psychic energizer by Knoll et al. (43, 44).

In contrast to the MAO inhibitors in medicinal use, like tranylcypromine, phenelzine, pargyline, isocarboxazide, etc., which strongly potentiate the effect of tyramine, (-)deprenyl was found to inhibit the uptake of tyramine and was predicted to be in man an MAO inhibitor without the 'cheese effect' (45, 46). Clinical studies confirmed this claim and (-)deprenyl is now considered to be a safe MAO inhibitor for human use (for review see 47, 48, 49, 50, 51).

It is well known that the 'cheese effect' is the most serious side reaction of the MAO inhibitors in clinical use. Soon after the introduction of MAO inhibitors as antidepressants, serious hypertensive crises, similar to a paroxysm induced by pheochromocytome, leading in certain instances to fatal intracranial bleeding, were observed (for review see 52). Potentiation of the pressor effect of tyramine is likely to be the main cause of dangerous hypertensive reactions which supervene after the intake of certain food materials containing high amounts of free amine (e.g. cheeses, yeast products, beans, chianti vines, pickled herring, chicken liver, etc.) in patients treated with MAO inhibitors. This 'cheese reaction' seriously discredited the MAO inhibitors and restricted their therapeutic use, which requires careful medical control. The 'cheese effect' first described by Blackwell (53) is thought to be primarily a consequence of inhibition of the intestinal enzyme (54).

(-)Deprenyl is devoid of this adverse effect for two reasons:

a/ it inhibits the uptake of tyramine (45, 46, 55), noradrenaline (56) and dopamine (57, 58),

b/ as a selective inhibitor of MAO-B (56) within the therapeutic dose range it leaves the MAO activity of the intestine practically unchanged (for review see 49).

The high selectivity of (-)deprenyl for inhibiting B-type MAO in vitro and in vivo. The discovery that two main forms of mitochondrial MAO exist and the development of our present knowledge concerning the dual nature of MAO is inseparable from the introduction of two substrate-selective highly potent irreversible inhibitors, deprenyl (44) and clorgyline (59).

Clorgyline (2,4-dichlorophenoxypropyl-N-methylpropargylamine), a compound similar to deprenyl, was found by Johnston to be a selective inhibitor of that type of MAO which deaminates 5-HT. To distinguish the two forms of MAO, one highly sensitive to clorgyline and one relatively insensitive to it, he introduced the terms 'type A' and 'type B' MAO. This nomenclature has become widely accepted, MAO-A is selectively inhibited by clorgyline, and MAO-B by (-)deprenyl (56).

MAO-A is thought to be specialized for binding and metabolizing the ethylamine side chain of the substrate if it is attached to a 5-hydroxy indole ring (serotonin oxidase), and MAO-B is specialized for recognizing and metabolizing phenylethylamine (phenylethylamine oxidase). There are many other amines that, because of structural similarities, are substrates of either MAO-A or MAO-B, or are common substrates of both enzymes (for review see 17, 47, 49, 56).

The high selectivity of (-)deprenyl to MAO-B in vivo was demonstrated in the cat by a special method developed for continuous monitoring of liver MAO-B activity (17). The metabolism of intravenously injected PEA was continuously monitored in anaesthetized cats using the nictitating membrane as detector. MAO-B in the liver was found to control the serum concentration of the injected amine. Neither the pretreatment of a cat with 10 mg/kg clorgyline nor the intravenous injection of high doses (5-10 mg/kg) of this MAO inhibitor changed the metabolism of intravenously injected PEA in the cat, as did 0.1 mg/kg of (-)deprenyl. Another selective inhibitor of MAO-A, Lilly 51641, was also found to be ineffective in the nictitating membrane test (60).

As the intestinal tissue contains, in many species, including man, mainly MAO-A (61), the finding that clorgyline was 60 times more potent than (-)deprenyl in blocking the oxidation of tyramine in intestines of the rat in vitro (55) and a similar difference in man (61) are of practical importance. It means that the main barrier controlling the access of tyramine to the circulation by effecting its degradation is practically unaffected in (-)deprenyl treated subjects but is blocked in clorgyline treated ones. Thus the selective MAO-A inhibitors have no advantage over non-selective MAO inhibitors (tranylcypromine, phenelzine, isocarboxazide, etc.), but the selective inhibition of MAO-B is more promising with respect to the hazards of combination with a variety of foods and drugs.

(-)Deprenyl has a higher affinity to the B form of MAO than to the A form (56). In high concentration, or when the enzyme is exposed to the inhibitor for a long time, the A form is also inhibited. On account of this the question must be considered whether (-)deprenyl loses its selectivity to the B form when patients are treated daily with the drug. We found that the selectivity of 0.25 mg/kg (-)deprenyl when rats were treated with daily doses for 21 days was the same as that in single dose experiments (62). The uptake of deprenyl in brain is a fast procedure reaching the peak concentration within seconds after an intravenous dose and almost all of the inhibitor is eliminated from the tissue after 20-30 min (63). Thus, it seems likely that the enzyme is not exposed to the inhibitor in brain for a long enough time and at a high enough concentration to establish irreversible bindings to the A form if the dose of (-)deprenyl is not higher than 0.25 mg/kg. At higher doses, however, (-)deprenyl reaches a concentration in the brain high enough to inhibit a portion of the A form too. The inhibition of both the A and B forms is higher in the brain than in the liver which may also be explained by the fast penetration of (-)deprenyl in the brain, rendering a higher concentration in this tissue in the initial phase of its distribution.

If (-)deprenyl was given in one single dose instead of in daily doses, but with the same total amount of the inhibitor, a higher degree of inhibition occurred, which means that a large proportion of both the A and B forms has been resynthetized during the period of treatment. No difference in the degree of inhibition with 0.25 mg/kg (-)deprenyl occurred when rats were treated for 14 or 21 days compared to the treatment for 7 days, which means that the daily synthesis of the enzyme was as high as the inhibition after each dose. The major portion of the inhibited activity was restored one week after treatment with three weekly injections of (-)deprenyl (62), which shows a great fluctuation of the enzyme activity when weekly doses are given instead of daily doses.

*References p. 132*

As (-)deprenyl is usually administered in daily oral doses of 5-10 mg (for review see 50) the dose range in man seems to be in accordance with the selective dose range of the drug in animal studies. It is worth mentioning that (-)deprenyl inhibits MAO-B activity with a very good safety margin. Only 0.17-0.26% of the $LD_{50}$ was needed in different species (mouse, rat, cat, dog) to block completely MAO-B activity in the brain (see 57, Table IV).

The action of low doses of (-)deprenyl on the selective inhibition of MAO-B in human brain was demonstrated by Riederer et al. (64). They compared the sensitivity of human brain mitochondrial MAO to (-)deprenyl and clorgyline in 15 brain areas *in vitro*. (-)Deprenyl was found to be many thousand times more powerful an inhibitor than clorgyline. For (-)deprenyl the $ID_{50}$ varied between 0.05 μM (hypothalamus) and 0.95 μM (caudate nucleus); values for clorgyline varied between 500 μM (pineal gland) and 3200 μM (raphe+reticular formation). They also demonstrated that the deamination of dopamine was almost completely inhibited in the brain of seven patients with Parkinson's disease treated with 10 mg of (-)deprenyl daily, $6.0 \pm 1.8$ days before death, whilst 34 per cent of MAO activity against 5-HT still remained present.

*Inhibition of the uptake of monoamines in vitro and in vivo by (-)deprenyl*. (-)Deprenyl inhibits the uptake of monoamines into the nerve endings of catecholaminergic neurons and the effect is independent from the MAO inhibiting property of the compound.

That deprenyl is a potent inhibitor of the uptake of tyramine *in vivo* and *in vitro* was first demonstrated by Knoll et al. in 1967 (45) and studied in detail in a number of papers (17, 46, 47, 55, 56, 57). (-)Deprenyl proved to be highly efficient in blocking the uptake of tyramine into the noradrenaline nerve terminals in different isolated organs (nictitating membrane of the cat, central ear artery and main pulmonal artery strip of the rabbit, rat vas deferens, etc.).

Studies with structural relatives of deprenyl revealed that inhibition of MAO and the effect on the uptake of monoamines are completely independent from each other. An example: TZ-650, which differs from deprenyl only in the lack of a methyl group at the beta-carbon and is as potent as deprenyl in inhibiting MAO-B, was found to be in contrast to deprenyl, a potent releaser of noradrenaline and this effect could be blocked by deprenyl (55). Thus, (-)deprenyl, in contrast to the non-selective and A-selective MAO inhibitors, as well as to many selective MAO-B inhibitors, is unique in its ability to inhibit tyramine uptake in different tests.

Deprenyl was found to inhibit also the uptake of noradrenaline. This was first demonstrated by Knoll and Magyar in 1972 (56), using mouse cortical slices and corroborated in studies performed with rat cortex (65) and heart tissue (66).

The ability of deprenyl to influence the release of acetylcholine in the striatum by inhibiting the uptake of dopamine was demonstrated by Knoll and his coworkers using isolated rat striatum slices. Neither clorgyline, the selective inhibitor of MAO-A, nor newly developed selective inhibitors of MAO-B, e.g. U-1424, (67), were able to inhibit the uptake of dopamine in the isolated striatal slices of the rat, whereas deprenyl facilitated dopaminergic neurotransmission in this test exclusively through this mechanism (57, 58).

Effect of (-)deprenyl on the brain content and turnover rate of catecholamines. To better understand the mechanism of the effect of (-)deprenyl on the catecholaminergic system, we have measured the content and turnover rate of dopamine in the striatum and noradrenaline in the brainstem of the rat under the influence of the subcutaneous injection of 0.25 mg/kg (-)deprenyl. We found that 24 hours after the injection of a single dose of 0.25 mg/kg (-)deprenyl, which is known to inhibit MAO-B activity selectively in the brain, the contents and turnover rates of the catecholamines remained unchanged. We were able, however, to detect important changes in the metabolism of monoamines after daily subcutaneous injections of 0.25 mg/kg (-)deprenyl for 14 days (68).

Table 1 shows that the repeated administration of small daily doses of (-)deprenyl increased significantly the turnover rate of dopamine in the rat striatum, whereas no significant change in the teldiencephalon-striatum was to be detected, as measured 24 hours after the last injection. The increase in the turnover rate of dopamine in the striatum was due to the enhancement of the fractional rate constant of dopamine efflux and the slight, but significant, increase in the dopamine content (60.3 versus 52.7 nmoles/g). With regard to noradrenaline, a significant decrease in the turnover rate and unchanged level of this amine in the brainstem was found. No change in the turnover rate of noradrenaline was to be detected in the teldiencephalon-striatum (Table 2).

This finding substantially supports our view (12) that (-)deprenyl facilitates dopaminergic modulation in the brain.

An increase in the turnover rate of dopamine due to a change in the efflux rate of this amine from its storage is in keeping with the possibility that (-)deprenyl, which increases the content of dopamine by

References p. 132

TABLE 1

The effect of (-)deprenyl on dopamine (DA) content, turnover rate of dopamine ($TR_{DA}$) and fractional rate constant ($k_b$) of dopamine efflux

| Striatum | DA | $TR_{DA}$ | $k_b$ |
|---|---|---|---|
| | nmoles/g | nmoles/g/hr | $hr^{-1}$ |
| Control (saline) | 52.7±1.6 | 13.7±1.3 | 0.26 |
| Deprenyl 14x0.25 mg/kg daily | 60.3±2.2* | 20.4±0.98* | 0.34 |
| Teldiencephalon-striatum | | | |
| Control (saline) | 2.8±0.1 | 1.3 | 0.45 |
| Deprenyl 14x0.25 mg/kg | 3.5±0.2* | 1.6 | 0.46 |

*$p < 0.05$

Animals were injected subcutaneously with 0.25 mg/kg (-)deprenyl daily for 14 days. Controls were treated with saline. Animals were killed 24 hours after the last injection of (-)deprenyl and saline, respectively. Rats were injected with 250 mg/kg i.p., α-methyl-p--tyrosin methyl ester HCl 1 and 2 hours before decapitation. Each time point had six values. TR=(steady state)x $k_b$. Brains were dissected according to Glowinski and Iversen (69). Catecholamine contents were determined fluorimetrically according to Carlsson and Waldeck (70). Turnover rates were measured according to Tozer et al.(71

TABLE 2

The effect of (-)deprenyl on noradrenaline (NA) content, turnover rate of noradrenaline ($TR_{NA}$) and fractional rate constant ($k_b$) of noradrenaline efflux

| Brainstem | NA | $TR_{NA}$ | $k_b$ |
|---|---|---|---|
| | nmoles/g | nmoles/g/hr | $hr^{-1}$ |
| Control (saline) | 3.1±0.2 | 0.81 | 0.26 |
| Deprenyl 14x0.25 mg/kg | 3.2±0.1 | 0.39 | 0.12 |
| Teldiencephalon -striatum | | | |
| Control (saline) | 1.2±0.1 | 0.30 | 0.26 |
| Deprenyl 14x0.25 mg/kg | 1.5±0.1* | 0.36 | 0.24 |

*$p < 0.05$

For details see Table 1

inhibiting MAO-B, also increases the rate of the utilization of this important modulator in the striatum. Presumably an increase in the rate of utilization is due to an increase in the firing rate of dopaminergic neurons. As, in contrast to the rat, MAO-B seems to be the main form of the enzyme in the nigrostriatal dopaminergic neurons in man (72), the conditions for (-)deprenyl to facilitate dopaminergic modulation in human brain are particularly favourable.

The effect of (-)deprenyl on the release of catecholamines from nerve terminals and the potential releasing effect of the metabolites of (-)deprenyl in vivo. We studied first the effect of (-)deprenyl on the release of noradrenaline in the microsomal fraction of rat heart homogenate (56). We were able to demonstrate that in contrast to MAO inhibitors in clinical use (nialamide, tranylcypromine, pargyline), which facilitated the outflow of the transmitter from the nerve terminals, deprenyl strongly inhibited the efflux of labelled noradrenaline.

We later found that in the rat heart preparation clorgyline, the selective inhibitor of MAO-A, enhanced the release of noradrenaline (17). Clorgyline enhanced the release of dopamine, too, from the synaptosomes of the striatum and acted in this test like tyramine, whereas (-)deprenyl left the efflux of labelled dopamine unchanged (55).

We concluded that (-)deprenyl per se is devoid of catecholamine releasing effect, it may even, as in the heart tissue, inhibit the efflux of noradrenaline from the nerve terminals. The in vivo effect of (-)deprenyl on the release of catecholamines, should be noted, as the propargyl group seems to be split off in the liver and the main metabolites of (-)deprenyl are amphetamine and methamphetamine (51), although with high probability these are the pharmacologically less active levo-rotatory forms of these compounds.

As we usually measure the effects of (-)deprenyl 24 hours after the injection of the drug, only traces of either the unchanged drug molecule or the metabolites can be present in the organism, as the elimination of (-)deprenyl and its metabolites is practically complete within a day (63). The possibility, however, of the retention of trace amounts of the metabolites of (-)deprenyl in brain tissue, which might still exert a small continuous release of dopamine and noradrenaline, respectively, from the nerve terminals, cannot be ruled out completely. The assumption of a certain share of traces of amphetamine-like metabolites of (-)deprenyl in the complex pharmacological effects of the drug is not necessarily inconsistent with the congruent experimental and clinical observations of the complete lack of amphetamine-like symptoms during the long-term administration of the usual daily doses of (-)deprenyl. It must be borne in mind, however, that even if we do not rule out the possibility of the accumulation of traces of amphetamine-like metabolites of (-)deprenyl and also take their releasing effect into account; the well known accumulation of PEA, an endogenous trace amine with higher catecholamine-releasing potency than (-)amphetamine in the (-)deprenyl-treated animal or man, will evidently surpass the releasing effect of the respectable traces of (-)deprenyl metabolites.

As the facilitation of the dopaminergic modulation in the brain by (-)deprenyl seems to be of high therapeutic importance, we checked the possible share of the accumulation of amphetamine-like metabolites in this effect.

As was demonstrated in Table 1, the daily administration of 0.25 mg/kg (-)deprenyl for 14 days increased significantly the turnover rate of dopamine in the rat striatum. Therefore we checked also the effect of (±)amphetamine on the striatal dopaminergic system, by injecting 0.25 mg/kg of this drug daily for 14 days. Table 3 shows the results. In contrast to (-)deprenyl, amphetamine decreased significantly the content of dopamine in the striatum and even the turnover rate showed a decreasing tendency. (±)Amphetamine influenced the turnover rate of noradrenaline in the brainstem (Table 4) like (-)deprenyl (Table 2). Thus, we may conclude that the metabolites of (-)deprenyl cannot play a substantial role in the facilitation of the dopaminergic modulation in the brain induced by this drug.

<u>The effect of (-)deprenyl on monoamine receptors</u>. The effect of clorgyline and deprenyl, the selective inhibitors of MAO-A and MAO-B, respectively, on postsynaptic noradrenaline and serotonin receptors were studied on isolated organs (17). In striking contrast to (-)deprenyl, clorgyline proved to be a very potent, selective, non-competitive inhibitor of the 5-HT receptor, leaving the acetylcholine and histamine receptors unaltered. In some preparations clorgyline itself stimulated the 5-HT receptors before blocking it. In the guinea pig vas deferens (-)deprenyl usually stimulated and clorgyline inhibited motor transmission. In this test, too, clorgyline was found to be a potent, non-competitive and selective inhibitor of the 5-HT receptor.

On the other hand, very high doses of (-)deprenyl proved to interact with dopamine receptors and inhibit the effect of apomorphine in the rat (57). To exert such an effect on postsynaptic dopamine

TABLE 3

The effect of (±)amphetamine on dopamine (DA) content, turnover rate of dopamine ($TR_{DA}$) and fractional rate constant ($k_b$) of dopamine efflux

| | DA | $TR_{DA}$ | $k_b$ |
|---|---|---|---|
| Striatum | nmoles/g | nmoles/g/hr | $hr^{-1}$ |
| Control (saline) | 53.9±1.8 | 23.9 | 0.45 |
| Amphetamine 14x0.25 mg/kg | 47.7±1.5* | 17.8 | 0.37 |
| Teldiencephalon -striatum | | | |
| Control (saline) | 2.4±0.2 | 0.9 | 0.38 |
| Amphetamine 14x0.25 mg/kg | 2.6±0.2 | 1.1 | 0.41 |

*$p < 0.05$

Animals were injected subcutaneously with 0.25 mg/kg (±)amphetamine (base) daily for 14 days. For other details see Table 1

TABLE 4

The effect of (±)amphetamine on noradrenaline (NA) content, turnover rate of noradrenaline ($TR_{NA}$) and fractional rate constant ($k_b$) of noradrenaline efflux

| | NA | $TR_{NA}$ | $k_b$ |
|---|---|---|---|
| Brainstem | nmoles/g | nmoles/g/hr | $hr^{-1}$ |
| Control (saline) | 3.4±0.2 | 0.85 | 0.25 |
| Amphetamine 14x0.25 mg/kg | 3.3±0.2 | 0.41 | 0.12 |
| Teldiencephalon -striatum | | | |
| Control (saline) | 2.2±0.1 | 0.83 | 0.38 |
| Amphetamine 14x0.25 mg/kg | 2.4±0.2 | 0.96 | 0.41 |

Animals were injected subcutaneously with 0.25 mg/kg (±)amphetamine (base) daily for 14 days. For other details see Table 1 receptors *in vivo*, doses 40-100 times higher than those needed for the selective inhibition of MAO-B were needed. Thus it may be concluded that (-)deprenyl leaves the function of the postsynaptic monoamine receptors in the therapeutic dose range unchanged. The fact, however, that (-)deprenyl has an affinity to the dopamine receptors and its binding results in a blockade of the receptors led to the proposition that the drug may, even in the doses used in therapy, inhibit the presynaptic dopamine receptors which are known to be more sensitive to inhibitors. As the presynaptic dopamine receptors serve as regulators of the release of dopamine, an inhibition of these receptors may represent an additional factor in the facilitation of dopaminergic modulation by (-)deprenyl (57).

The effect of long-term treatment with low doses of (-)deprenyl on postsynaptic catecholamine receptors, however, needs further careful analyses in the future. Especially receptor binding studies following (-)deprenyl treatment with different doses and different durations are needed to get final informations regarding the effects of (-)deprenyl on the metabolism and function of the catecholamine receptors.

*The use of (-)deprenyl in current therapy and new aspects for its clinical application in the future*. Deprenyl was originally described as a new spectrum MAO inhibitor, essentially differing from the previously known MAO inhibitors in its ability to block the uptake of tyramine (45, 46), the substance culpable for the 'cheese effect' (53)

Our claim that (-)deprenyl is an MAO inhibitor without the 'cheese effect' was substantially supported by the clinicians, who, even during long term administration of the drug, never observed hypertensive reactions and there was no need for any dietary restriction. In some volunteers treated with (-)deprenyl, Varga tried to provoke the 'cheese reaction' in his first clinical trial in 1966, by administering huge amounts of tyramine-rich cheeses, but no significant change in the blood pressure could be detected (E. Varga, unpublished results). Elsworth et al. (73) and Sandler et al. (74) demonstrated that subjects were able to consume up to 200 mg of tyramine during (-)deprenyl treatment before a rise of blood pressure and slowing puls occurred. This amount of tyramine is unlikely to be encountered during the course of a normal diet.

The safeness of (-)deprenyl was further demonstrated by Pare et al. (75) and Mendis et al. (76) in patients. The authors used the tyramine pressor test (77) and found that even high doses of (-)deprenyl failed to increase the sensitivity to intravenous tyramine in the patients, whereas moderate doses of standard MAO inhibitors increased it considerably. Clinical advantage of the peculiar pharmacological spectrum of (-)deprenyl was first taken in the levodopa treatment of parkinsonian patients.

The discovery of Ehringer and Hornykiewicz in 1960 (42) that striatal dopamine is dramatically decreased in Parkinson's disease led to the levodopa treatment of the disease, a kind of very efficient substitution therapy with unfortunately high incidence of side effects. The first clinical trial to improve parkinsonian symptoms by administering levodopa, the precursor of dopamine, which passes the blood-brain barrier, was performed by Birkmayer and Hornykiewicz in 1961 (78) who injected levodopa intravenously. The dramatic effect of levodopa in Parkinson's disease proved the significance of the new therapy in this degenerative neurological disease, but the drug effect was of short duration and accompanied by various adverse effects. The possibility to potentiate the levodopa effect by concurrent administration of an MAO inhibitor was evident and it was soon checked by Birkmayer and Hornykiewicz in 1962 (79). MAO inhibitors, however, potentiated the unwanted effects of levodopa and also the danger of hypertensive crises made such combinations impossible.

To decrease the side effects of levodopa, the concurrent administration of peripheric decarboxylase inhibitors was introduced by Birkmayer and Mentasti in 1967 (80). The need, however, for the levodopa-sparing effect of a safe MAO inhibitor, devoid of the usual side effects, still remained. (-)Deprenyl, the MAO inhibitor without the 'cheese effect', lent itself particularly well to this purpose because it could be safely combined with levodopa. Birkmayer et al. (81) demonstrated the clinical benefits of the concurrent administration of levodopa plus a decarboxylase inhibitor plus deprenyl. Their finding was corroborated by many authors (82, 83, 84, 85, etc., for review see 50 and 86). Deprenyl proved to potentiate the therapeutic effect of levodopa without increasing the side effects. The drug was found to be of peculiar clinical benefit in patients on long term levodopa treatment who had developed the 'on-off' phenomenon. The use of (-)deprenyl allowed the beginning of levodopa therapy with smaller doses.

A considerable decrease of the clinical efficiency of levodopa is regularly observed in parkinsonian patients treated continuously for years with levodopa plus a decarboxylase inhibitor. A raise of the dose of levodopa in such patients usually increases the frequency of adverse effects without further therapeutic benefit. The addition of (-)deprenyl to the regimen, however, proved to lead in most of the

*References p. 132*

cases to significant improvement. For such reasons it is now proposed that (-)deprenyl be administered from the beginning as a useful consti- tuent of the combined levodopa-therapy of Parkinson's disease (for review see 49).

The effect of (±)deprenyl in endogenous depression was first studie by Varga and Tringer in 1967 (87) and that of (-)deprenyl by Tringer et al. in 1971 (88). According to these clinical trials both the racem form and the (-)isomer of deprenyl exerted an antidepressant effect with a rapid onset. These authors used relatively high daily doses of deprenyl (up to 40 mg) without observing important side effects. The complete lack of hypertensive reactions despite of the lack of any dietary restriction was the first proof for the safeness of deprenyl in man.

In 1980 Mann and Gershon (89) published the first report on the effect of (-)deprenyl on depressed patients using the compound in a dose which inhibits MAO-B selectively. The drug improved significantly the scores in all subcategories of the Hamilton depression scale. Mann and Gershon emphasized that the anxiety-relieving effect of (-)depreny is of particular interest. In the placebo period before treatment, the score for anxiety-somatization was found to be $7.3 \pm 0.5$ in their group of patients. This was reduced to $2.7 \pm 0.8$ ($p < 0.01$) after the daily administration of 10 mg (-)deprenyl for 21 days.

The hypothesis that serotonin (5-HT) deficiency in the brain may also be one of the causative factors in endogenous depression led to the clinical trials of the antidepressant effect of precursors of 5-HT tryptophan and 5-hydroxytryptophan (5-HTP). 5-HTP was claimed to posse antidepressant properties in certain cases (for review see 90). Becaus of the safeness of (-)deprenyl in humans, this drug was used in combi- nation with 5-HTP in affectively ill patents (91, 92). According to these authors 5-HTP plus (-)deprenyl was more effective than any one ( the compounds alone. The rapid onset of the therapeutic effect with the combination and the absence of hypertensive reactions were empha- sized.

In a double blind study Mendis et al. (76) found that 2 out of 11 patients on (-)deprenyl attained marked improvement after three weeks of treatment, whereas 50 per cent of patients became symptom free in a trial of tricyclic antidepressants conducted in similar patients. Mendis et al. (76) mentioned the complete absence of the well kown side effects of MAO inhibitors in the patients treated with (-)depren There was no evidence, either subjective or objective, of postural hypotension, no impotence, no delay in ejaculation and no hesitancy in micturition.

As depression is a very complex syndrome and different disorders of amine metabolism as well as other known and unknown factors probably contribute to the pathogenesis of the illness, (-)deprenyl which facilitates dopaminergic tone in the brain might be of therapeutic value in one category of depression only, that of patients with a deficient dopaminergic activity.

The pharmacological properties of (-)deprenyl, the peculiar activation of the dopaminergic neuron by this drug seem to be essentially different from the effects of drugs which are used in the clinic as stimulants of the dopaminergic system. At present levodopa and bromocriptine are mainly used for this purpose. The effect of levodopa is complex. It is thought to be an agonist acting through the uptake and release mechanisms in the presynaptic neuron. However, because of the rapid conversion of levodopa to dopamine in the brain, the possibility for a stimulation on the postsynaptic dopamine receptors and, when high doses are given, even a stimulation of the presynaptic dopamine receptors, thereby an inhibition of the dopaminergic neuronal activity, cannot be ruled out. Such a mechanism may play a considerable role in the parkinsonian patients on long-lasting levodopa treatment.

Bromocriptine acts as a pure postsynaptic dopamine-receptor agonist. (-)Deprenyl acts differently. By itself it does not elicit an acute increase in dopaminergic activity as would levodopa or bromocriptine. It seems to make only the dopaminergic neurons, by blocking MAO-B and the uptake of dopamine, more sensitive to a physiological stimulus. The clinical experiences with (-)deprenyl support this view. In parkinsonians it potentiates the effect of levodopa without increasing the side effects. When given with (-)deprenyl, a smaller amount of levodopa is sufficient to exert the same therapeutic effect, whereas (-)deprenyl by itself is ineffective.

A further support to this peculiar type of effect of (-)deprenyl on the dopaminergic system is given in a recent study by Koulu and Lammintausta (93). They investigated the effect of (-)deprenyl on human growth hormone secretion in healthy volunteers. 5 mg (-)deprenyl was given orally 24 hours before the tests and an additional 10 mg of (-)deprenyl 10 hours before the tests. (-)Deprenyl did not change the basal growth hormone secretion but significantly enhanced the levodopa--stimulated hormone release. 200 mg levodopa plus 50 mg benserazide, given per os, increased the hormone secretion from $1.8 \pm 0.2$ ng/ml to a maximum of $11.3 \pm 4.88$ ng/ml. After (-)deprenyl premedication levodopa raised the basal value of $1.8 \pm 0.3$ ng/ml to $23.3 \pm 6.14$ ng/ml and the

*References p. 132*

TABLE 5

The age-related decrease of sexual vigor in male CFY rats

| Age of animals (months) | No. of animals | Number, in parantheses per cent, of males showing in 4 consecutive mating tests | | | | |
|---|---|---|---|---|---|---|
| | | complete sexual inactivity | mountings only | mountings and intromissions ('sluggish males') | ejaculation in one test only | full scale sexual activity |
| 3-6 | 381 | 21 (5.70) | 20 (5.24) | 140 (36.75) | 80 (20.47) | 120 (31.80) |
| 12-18 | 137 | 27(19.71) | 27(19.71) | 76 (55.47 | 5 ( 3.65) | 3 ( 2.19) |

Differences between the two groups were significant in all categories, using the t test for two means, at $p < 0.01$ level. The copulatory patterns (mounting, intromission and ejaculation) of the male in the presence of the receptive female were scored in the light phase between 11.00 a.m. and 14.30 p.m., according to Beach (94).

growth hormone levels remained significantly higher during the 150 min observation period. (-)Deprenyl, however, did not change the effect of bromocriptine on growth hormone secretion. These findings support the view that (-)deprenyl renders the dopaminergic neuron, more sensitive to physiological and pharmacological influences.

The continuous administration of (-)deprenyl as a proposed method of treatment for the prevention or the counteraction of age-related decay of dopaminergic tone in the brain is promising.

To facilitate dopaminergic modulation in the brain by sensitizing the dopaminergic neurons to physiological and pharmacological influences with a safe, well tolerated drug, which can be administered for years without adverse effects, seems to be highly desirable for improving the quality of life in senescence. (-)Deprenyl may serve as the first experimental tool for checking the validity of this approach.

## The restitution of sexual vigor in aged male rats by (-)deprenyl. An experimental model illustrative of the possibility to counteract the age-dependent decline of a physiological function by appropriate medication

Sexual performance of male rats represents a quantifiable function decreasing with age. As an experimental model, it is hoped to possess good predictive value for man, as the similarities in the decay of sexual vigor in male rats and man with increasing age are conspicuous.

The study of Martin (37), who analysed the coital activity as function of age interviewing 628 subjects between ages 20-95, has been mentioned previously. He demonstrated on the one hand, the remarkable age-related decline of sexual potency in man, and on the other hand, also the great individual differences in all age groups. Essentially the same was observed in a series of experiments performed with J. Dallő and T.T.Yen in our laboratory in male rats.

Table 5 shows the striking difference in the sexual performance among less than 6 months' and more than 12 months' old male rats. For example, out of 381 males between ages of 3-6 months 120 (31.8%) showed full scale sexual activity, i.e. they were capable of ejaculating regularly in four consecutive mating tests, whereas only 3 (2.19%) out of 137 males between ages of 12-18 months performed similarly. On the other hand about 11 per cent (41 out of 381) of the males in the younger group proved to be either completely inactive (no mount, no intromission, no ejaculation in the four consecutive mating tests) or showed only mounting, whereas in the 'old group' nearly 40 per cent

References p. 132

(54 out of 137) of the males behaved similarly. Thus, comparing all categories in the two groups of rats in Table 5, we may conclude that the age-related decline of sexual activity in the male rats of the CFY strain is both biologically and statistically highly significant.

We found that the continuous administration of low doses of (-)deprenyl increased significantly the sexual vigor of aged male rats. Fig. 1 shows an example. Out of the 76 males of the 'old group' which

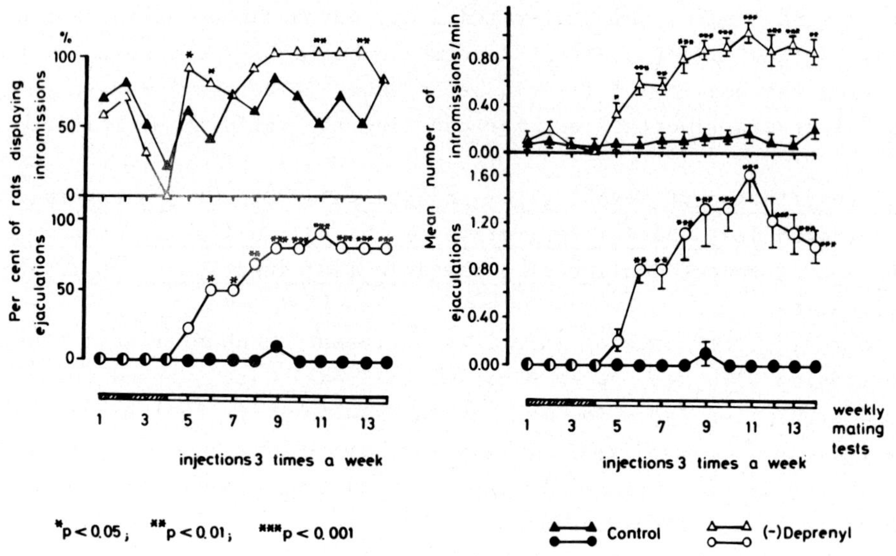


Fig. 1. The true aphrodisiac effect of the repeated administration of 0.25 mg/kg, s.c., (-)deprenyl for 10 weeks on sexually sluggish male rats.
Male CFY rats (LATI, Godollo, Hungary) weighing 650-750 g, which showe at least one intromission without any ejaculatory patterns out of 4 mating untreated tests were chosen as sexually sluggish ones for the experiment. Copulatory tests were performed once a week on Tuesdays. For each test a female in oestrus, showing high receptivity, brought into heat by subcutaneous injection of 30 µg of oestradiol monopropionate, followed 48 hours after by 0.5 mg progesterone, was used 4-7 hours after the progesterone injection. The copulatory patterns (mounting, intromission, and ejaculation) of the male in the presence of the female were scored, in the light phase between 11.00 a.m. and 14.30 p.m., according to Beach (94) by an experimenter during a 30 mi period.
Statistics: Student's t test for two means.
(-)Deprenyl (Jumex[R], Chinoin, Budapest) 0.25 mg/kg, dissolved in saline, was injected subcutaneously in a volume of 1 ml/kg, on Monday Wednesdays and Fridays (N=20). The control group (N=10) was treated similarly with 1 ml/kg saline.

were selected according to their behavior in the first four consecutive weekly mating tests as 'sexually sluggish' (see Table 5) 20 were injected subcutaneously with 0.25 mg/kg of (-)deprenyl and 20 with saline 3 times a week and their sexual activity was tested weekly during a period of 10 weeks. The data in Fig. 1 clearly demonstrate that no change in the sexual performance of the saline-treated rats was to be observed during the long-lasting experiment. (-)Deprenyl, however, facilitated sexual activity enormously. A highly significant increase in the mean number of intromissions/min and the appearance of ejaculations characterized the immediate consequences of drug treatment. The full scale sexual activity persisted during the 10 weeks of observation.

(-)Deprenyl is not only a highly potent inhibitor of MAO but, as it has been discussed previously, it possesses a highly complex pharmacological spectrum of activity. Is the strong aphrodisiac effect of (-)deprenyl due solely to its MAO-inhibitory effect?

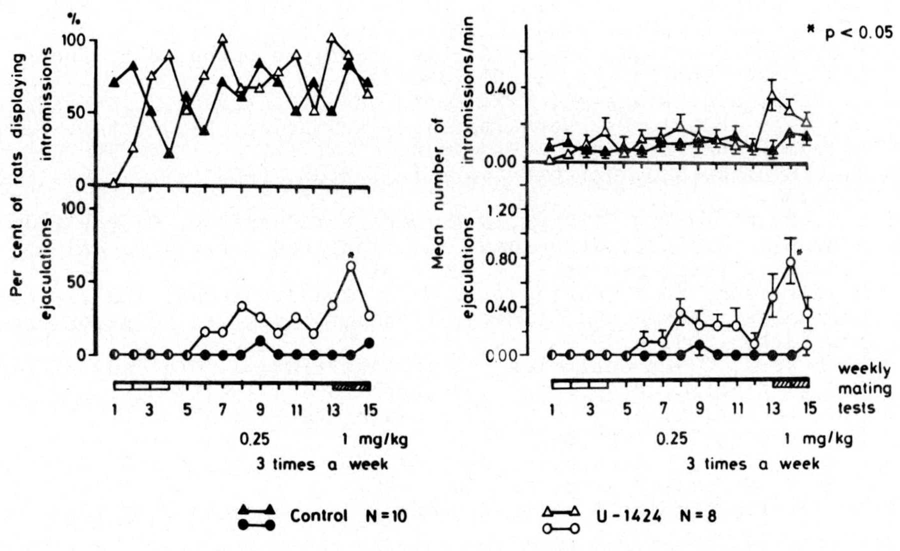


Fig. 2. The ineffectiveness of the repeated administration of U-1424 for 10 weeks on sexually sluggish male rats.
U-1424, dissolved in saline, was injected subcutaneously in a volume of 1 ml/kg, on Mondays, Wednesdays and Fridays. The control group was treated similarly with saline. Mating tests were performed on Tuesdays. For details see Fig. 1.

As structure-activity relationship studies revealed the requirement for developing selective inhibitors of MAO-B with and without differen other actions on the monoamine systems (48, 60, 67, 95), we selected U-1424, a 'pure' inhibitor of MAO devoid of either catecholamine releasing or monoamine uptake inhibitory effects, to answer the question. Fig. 2 shows the ineffectiveness of U-1424 in restoring full scale sexual activity in the 'sluggish rats', proving that (-)deprenyl exerts its aphrodisiac effect by more than one mechanism.

The possibilities to elevate mood, to increase sexual vigor and to counteract the motoric changes in the elderly, by the continuous admin istration of small doses of (-)deprenyl, deserve careful investigation in the future, as it could be a model for improving the quality of lif in senescence by the administration of a drug, which, due to its complex pharmacological spectrum of activity, works against the change attributable to the age-dependent loss of dopamine in the aging brain.

## REFERENCES


1 D.S. Robinson, J.M. Davis, A. Nies, C.L. Ravaris and D. Sylwester, Arch. Gen. Psychiat., 24(1971)536-539.
2 D.S. Robinson, J.M. Davis, A. Nies, J.R. Colburne, W.E. Runney and D.M. Shaw, The Lancet, i(1972)290-291.
3 A. Nies, D.S. Robinson, J.M. Davis and C.L. Ravaris, in Eisdorfer and Fann (Eds.), Psychopharmacology and Aging: Adv. Behav. Biology Plenum Press, New York, 1973, p.41.
4 T.J. Mantle, N.J. Garrett and K.F. Tipton, FEBS Letts., 64(1976) 227-230.
5 J.C. Shih, in T.P. Singer, R.W. von Korff and D.L. Murphy (Eds.), Monoamine Oxidase, Structure, Function, and Altered Functions, Academic Press, New York, 1979, p.413.
6 A. Carlsson, in E. Usdin, I.J. Kopin and J. Barchas (Eds.), Catecholamines: Basic and Clinical Frontiers, Vol. 1, Pergamon Press, New York, 1979, p.4.
7 B. Eckert, C.-G. Gottfries, L. von Knorring, L. Oreland, Å. Wiberg and B. Winblad, Progr. Neuropsychopharmacol., 4(1980)57-68.
8 C.J. Fowler, L. Oreland, J. Marcusson and B. Winblad, N. S. Arch. Pharmacol., 311(1980)263-272.
9 C.J. Fowler, Å. Wiberg, L. Oreland, J. Marcusson and B. Winblad, J. Neural Transmission, 49(1980)1-20.
10 M. Strolin Benedetti and P.E. Keane, J. Neurochem., 35(1980)1026-1032.
11 A.K. Student and D.J. Edwards, Biochemical. Pharm., 26(1977)2337-2342.
12 J. Knoll, in M.B.H. Youdim and E.S. Paykel (Eds.), Monoamine Oxidase Inhibitors - The State of Art, John Wiley and Sons Ltd., Chichester-New York-Brisbane-Toronto, 1981. p.45.
13 J. Knoll, in T.P. Singer and R.N. Ondarza (Eds.), Molecular Basis of Drug Action, Elsevier North Holland, New York, 1981, p.185.
14 H. Brody, D. Harman and J.M. Ordy, Clinical, Morphological and Neurochemical Aspects in the Aging Central Nervous System, Excerpta Medica, Amsterdam-Oxford-New York, 1976.

15 M.J. Ball, Acta Neuropathol.(Berlin), 37(1977)111-118.
16 H.C. Sabelli and W.J. Giardina, in H.C. Sabelli, (Ed.), Chemical Modulation of Brain Function, Raven Press, New York, 1973, p.225.
17 J. Knoll in G.E.W. Wolstenholme and J. Knight (Eds.), Monoamine Oxidase and Its Inhibition. Ciba Foundation Symposium 39(new series) Elsevier, Amsterdam, 1976, p.135.
18 A. Bertler, Acta Physiol. Scand., 51(1961)97-107.
19 P. Riederer and S. Wuketich, J. Neural Transm., 38(1976)277-301.
20 E.G. McGeer, P.L. McGeer and J.A. Wada, J. Neurochem., 18(1971) 1647-1658.
21 E. Kraepelin, Psychiatrie. Ein Lehrbuch fur Studierende und Aerzte, 5. Aufl., Abel, Leipzig, 1896.
22 R.N. Butler, Am. J. Psychiatry, 132(1975)893-900.
23 C. Leering, H.W. Hilhorst and M.J. Verhoef, Akt. Gerontol., 9(1979) 289-298.
24 J. Nielsen, Acta Psychiat. Scand., 38(1963)307-330.
25 D.W.K. Kay, P. Beamish and M. Roth, Brit. J. Psychiat., 110(1964) 146-158.
26 A. Stenback, Akt. Gerontol., 9(1979)277-282.
27 J.F.J. Cade, Med. J. Aust., 2(1949)349-352.
28 J. Delay and P. Deniker, in Compte rendu du Congres des Al. et Neurol. de Langue Fr., Masson et Cie, Paris, 1952.
29 F.M. Berger, J. Pharmacol. Exp. Ther., 112(1954)413-423.
30 R. Kuhn, Am. J. Psychiatry, 115(1958)459-464.
31 G.E. Crane, Psychiatr. Res. Rep., 8(1959)142-152.
32 L.H. Sternbach, in S. Garattini, E. Mussini and L.O. Randall (Eds.), The Benzodiazepines, Raven Press, New York, 1973, p.1.
33 P.A. Janssen, in M. Gordon (Ed.), Psychopharmacological Agents, Vol. 3., Academic Press, New York, 1974, p.128.
34 T.H. Svensson and A. Carlsson, (Eds.), Acta Psychiat. Scand. Suppl. 280, Vol. 61, 1980, p.280.
35 A.C. Kinsey, W.B. Pomeroy and C.E. Martin (Eds.), Sexual Behavior in the Human Male, W. B. Saunders, Philadelphia, 1948.
36 J. Money and H. Musaph (Eds.), Handbook of Sexology, Elsevier/North Holland Biomedical Press, Amsterdam-New York-Oxford, 1977.
37 C.E. Martin, in J. Money and H. Musaph (Eds.), Handbook of Sexology, Elsevier/North Holland Biomedical Press, Amsterdam-New York-Oxford, 1977, p.813.
38 J.M. Charcot, Leçons sur les maladies du system nerveux faites à la Salpérière. Recueillies et publiées par A. Bourneville, S. 155, Paris, Delahaye et Lecrosnier, 1892.
39 K.A. Montagu, Nature, 180(1957)244-245.
40 A. Carlsson, M. Lindqvist and T. Magnusson, Nature, 180(1957)1200.
41 A Bertler and E. Rosengren, Experientia, 15(1959)10-11.
42 H. Ehringer and O. Hornykiewicz, Klin. Wochenschr., 38(1960)1236-1239.
43 J. Knoll, Z. Ecsery, J.G. Nievel and B. Knoll, MTA V. Oszt. Közl., 15(1964)231-239.
44 J.Knoll, Z. Ecsery, K. Kelemen, J.G. Nievel and B. Knoll, Arch. int. Pharmacodyn. Ther., 155(1965)154-164.
45 J. Knoll, E.S. Vizi and G. Somogyi, MTA V. Oszt. Közl., 18(1967) 31-37.
46 J. Knoll, E.S. Vizi and G. Somogyi, Arzneim.-Forsch., 18(1968) 109-112.
47 J. Knoll, Horizons Biochem. Biophys., 5(1978)37-64.
48 J. Knoll, TINS, 2(1979)111-113.
49 J. Knoll, in M. Sandler (Ed.), Enzyme Inhibitors as Drugs, Macmillan, London, 1980, p.151.
50 W. Birkmayer and P. Riederer, Die Parkinson-Krankheit. Biochemie, Klinik, Therapie, Springer-Verlag, Wien-New York, 1980.

51 G.P. Reynolds, J.D. Elsworth, K. Blau, M. Sandler, A.J. Lees, and G.M. Stern, Br. J. clin. Pharmac., 6(1978)542-544.
52 F.J. Ays. B. Backwell (Eds.), Discoveries in Biological Psychiatry. J.B. Lippincott Co, Philadelphia, 1970.
53 B. Blackwell, Lancet, ii(1963)849-851.
54 B. Blackwell, E. Marley, J. Price and D. Taylor, Br. J. Psychiat., 113(1967)349-365.
55 J. Knoll, in N. Seiler, M.J. Jung and J. Koch-Weser (Eds.), Enzyme-Activated Irreversible Inhibitors, Elsevier/North-Holland Biomedical Press, Amsterdam-New York-Oxford, 1978, p.253.
56 J. Knoll and K. Magyar, Adv. Biochem. Psychopharmacol., 5(1972) 393-408.
57 J. Knoll, J. Neural Transm., 43(1978)177-198.
58 L.G.Hársing Jr., K. Magyar, K. Tekes, E.S. Vizi and J. Knoll, Pol. J. Pharmacol. Pharm., 31(1979)297-307.
59 J.P. Johnston, Biochem. Pharmacol., 17(1968)1285-1297.
60 J. Knoll, in T.P. Singer, R.W. von Korff and D.L. Murphy (Eds.), Monoamine Oxidase: Structure, Function, and Altered Functions, Academic Press, New York, 1979. p.431.
61 R.F. Squires, Adv. Biochem. Psychopharmac., 5(1972)355-370.
62 B. Ekstedt, K. Magyar and J. Knoll, Biochem. Pharmacol., 28(1978) 919-923.
63 K. Magyar, J. Skolnik and J. Knoll, in E.P. Leszkovszky (Ed.) V. Conferentia Hungarica pro Therapia et Investigatione in Pharmacologia, Akadémiai Kiadó, Budapest, 1971, p.103.
64 P. Riederer, M.B.H. Youdim, W. Birkmayer and K. Jellinger, Adv. Biochem. Psychopharmacol., 19(1978)377-381.
65 C. Braestrup, H. Andersen and A. Randrup, Eur. J. Pharmacol., 34(1975)181-187.
66 L.L. Simpson, Biochemical. Pharmacol., 27(1978)1591-1595.
67 J. Knoll, Z. Ecsery, K. Magyar and E. Sátory, Biochem. Pharmacol., 27(1978)1739-1747.
68 G. Zsilla, and J. Knoll, in E. Costa and G. Racagni (Eds.), Typical and Atypical Antidepressants, Raven Press, New York, 1981, in press.
69 J. Glowinski and L.L. Iversen, J. Neurochem., 13(1966)655-669.
70 A. Carlsson and B. Waldeck, Acta Physiol. Scand., 44(1958)293-298.
71 T.N. Tozer, N.H. Neff and B.B. Brodie, J. Pharmacol. Pharm., 153 (1966)177-182.
72 V. Glover, M. Sandler, V. Owen and G. Riley, Nature, Lond., 265(197 80-81.
73 J.D. Elsworth, V. Glover, G.P. Reynolds, M. Sandler, A.J. Lees, P. Phuapradit, K.M. Shaw, G.M. Stern and P. Kumar, Psychopharmacology, 57(1978)33-38.
74 M. Sandler, V. Glover, A. Ashford and G.M. Stern, J. Neural Transm., 43(1978)209-215.
75 C.M.B. Pare, M. Sandler and G. Stern, Abstr. 11th CINP Congress Vienna, 1978, p.286.
76 N. Mendis, C.M.B. Pare, M. Sandler, V. Glover and G. Stern, in M.B.H. Youdim and E.S. Paykel (Eds.), Monoamine Oxidase Inhibitors. The State of the Art, John Wiley and Sons Ltd, Chichester-New York-Brisbane-Toronto, 1981, p.171.
77 K. Ghose, P. Turner and A. Coppen, The Lancet, i(1975)1317-1318.
78 W. Birkmayer and O. Hornykiewicz, Wien. klin. Wschr., 73(1961) 787-788.
79 W. Birkmayer and O. Hornykiewicz, Arch. Psychiat. Nervenkrh., 203(1962)560-740.
80 W. Birkmayer and M. Mentasti, Arch. Psych. u. Z. ges. Neurol., 210(1967)29-35.

81 W. Birkmayer, P. Riederer, L. Ambrozi and M.B.H. Youdim, The Lancet, i(1977)439-443.
82 M.D. Yahr, J. Neural Transm., 43(1978)227-238.
83 G.M. Stern, A.J. Lees and M. Sandler, J. Neural Transm., 43(1978) 245-251.
84 U.K. Rinne, T. Siirtola, V. Sonninen, J. Neural Transm., 43(1978) 253-262.
85 E. Csanda, J. Antal, M. Antony and A. Csanaky, J. Neural Transm., 43(1978)263-269.
86 K. Magyar (Ed.), Monoamine Oxidases and Their Selective Inhibitors, Pergamon Press-Akadémiai Kiadó, Budapest, 1980.
87 A. Varga and L. Tringer, Acta Med. Acad. Sci. Hung., 23(1967) 289-295.
88 L. Tringer, G. Haits and E. Varga, in E. P. Leszkovszky (Ed.), V. Conferentia Hungarica pro Therapia et Investigatione in Pharmacologia, Akadémiai Kiadó, Budapest, 1971, p.111.
89 J. Mann and S. Gershon, Life Sciences, 26(1980)877-882.
90 H.M. van Praag and S. de Haan, Acta Psychiat. Scand., Suppl. 280, 61(1980)89-96.
91 J. Mendlewicz and M.B.H. Youdim, J. Neural Transm., 43(1978)279-286.
92 J. Mendlewicz and M.B.H. Youdim, in M.B.H. Youdim and E.S. Paykel (Eds.), Monoamine Oxidase Inhibitors-State of the Art, John Wiley and Sons Ltd, Chichester-New York-Brisbane-Toronto, 1981, p.177.
93 M. Koulu and R. Lammintausta, J. Neural Transm., 1981, in press.
94 F.A. Beach, Exp. Zool., 97(1944)249-295.
95 J. Knoll in J. Szentágothai, J. Hámori and E.S. Vizi (Eds.), Neuron Concept Today, Akadémiai Kiadó, Budapest, 1976, p.109.

J.A. Keverling Buisman (Editor), *Strategy in Drug Research*



# SOFT DRUGS: STRATEGIES FOR DESIGN OF SAFER DRUGS

NICHOLAS BODOR
Department of Medicinal Chemistry, College of Pharmacy, University of Florida, Box J-4, JHMHC, Gainesville, Florida 32610

## ABSTRACT

Strategies for design of safer drugs are discussed. The various novel classes of "soft drugs" are designed to be active pharmacological agents and to avoid undesired metabolic disposition (primarily various oxidative routes, multiple metabolism leading to active and/or toxic intermediates, etc.), by simultaneous design of their predictable and controllable detoxification-metabolism. It can be demonstrated that the various soft drug design methods are general and the "soft analog", "inactive metabolite approach" or the "activated soft compounds", etc. methods can successfully be applied to antimicrobial agents, anticholinergics, anticancer drugs, steroidal antiinflammatory agents, β-blockers, etc.

---

## INTRODUCTION

Successful prediction on a rational (hopefully quantitative) basis of the biological activity of compounds leading to new drugs is the main objective of drug designers. This is generally achieved by considering a known bioactive molecule as the basis (lead compound) for structural modifications, either by the group or by the biofunctional moieties approach. Thus, after finding a promising lead structure, the main aim is to design, synthesize and test logical series of compounds in order to be able to quantitatively express and optimize the desired activity. The structural modifications should theoretically lead to clear structure-activity relationships, thus finding the compound with optimum therapeutic properties. The situation is not that simple, however. Some of the methods in which the various molecular manipulations can be performed in order to obtain drugs of increased potency or to alter some pharmacokinetic properties have been excellently outlined by Ariëns (refs. 1, 2).

More recently, some other types of considerations were also included in the drug design process, aiming to improve delivery, distribution and pharmacokinetic properties of drugs. Thus, the prodrug approach (refs. 3, 4, 5) generally starts with

*References p. 163*

a known drug and the main objective of the structural modifications is to improve delivery and/or elimination, pharmacokinetic properties of the drug using an inactive, transport form of it which is cleaved to the active species after its administration. Although originally aimed to improve currently marketed and known drugs, the prodrug approach should become an integral part of the early drug design process, particularly by developing new chemical methods useful in prodrug design (ref. 6).

As a noticeable gap, it is interesting to note that metabolism considerations were not included in the general drug design process. Although "vulnerable moieties have been identified as the ones whose role is the bioinactivation or metabolism-elimination of the drug after it has performed its role, little or no attention was paid in the design process to the rationale design of the metabolic disposition of the drugs. This is the case despite the fact that the toxicity of a number of bioactive molecules is due to their increased elimination half-life, stability or other factors introduced during the process of increasing their activity. In most cases by maximizing drug activity based on a structure-activity relationship, the related toxicity of the drug is also increased, not altering the therapeutic index or even resulting in new toxicity.

It is becoming well recognized that damage to DNA is the major cause of most cancer and genetic birth defects (ref. 7). Many drugs and particularly their metabolic activation-deactivation routes contribute to toxic processes via formation of active metabolites. The phenomenon, metabolic activation to highly reactive intermediates which covalently bind to tissue macromolecules is the initial step in cell damage. It is also evident that reactive metabolites will not survive long enough to be excreted and identified, thus the classical types studies of the stable metabolites may provide misleading information. Recent work indicates that a number of highly reactive intermediates are the result of oxidative metabolisms (ref. 8), for example by the microsomal P-450 oxygenase (ref. 9). The oxidative biotransformations can take place via epoxides, alcohols (phenols), through oxo- derivatives and carboxylic acids, involving aromatic rings, aliphatic chains, etc. Oxidative N-dealkylation can occur in the small intestine as well (ref. 10). It appears that the relative toxicity is related to the reactivity of the intermediates. Thus, it was suggested that the more stable epoxides are not carcinogens or mutagenic agents, such as the ones formed from carbamezapine (ref. 11) or trans-4-acetylaminostilbene (ref. 12). Understanding how metabolites form is extremely important in order to predict the possible side effects of drugs. New metabolites and metabolic pathways are constantly reported (ref. 13) which can be very useful not only in understanding toxicity, but also in drug design. The concept of dose-threshold (ref. 8) in explaining toxicity of certain drugs at a higher dose level due to depletion of glutathione is a very good example for useful novel concepts in metabolism. It certainly underlines the possibility of toxic side effects at a much lower dose level, as in the usual case of use of multiple different drugs, which, however, require the same oxidative-glutathione conjugation sequence. This so called "drug interaction" process is of extreme importance in therapeutics. It also serves as one of the basic guide lines in soft drug design: to avoid metabolic transformations which can lead to toxic intermediates and which are saturable and are involved in the metabolism of a large number of different compounds.

The basic idea of including metabolism considerations into the drug design process is not entirely new. In one of his excellent reviews, Ariëns has mentioned (ref. 14) the importance between structure and drug metabolism. One interesting thought to avoid drug toxicity was provided by Ariëns (ref. 15), who suggested design of nonmetabolizable drugs. At first sight this idea sounds quite attractive as one would in this way avoid unwanted toxicity due to reactive intermediates and the drug pharmacokinetics would be rather simple, controlled primarily by renal excretion. We would call these kinds of nonmetabolizable drugs "hard drugs". It is very unlikely, however, that one can ever succeed in designing ideal hard drugs. It is well recognized that the body can attack and alter chemically quite stable structures and even if a drug is 95 percent excreted unchanged, the unaccounted small portion can and most likely will cause toxicity: the harder it is to metabolize (i.e. oxidize) the structure, the more likely it is to form highly reactive intermediates. In addition, in order to achieve nonmetabolizable properties, one has to go to pharmacokinetic extremes: to design either highly lipophilic structures (for example by steric "packing" of the metabolically sensitive parts) or very water soluble compounds. The elimination half-life in the first case would be very long and only very small amounts of the drug would be in the free, available form, while in the latter case, the biological half-life would be very short. The suggestion of blocking structural parts (i.e. C-H bonds) sensitive to oxidative metabolism by replacing the H atom with F is also of questionable value: it will make it harder for the enzyme systems to get rid of the molecule, but nevertheless it will, by finding a different position to attack. An alternate suggestion (ref. 16) of using alkyl chains as safe metabolic oxidizable handles is of more value: it would direct the metabolism-elimination towards a predictable route. The deliberate use of the oxygenase systems for elimination of the drugs, however, is not the best, as it is subject to competition and saturation.

Predicting metabolism of the drugs is not only possible, but it can be done on a more rationale basis as more and more information on the various enzyme systems is obtained. It is also possible to control and direct metabolism. "Soft drugs" can be defined as biologically active chemical compounds (drugs) which might resemble structurally known active drugs (i.e. soft analogs) or could be entirely new types of structures, but which are all characterized by a predictable *in vivo* destruction (metabolism) to nontoxic moieties, after they achieve their therapeutic

*References p. 163*

role. The metabolic disposition of the soft drugs takes place with a controllable rate in a predictable manner.

It is evident from the above discussions that one of the primary concepts in soft drug design is to avoid most oxidative metabolisms. The various oxygenase systems have vital roles in numerous basic biochemical processes, they are saturable, many drugs metabolized by them can possibly go through highly reactive intermediates, and many compounds are competing for these enzymes. It is suggested to use as much as possible the hydrolytic mechanisms, for example the various esterases. It is important to note that nonspecific esterases have no important role in basic biochemical processes (except maybe in producing certain enzymes, such as some lipases), their main role is exactly to get rid of a variety of foreign substances. So let's use them in a rational way.

A simple formal comparison of a drug (D), prodrug (pD) and soft drug (sD) is given in Scheme 1, where M represents metabolites.

Scheme 1

a)

$k_I \rightarrow$ D

D $\xrightarrow{k_5}$ elimination of D (unchanged or conjugate)

D $\underset{k_2 \ldots k_m}{\xrightarrow{k_3 \ldots k_i}}$ $M_k \ldots M_p$ $\xrightarrow{k_9}$ elimination

D $\xrightarrow{k_1 \ldots k_n}$ $[I_1^*, I_2^* \ldots I_n^*]$ $\xrightarrow{k_4 \ldots k_j}$ $[D_1', D_2' \ldots D_m']$ $\xrightarrow{k_8}$ elimination

$[I_1^*, I_2^* \ldots I_n^*]$ $\xrightarrow{k_6 \ldots k_\ell}$ $M_1 \ldots M_{k-1}$

$[D_1', D_2' \ldots D_m']$ $\xrightarrow{k_7 \ldots k_p}$ $M_1 \ldots M_{k-1}$ $\rightarrow$ elimination

b)

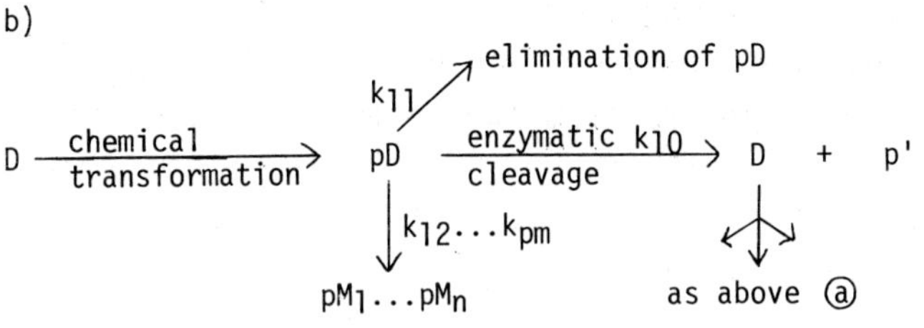


c)

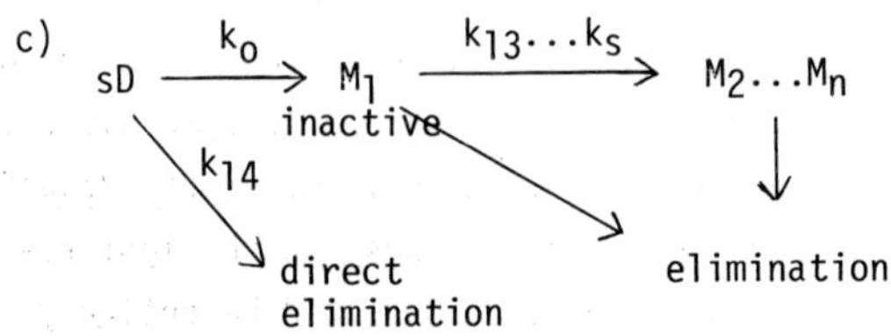

Thus, a drug D can undergo a wide variety of transformations, among them formation of reactive intermediates ($I_1^* \ldots I_n^*$) and active analogs ($D_1' \ldots D_m'$) are the highly unwanted ones. Transformation of the drug into a prodrug (pD) might alter some of the toxicity aspects by changing the relative rates of the various processes. An ideal prodrug is inactive and does not undergo any other transformations, but the one leading to the drug and some nontoxic carrier (p'), in other words $k_{10} \gg k_{11} + k_{12} + \ldots + k_{pm}$. Thus, the main role of a prodrug is that by altering the input rate ($k_I$) for the drug, as well as, by coordinating $k_{10}$ and $k_1$-$k_5$, an improved delivery of the D might be achieved.

Formally, the soft drug (sD) is just the opposite of a prodrug. While the prodrug is inactive and it is activated enzymatically, the soft drug is active and is deactivated enzymatically by a predictable and controllable process. The main point is, however, that the soft design deliberately simplifies the disposition processes of the D. Instead of possible multiple activation-deactivation processes, a simple, one step deactivation process is designed for the drug disposition. What is possibly achieved by this is: separation of desired activity from toxicity (improved therapeutic index) and avoidance of multiple active species systems. It is also important to note that the new soft drug does not necessarily have to be the most potent species if its metabolism is controllable, a higher dose of a less potent but nontoxic compound can be used.

There are a number of ways in which the rational design of soft drugs can be approached. Based on the various approaches developed during the past few years, the soft drugs can be classified at this stage in five distinct groups:

1. Soft analogs
2. Activated soft compounds (soft novel bioactive agents)
3. Active metabolite types
4. Controlled released endogenous agents
5. Inactive metabolite types

Examples for each of these, rather general approaches, are given in order to explain the techniques involved and to define their scope.

## SOFT ANALOGS

Compounds in this class are close structural analogs of known active drugs or bioactive compounds which, however, have a specific metabolically weak spot built into their structure which provides their one step detoxification. These weak spots are not oxidizable alkyl chains or other handles subject to conjugation. It is important to design the weak spot in such a manner that the detoxification will take place as soon as possible after the desired activity is achieved. The following basic properties characterize the soft analogs: 1) the weak spot is subject to certain <u>enzymatic</u> hydrolytic (or possibly other) cleavage, but it is stable enough chemically to provide formulation stability; 2) the compounds are

*References p. 163*

close structural analogs, isosteric and/or isoelectronic with the lead drugs; 3) the metabolically weak spot is built in a noncritical structural part which results in little or no effect on the transport, affinity and activity of the drug; 4) the built in metabolism is the major or preferentially the only metabolic route for deactivation of the drug; 5) the rate of the predictable metabolism can be controlled by molecular manipulations; 6) the products resulting from the metabolism are non-toxic and lack significant biological activity; 7) the predicted metabolism does not require enzymatic processes leading to highly active intermediates.

Ideally, the metabolism of this type of soft drug results in profound structural changes leading to complete destruction of the binding and affinity properties and of the active sites of the molecule.

Our research towards soft analogs started after the discovery of the "soft quaternary salts" (ref. 16), simply described as structure **1** and characterized by a chemical or enzymatic hydrolytic cleavage process leading to the simultaneous destruction of both the ester and of the quaternary ammonium head:

$$\underset{\mathbf{1}}{R\text{-}\overset{\displaystyle O}{\overset{\|}{C}}\text{-}O\text{-}\overset{\displaystyle R_1}{\overset{|}{C}H}\text{-}\overset{+}{N}\lessgtr} \xrightarrow{H_2O} RCOOH + R_1CHO + N\lessgtr$$

This profound change in the molecular structure effectively cuts the compound into three small pieces: one acid, one aldehyde and a tertiary amine. Compounds of type **1** were first used for improved delivery of some tertiary amine type drugs such as pilocarpine (ref. 17) and more recently erythromycin (ref. 18).

The soft quaternary salts can easily be synthesized by reacting the tertiary amine with the corresponding "soft alkylating" agent **2**, which can be obtained from an acyl halide and aldehyde:

$$RCOX + R_1CHO \longrightarrow \underset{\mathbf{2}}{R\text{-}\overset{\displaystyle O}{\overset{\|}{C}}\text{-}O\text{-}\overset{\displaystyle R_1}{\overset{|}{C}H}\text{-}X}$$

$$R\text{-}\overset{\displaystyle O}{\overset{\|}{C}}\text{-}O\text{-}\overset{\displaystyle R_1}{\overset{|}{C}H}\text{-}X + N\lessgtr \longrightarrow \underset{\mathbf{1}}{R\text{-}\overset{\displaystyle O}{\overset{\|}{C}}\text{-}O\text{-}\overset{\displaystyle R_1}{\overset{|}{C}H}\text{-}\overset{+}{N}\lessgtr}$$

X = Cl, Br, I
R = alkyl, aryl, etc.
$R_1$ = H, $CH_3$, $C_6H_5$, $CCl_3$, etc.

The basic difference in the metabolic disposition of the "soft" quaternary salts (hydrolysis) compared to the conventional "hard" quaternary salts (multiple oxidation) suggested, however, a direct usefulness of the soft quaternary salts as active species.

Soft quaternary antimicrobial agents

The first application of the soft quaternary salts type soft analogs is provided by the isosteric analogs of cetylpyridinium chloride (3) and some corresponding homologs and analogs (ref. 19). Thus, the soft quaternary salt 4 is a close isosteric analog of 2, both side chains contain essentially sixteen atoms:

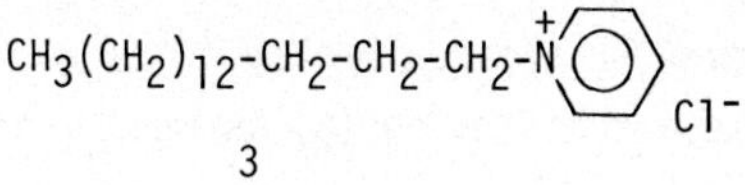

$CH_3(CH_2)_{12}$-$CH_2$-$CH_2$-$CH_2$-$\overset{+}{N}$(pyridinium) $Cl^-$ (3)

$CH_3(CH_2)_{12}$-C(=O)-O-$CH_2$-$\overset{+}{N}$(pyridinium) $Cl^-$ (4)

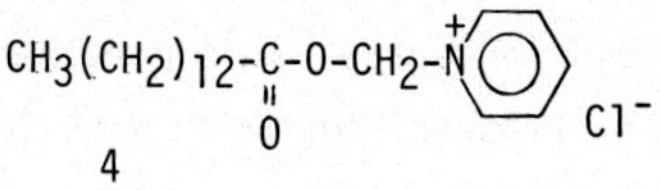

The physical properties of the soft analog 4 are close to those of 3 as demonstrated by their almost similar critical micelle concentrations (CMC), Table 1.

TABLE 1

Comparative critical micelle concentrations (CMC) of selected quaternary salts[a]

| Compound Nr. | Structure | CMC |
|---|---|---|
| 3 | $CH_3(CH_2)_{15} \cdot Py^+ \cdot Cl^-$ | $1.3 \times 10^{-4}$ M |
| 4 | $CH_3(CH_2)_{12}COOCH_2 \cdot Py^+ \cdot Cl^-$ | $1.7 \times 10^{-4}$ M |
| 5 | $CH_3(CH_2)_{10}COOCH_2 \cdot Py^+ \cdot Cl^-$ | $6.5 \times 10^{-4}$ M |
| 6 | $CH_3(CH_2)_{10}COOCH_2$-$\overset{+}{N}$(imidazolium)N-$CH_3 \cdot Cl^-$ | $6.0 \times 10^{-4}$ M |

[a]Using molecular light scattering method, in 0.1 M $NaH_2PO_4$. pH 7.08, $\mu = 0.5$; T = 25±0.2°.

TABLE 2

Contact germicidal efficiency of some soft quaternary ammonium compounds[a]

| Nr. | Structure | Conc. (ppm) | Sterilization Time (min)[b] S. Aureus | P. Aeruginosa | S. Pyogenes |
|---|---|---|---|---|---|
| 3 | $CH_3(CH_2)_{15} \cdot Py^+ \cdot Cl^-$ | 1018 | 0.5 | 0.5 | 0.5 |
| 5 | $CH_3(CH_2)_{10} \cdot COOCH_2 \cdot Py^+ \cdot Cl^-$ | 1016 | 1 | 0.5 | 0.5 |
| 6 | $CH_3(CH_2)_{10} \cdot COOCH_2 \cdot Im^+ \cdot Cl^-$ | 1066 | 0.5 | 0.5 | 0.5 |
| 7 | $CH_3(CH_2)_{15} \cdot \overset{+}{N}(CH_3)_3 \cdot Br$[c] | 1007 | 0.5 | 0.5 | 0.5 |
| 8 | $CH_3(CH_2)_{10} \cdot COOCH_2$-N(bicyclic)$ \cdot Cl^-$ | 1016 | 1 | 0.5 | 0.5 |
| 9 | $CH_3(CH_2)_{10} \cdot COOCH_2$-N(bicyclic)N$ \cdot Cl^-$ | 1009 | 7 | 0.5 | 0.5 |

[a]In 0.1 M $NaH_2PO_4$, pH 6.0; 25°C

[b]Time intervals screened: 0.5, 1, 2, 3, 4, 5, 6, 7, 8, 9, 10, 15 and 30 min.

[c]CTAB

Close similarity in the properties of analogs 5 and 6 can also be seen (N-methylimidazole (Im) was preferred to pyridine because of its lower toxicity). All these compounds are good germicidal agents. At a concentration of about 0.1 percent completely sterilize a variety of bacteria as shown in Table 2.

A comparison of the relative toxicities of cetylpyridinium chloride and one of the soft analogs very clearly supports the concept of soft analog design. As Table 3 indicates, 3 is a rather toxic compound even when taken orally (3 is a usual component of mouth wash formulations), while a soft analog (6) is much less toxic.

TABLE 3

Relative toxicity of hard and soft quaternary salts

| | $LD_{50}$ mg/kg (white Swiss male mice) | |
|---|---|---|
| Route | $CH_3(CH_2)_{10}COOCH_2 \cdot Im^+ \cdot Cl^-$ (6) | $CH_3(CH_2)_{15} \cdot Py^+ \cdot Cl^-$ (3) |
| I.V. | 75-100 | |
| I.P. | 140-160 | 10 |
| Oral | 4110 | 108 |

The contact germicidal efficiency of 3 and 6 are comparable, although the minimum inhibitory concentrations of 3 are somewhat lower. This, however, is more than offset by the very significant difference in their relative toxicities. The

TABLE 4

Hydrolysis kinetics for $CH_3(CH_2)_{10}COOCH_2 \cdot Py^+ \cdot Cl^- \rightarrow CH_3(CH_2)_{10}COOH + CH_2O + Py$

| Conditions | Rate Constant, k ($min^{-1}$) | $t_{\frac{1}{2}}$ (min) |
|---|---|---|
| pH 9.3; $\mu$ = 0.5, 25±0.1° | | |
| $-\frac{d(5)}{dt}$ | $4.3 \times 10^{-2}$ | 16 |
| $+\frac{d(Py)}{dt}$ | $4.3 \times 10^{-2}$ | 16 |
| pH 7.0; $\mu$ = 0.5, 25±0.1° | $1.5 \times 10^{-3}$ | 450 |
| 40±0.1° | $4.2 \times 10^{-3}$ | 166 |
| 50±0.1° | $1.1 \times 10^{-2}$ | 64 |
| pH 4.6; $\mu$ = 0.5, 50±0.1° | $5.2 \times 10^{-4}$ | 1325 |

low toxicity of 6 is due to its very facile hydrolytic deactivation. Kinetic studies of the hydrolysis of analog 5 (Table 4) show its base catalyzed hydrolysis, while the identical rate constants obtained by following the disappearance of 5 and appearance of pyridine support the mechanism for the instantaneous cleavage of the hydroxymethyl intermediate to the amine and formaldehyde.

It is important to note that the $t_{\frac{1}{2}}$ for hydrolysis at 37° in human plasma is only about 6 minutes.

Soft anticholinergic agents

Among the many chemically useful effects of antimuscarinic type compounds (antispasmodic, antisecretory, mydriatic, etc.) the local antisecretory activity was for long thought to be beneficial in inhibiting eccrine sweating. Indeed, the known anticholinergics are very effective for locally reducing sweating, including the quaternary ammonium type derivatives. Thus, in an order of potency established by Kilmer-McMillan (ref. 20) of atropine (10) > scopolamine (11) > antrenyl (12) > probanthine (13) > banthine > scopolamine·HBr > atropine methyl nitrate > homatropine methyl bromide, the quaternary salts 12 and 13 were found to be very effective.

$HOCH_2$, $C_6H_5$ >CH-COO–, N-$CH_3$

10

$HOCH_2$, $C_6H_5$ >CH-COO, N-$CH_3$, O

11

$C_6H_5$, HO, cyclohexyl >C-$COOCH_2CH_2$-$\overset{+}{N}$($C_2H_5$)($CH_3$)($C_2H_5$)

12

xanthene(O)-$COOCH_2CH_2$-$\overset{+}{N}$($CH(CH_3)_2$)($CH_3$)($CH(CH_3)_2$) · $Br^-$

13

All attempts, however, to develop a useful drug based on one of these antimuscarinic agents have failed since their effects could not be localized to the place of application: even the quaternary salts exhibited unwanted systemic anticholinergic activity, such as dry mouth, mydriasis, etc.

The quaternary anticholinergics thus appeared to be ideal candidates for a "soft analog" type design. All known anticholinergics based on aminoalcohol esters contain at least two carbon atoms separating the ester function and the quaternary head, as shown by structures 14 and 15, which implied that a distance of about 7 Å between these two functions is necessary for activity. On the other hand, even a hydrolytic cleavage of such esters would not destroy the quaternary head, providing a source for other anticholinergic agents. A soft quaternary analog

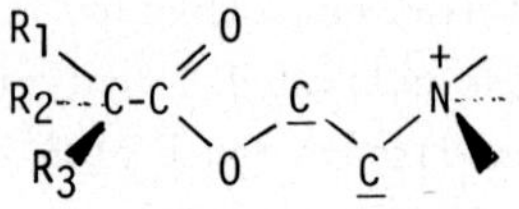

14

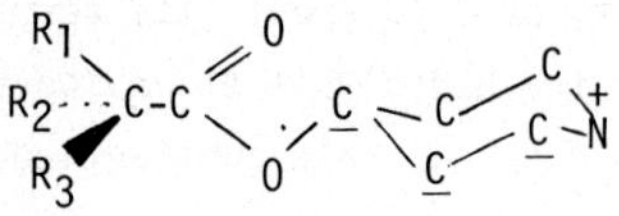

15

(16) of 14 and 15 would contain only <u>one</u> carbon atom separating the ester and the positive charge, providing again a facile way to fully deactivate the compound as shown by the hydrolysis of 16:

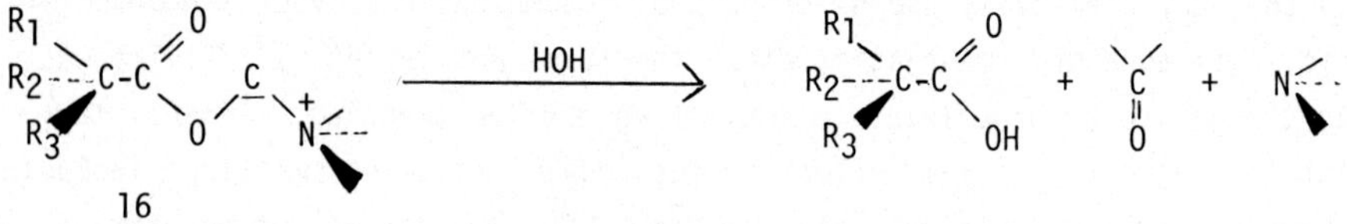

HOH

16

The design of the novel potential "soft" anticholinergics involved thus, three basic components: an acid, an aldehyde and a tertiary amine. The aim of the variations used was to develop some feel for a structure-activity relationship involving these components (ref. 21). There were some basic questions to be answered first: can these, particularly the sterically hindered acid containing compounds, be made, are they stable enough, and finally, will they be active, since based on the generally accepted structural requirements and in view of the fact that acetylnorcholine (17) the "soft" analog of acetylcholine (18) is about 5,000 times less potent than 18 (ref. 22), one would expect significantly lower activity.

$CH_3COOCH_2\overset{+}{N}(CH_3)_3$

17

$CH_3COOCH_2CH_2\overset{+}{N}(CH_3)_3$

18

A large variety of compounds were synthesized and tested first for their intrinsic anticholinergic (and/or cholinergic) and antihistaminic acitivities. The results are shown in Table 5.

TABLE 5

Acetylcholine and histamine antagonist potency of some "soft analogs"

$$R_2-\overset{R_1}{\underset{R_3}{C}}-\overset{O}{\overset{\|}{C}}-O-CH_2-\overset{+}{N}\lessgtr$$

| Nr | Structure $R_1$ | $R_2$ | $R_3$ | $\geqq N$ | anti-cholinergic[a] $pA_2$ | anti-histaminic[b] $pA_2$ | cholinergic[c] potency |
|---|---|---|---|---|---|---|---|
| 19 | $C_6H_5$ | 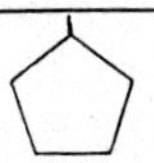 | H | $-N(CH_2CH_3)_3$ | 8.1 | No | -- |
| 20 | $C_6H_5$ | | H | 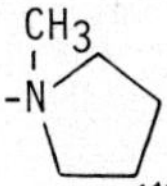 $CH_3$ -N | 8.4 | No | -- |
| 21 | $C_6H_5$ | 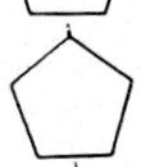 | H | 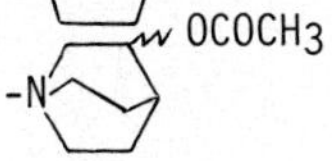 -N $OCOCH_3$ | 8.6 | 5.7 | -- |
| 22 | $C_6H_5$ | 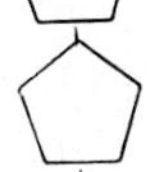 | H | 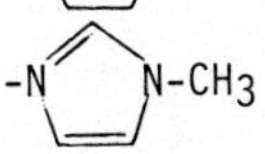 -N N-$CH_3$ | 7.8 | 6.3 | -- |
| 23 | $C_6H_5$ | 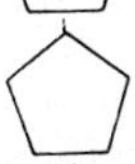 | H | $-N(CH_2CH_2OCH_2CH_2CH_3)_3$ | -- | -- | -- |
| 24[d] | $C_6H_5$ | 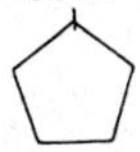 | H | $-CH_2-\overset{+}{N}(CH_2CH_3)_3$ | 8.5 | 7.3 | -- |
| 25 | $C_6H_5$ | | H | 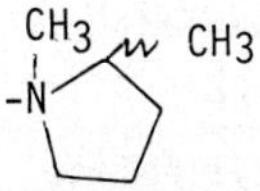 $CH_3$ -N $CH_3$ | 9.3 | 7.9 | -- |
| 26 | $C_6H_5$ | 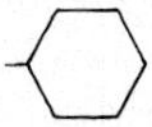 | H | $-N(CH_2CH_3)_3$ | 8.6 | 5.7 | -- |
| 27 | $C_6H_5$ | H | H | 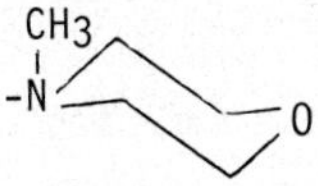 $CH_3$ -N O | nonspecific depressant | | |
| 28 | $C_6H_5$ | $-CH_2CH_3$ | H | $-N(CH_2CH_3)_3$ | 6.6 | 6.5 | -- |
| 29 | $C_6H_5$ | $-CH_2CH_3$ | H | 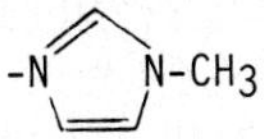 -N N-$CH_3$ | 5.9 | 5.9 | -- |
| 30 | $C_6H_5$ | $C_6H_5$ | $CH_3$ | 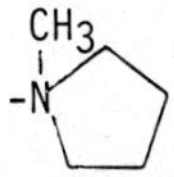 $CH_3$ -N | 8.4 | -- | -- |
| 31 | $CH_3CH_2$ | $CH_3$ | H | 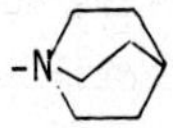 -N | -- | -- | 1:5 Bl: hexamethonium |
| 32 | $CH_3CH_2$ | $CH_3$ | H | 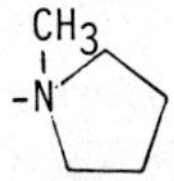 $CH_3$ -N | -- | 5.6 | -- |
| 33 | $CH_3CH_2$ | $CH_3$ | H | 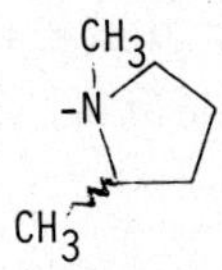 $CH_3$ -N $CH_3$ | 4.9 | -- | -- |
| 34 | H | H | H | $-N(CH_2CH_3)_3$ | -- | -- | $1:10^4$ Bl: atropine not hexamethonium |

| | | | | | | |
|---|---|---|---|---|---|---|
| 35 | | 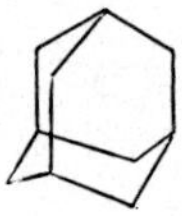 | 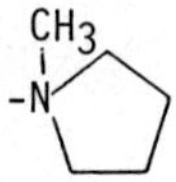 $CH_3$ -N | 6.9 | -- | -- |
| 36 | | 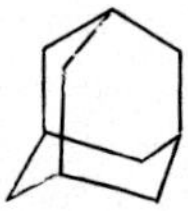 | 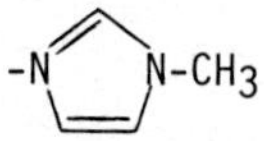 -N N-$CH_3$ | 5.7 | 5.3 | -- |
| 37 | $C_6H_5$ | 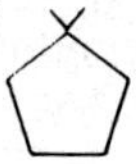 | -$N(CH_2CH_3)_3$ | 7.1 | -- | -- |
| 38 | $C_6H_5$ | 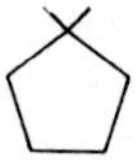 | 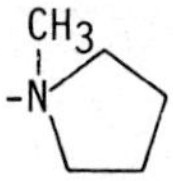 $CH_3$ -N | 7.3 | -- | -- |
| 39 | $C_6H_5$ | | 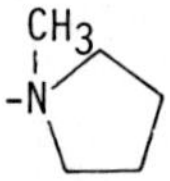 $CH_3$ -N | 5.8 | -- | -- |
| 40 | $C_6H_5$ | 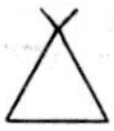 | 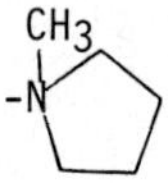 $CH_3$ -N | 6.6 | 6.2 | -- |

[a]Anticholinergic activity was assessed using the guinea-pig ileum test: strips of whole ileum were used in McEwen's solution at 37°C. 1 g tension was applied and cumulative concentration response curves were recorded to acetylcholine, then in the presence of antagonists at different concentrations. $pA_2$ values were then calculated from the dose-ratio obtained.

[b]As a, using histamine instead of acetylcholine.

[c]Cholinergic potency compared to that of acetylcholine. It was checked whether activity could be blocked by hexamethonium or by atropine.

[d]The "hard quaternary" analog of 19.

The $pA_2$ value for atropine obtained in the same test was 8.5. This and the direct comparison to the "hard" analog 24 answered the first question: the designed soft analogs are very potent anticholinergics, comparable to the known compounds. The analog 25 is even significantly more potent than atropine. Clear cut structure-activity relationships for the acid and the tertiary amine parts could be also established. But the next, most important question was the relative systemic _in vivo_ activity: are these new types of antimuscarinic agents "soft", indeed? The initial _in vivo_ experiments were carried out using anesthetized rats. Arterial blood pressure and heart rate were constantly recorded, while the drugs were administered into a cannulated brachial vein. A dose of acetylcholine producing 70-80 percent of the maximum vasopressor effect was chosen and used throughout the experiment. After a dose of the test drug was injected, the established acetylcholine dose was injected at 1, 3, 5 ... minutes and the response recorded. In this way, a measure of both the activity and duration of action of the test drug could be assessed. The results obtained for a selected soft anticholinergic, the potent 19 are given in Table 6.

TABLE 6

Acetylcholine antagonist effect on the cat blood pressure of the soft anticholinergic 19

| Concentration ($mol\ kg^{-1}$) | Activity | | | | | | | | | | |
|---|---|---|---|---|---|---|---|---|---|---|---|
| $5.7 \times 10^{-8}$ | 1<br>0 | 3<br>18 | 5<br>55 | 7<br>82 | 9<br>100 | | | | | | Time (min)<br>% Response[a] |
| $5.7 \times 10^{-7}$ | 1<br>0 | 3<br>0 | 6<br>0 | 12<br>18 | 15<br>36 | 18<br>55 | 22<br>65 | 27<br>73 | 31<br>95 | 37<br>100 | Time (min)<br>% Response[a] |

[a]Percent response to a dose of acetylcholine (0.05 μg/kg) compared to the same dose in absence of the antagonist.

The above data clearly demonstrate that the potent soft anticholinergic 19 is short acting. At the same concentration, atropine completely inhibits acetylcholine response for several hours. Moreover, a lower dose of 19 ($1 \times 10^{-9}$ mol $kg^{-1}$) could not produce any anticholinergic activity upon slow infusion for 4 hours, while atropine did accumulate quickly, producing increasing activity. All these results indicate the high intrinsic activity but fast deactivation properties of the soft anticholinergics. Preliminary human studies have supported both the positive local effect and the lack of systemic activity.

## Conclusions

The above two examples clearly demonstrate the soft analog design technique. The method, however, is rather general, it is not restricted to these quaternary salts only. It was successfully applied to compounds designed to reduce specifically low density lipoproteins (LDL), as well as, to some cardiovascular agents (ref. 23).

## ACTIVATED SOFT COMPOUNDS

Drugs in this class are not analogs of known drugs. The design process of these compounds starts with a known or designed nontoxic compound which is then activated to perform a certain role by introducing in the structure a group which is then responsible for its pharmacological activity. The activated form will loose the activating group and revert to the original nontoxic compound or fall further apart to nontoxic moieties during the process of performing its role. The following examples will illustrate this design method.

## N-chloramine type antimicrobial agents

During the search for locally active antimicrobial agents of low toxicity, N-chloramines based on aminoacids, aminoalcohol esters and related compounds were identified as good candidates (refs. 24-28). The idea was to have a source of positive chlorine ($Cl^+$) of low chlorine potential ($K_{cp}$) (ref. 28), but with good activity. The release of the positive chlorine would result in regenerating the original amines:

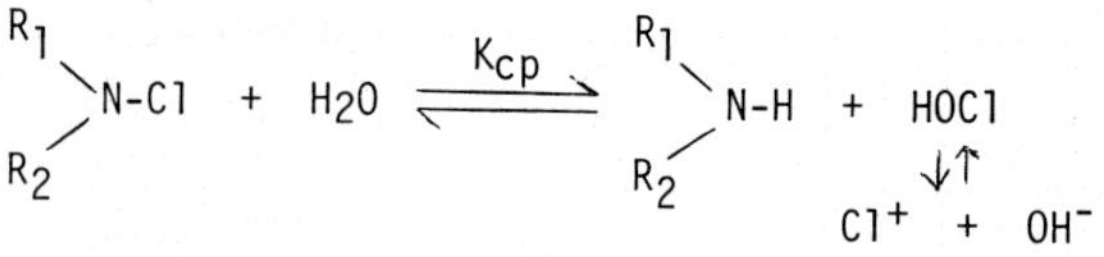

$$R_1R_2N\text{-}Cl + H_2O \underset{}{\overset{K_{cp}}{\rightleftharpoons}} R_1R_2N\text{-}H + HOCl \quad (HOCl \rightleftharpoons Cl^+ + OH^-)$$

Chloramines are, however, generally too unstable to have them formulated or to keep them unchanged for a prolonged time. The mechanism of their decomposition was, however, established as α,β dehydrohalogenation (ref. 25) and it was found that highly stable but potent chloramines can be obtained if the α-carbon does not contain any H atom. Examples for stable, noncorrosive N-chloramines derived from a nontoxic aminoacid and corresponding aminoalcohol are the structures 41-44.

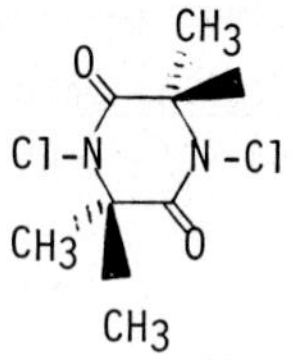

41 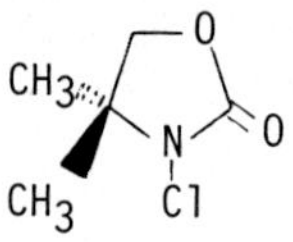 42 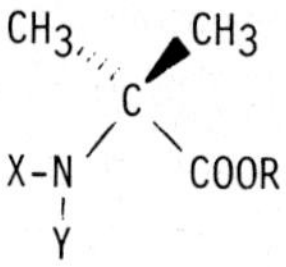 43 44

X=Cl
Y=H or Cl
R=alkyl, alkoxyalkyl, etc.

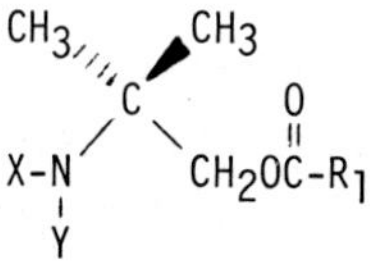

$R_1$ = as R or aryl, N-methylpyridinium, etc.

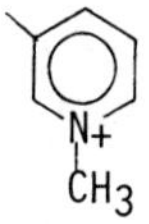

The stable 42 was compared to the more reactive N-chlorosuccinimide (45) and it was found, as an additional advantage, that it is not denatured by materials such as horse serum (Table 7).

TABLE 7

Contact germicidal efficiency of some N-chloramines[a]

| Compound | Conc. ppm | Horse serum % | Sterilization time[b], (min) Staph. epidermis | E. coli | K. pneumoniae | P. aeruginosa | Staph. aureus | B. bronchi-septica |
|---|---|---|---|---|---|---|---|---|
| 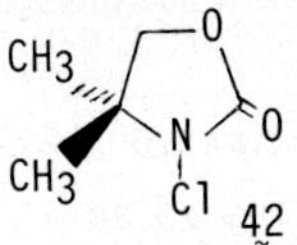 42 | 298 | 0 | 0.5 | 0.5 | 0.5 | 0.5 | 1 | 0.5 |
| | 298 | 5 | 1 | 0.5 | 0.5 | 0.5 | 3 | 0.5 |
| 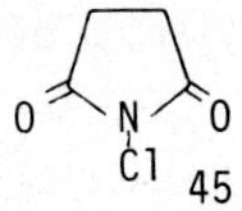 45 | 301 | 0 | 0.5 | 0.5 | 0.5 | 0.5 | 0.5 | 0.5 |
| | 301 | 5 | 7 | 3 | 8 | 9 | 10 | 5 |

[a]pH 4.6 at 25°C

[b]Time intervals screened: 0.5, 1, 2, 3, 4, 5, 6, 7, 8, 9 and 10 min. A time of 0.5 min could thus mean much less.

The mechanism of action of 42 was found to involve inhibition of bacterial growth by inhibiting DNA, RNA and protein synthesis. It was found (ref. 29) that the initial precursor was regenerated while the $Cl^+$ did interact primarily with -SH containing enzymes as shown in Table 8.

TABLE 8

Inhibition of enzyme activity by 3-chloro-4,4-dimethyl-2-oxazolidinone

| Conc. of 42 (M) / Enzyme | Inhibition[a], % Malic Dehydro-genase | Lactic Dehydro-genase | Creatine Phospho-genase | Fumarase | Ribo nuclease |
|---|---|---|---|---|---|
| $5.34 \times 10^{-5}$ | 16 | 10 | 0 | | 0 |
| $1.07 \times 10^{-4}$ | 20 | 15 | 5 | 100 | 0 |
| $4.28 \times 10^{-4}$ | 54 | 40 | 30 | 100 | 0 |
| $8.56 \times 10^{-4}$ | 62 | 50 | 53 | 100 | 0 |
| $1.28 \times 10^{-2}$ | 100 | 100 | 85 | 100 | 0 |
| $1.72 \times 10^{-2}$ | 100 | 100 | 100 | 100 | 0 |

[a]No inhibition was found if the enzymes were pretreated with dithiothreitol at the concentration of 42.

## Soft alkylating compounds

During the development of the soft quaternary salts, a number of "soft" alkylating agents were prepared. These compounds can formally be derived from simple alkanol esters of aliphatic or aromatic acids which then are activated by introducing a halogen atom to the α carbon of the alcohol portion. These α-halo esters are relatively weak alkylating agents; thus it was assumed that many of them could have antitumor activity as their lower alkylating potency would allow their transport to tumor cells without indiscriminant alkylation. On the other hand, as activated esters, all these compounds are subject to hydrolytic cleavage-deactivation, hence, their overall toxicity should be lower than that of conventional alkylating agents, which can only be deactivated by the alkylating process.

A variety of α-halo esters were synthesized (ref. 30) and their relative alkylating potency was determined by a competitive alkylation method, using as an arbitrary standard, chloromethyl pivalate (46) competing for the alkylation of a tertiary amine of low steric hindrance, 3-acetoxyquinuclidine (47). The analysis of the product composition allowed expressing the relative alkylating reactivity (RAR), as shown in Table 9.

TABLE 9

Relative alkylating reactivity (RAR) of selected soft alkylating agents

$$\underset{2}{R\text{-}COOCH(R_1)\text{-}Y} + \underset{46}{t\text{-}BuCOOCH_2Cl} + \underset{47}{N\text{(3-OAc-quinuclidine)}} \xrightarrow[CH_3CN]{70\ 0.1^\circ} \underset{48}{R\text{-}COOCH(R_1)\text{-}N^{+}\text{(3-OAc-quinuclidinium)}} + \underset{49}{t\text{-}BuCOOCH_2N^{+}\text{(3-OAc-quinuclidinium)}}$$

| Nr | R | $R_1$ | Y | Product Composition % 48 | 49 | RAR (48/49) |
|---|---|---|---|---|---|---|
| 2a | $CH_3(CH_2)_4$ | H | Cl | 35 | 65 | 0.54 |
| 2b | $C_5H_9$-$CH_2$ (cyclopentyl-$CH_2$) | H | Cl | 40 | 60 | 0.67 |
| 2c | $C_6H_5CH_2$ | H | Cl | 73 | 27 | 2.70 |
| 2d | $C_6H_5$ | H | Cl | 40 | 60 | 0.67 |
| 2e | $C_6H_5$ | H | Br | 93 | 7 | 13.29 |
| 2f | $CH_3(CH_2)_4$ | $CH_3$ | Cl | -- | >99 | 0 |

The very hindered 2f is much less reactive than its previous homolog, chloromethyl hexanoate 2a. Biological studies revealed no activity of 2f, while 2a was active in the P388 leukemia test (Table 10).

TABLE 10

Activity of the soft alkylating agent 2a in P388 lymphocytic leukemia[a]

| dose, mg/kg | no. of animals | % ILS[b] |
|---|---|---|
| 400 | 5 | 109 |
| 200 | 6 | 127[c] |
| 100 | 6 | 120 |
| 50 | 6 | 107 |

[a]One daily dose; total number of doses = 9.

[b]Percent increase in median survival time as compared to the control group.

[c]Activity confirmed by second test.

It is believed that this novel type of mild alkylating agent has good potential to be useful in cancer treatment: it is small, thus its incorporation in transport molecules will not alter significantly the affinity-binding and transport properties of the carrier molecule, while the circulating free part can be deactivated by esterases, resulting in a more favorable separation of the desired activity from toxicity.

ACTIVE METABOLITES

It is well-known that a wide variety of drugs undergo step-wise metabolic degradation yielding intermediates and structural analogs which have similar activity to the original drug molecule. (For example, oxyphenbutazone, 4-hydroxypropranolol and many other active drug metabolites belong to this class). The point is that these generally oxidative metabolic transformations will put, on one hand, a burden on the oxidative enzyme systems, and even more importantly, will result in a number of potentially active compounds which have, however, different pharmacokinetic, binding, distribution and elimination properties. The overall result is that depending on the presence of other compounds requiring the same enzyme system, as well as, on the activity level of the specific individual's enzymes, a variety of combinations of the active species will be present in different individuals, making practically impossible the safe and effective general dosing of these compounds. A good illustration of the situation is given by the metabolism of bufuralol (50) (ref. 31) (Table 11), one of the many β-blockers which undergo metabolic transformations leading to compounds of the same type of activities, but different selectivity and rather different pharmacokinetic properties.

TABLE 11

Metabolism and pharmacokinetic properties of bufuralol (50) and its metabolites (51-53)

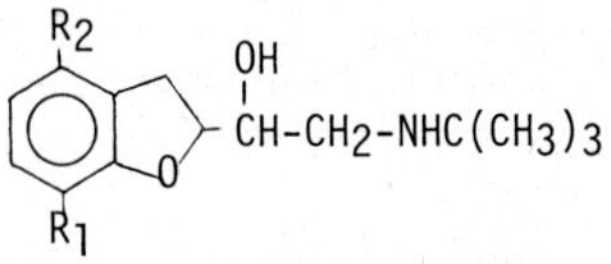

|  | $R_1$ | $R_2$ | Conc.[a] (μg/ml) | $t_{\frac{1}{2}}$[b] (hr) |
|---|---|---|---|---|
| 50 | $-CH_2CH_3$ | H | 22 | 4 |
| 51 | $-CH(OH)CH_3$ | H | 19 | 7 |
| 52 | $-COCH_3$ | H | 8 | 12 |
| 53 | $-CH_2CH_3$ | OH | <2 | 4 |

[a]Blood concentration at 9.5 hr after administration to humans (20 mg oral dose)
[b]Biological half-life

Interestingly, the oxidized metabolites 51 and 52 have longer half-lives than the basic compounds. All 51-53 are potent β-blockers. Evidently, their relative *in vivo* ratios will vary with time, individual enzyme levels, etc.

This is clearly a general problem. In many instances, it is not even clear which is the main active drug form, the drug or its metabolite(s). In the latter case, the drug is only a prodrug. It is important to realize, however, that in a large number of cases, based on our present knowledge, many metabolites can be *predicted* and one does not have to wait for the classical metabolism studies to synthesize, identify and test these candidates.

According to the basic soft drug design concept, it is preferred to use an active species which undergoes a *one step*, *singular* metabolic deactivation. Thus, the *active metabolite theorem* of the soft drug design suggests that whenever oxidative metabolic transformations of a drug take place going through possibly toxic, highly reactive intermediates or through pharmacologically active species, *if activity and pharmacokinetic conditions permit it, the drug of choice should be the active metabolite which is in the highest oxidized state*.

The theorem can and certainly should be expanded to *other metabolic transformations* besides the oxidative ones.

## ENDOGENOUS SUBSTANCES AS NATURAL SOFT DRUGS

Endogenous substances, such as steroid hormones (hydrocortisone, progesterone, testosterone, estradiol) or dopamine and others can be considered as *natural soft drugs*, since the body has developed efficient, fast metabolic ways for their disposition without going through highly reactive intermediates. Thus, their metabolism is *predictable* and it is certain that if used at *concentrations close to their normal levels*, they will not cause unexpected toxicity. The metabolism of many of these compounds is often so fast that they cannot efficiently be used as drugs. The situation can possibly be controlled by a prodrug-soft drug combination. This kind of combination appears to be ideal for delivery of such natural soft drugs as hydrocortisone. Although hydrocortisone (54) is an endogenous glucocorticoid, its topical application, resulting in higher than normal *in vivo* levels, can cause side effects such as dermal atrophy, thymus involution and suppression of adrenal, hypothalamus and pituitary functions. Formulations of hydrocortisone which only increase the efficiency of its delivery cannot realistically be expected to alleviate any of these problems. Improved separation of activity from toxicity should result from a derivative of hydrocortisone, that is (1) not active itself, but (2) accumulates in the skin and (3) hydrolyzes slowly to release the parent drug, 54, at such a rate that the rate of the systemic metabolism of the released parent drug to inactive normal metabolites more closely matches the rate of release of the drug from the skin. In this way, due to the natural soft drug properties of 54, local activity should be separated from unwanted side effects. No known derivative of hydrocortisone appeared, however, to satisfy these criteria. Since the α,β-unsaturated ketone group is essential for binding and activity of the glucocorticoids, this group became our primary target. Spirothiazolidine type derivatives were selected as the best candidates, although they were unknown, and even suggested to be unobtainable via the known methods of synthesis. Thiazolidines offered some unique advantages, as the natural aminoacid, cysteine and its derivatives could be used to obtain them, while the compounds should be subject to biological cleavage (of the imine formed after spontaneous cleavage of the carbon-sulfur bond (ref. 32)). Appropriate conditions were found and a large number of 3-spirothiazolidines of hydrocortisone and its derivatives were synthesized (ref. 33), such as 56-60.

$CH_2OCOCH_3$, C=O, HO, OH, O — 55 —[Pyridine / cysteine ethyl ester]→ $CH_2OCOCH_3$, C=O, HO, OH, S, NH, $COOC_2H_5$ — 57

Several important structural features in the molecule had to be established, such as the location of the double bond (4,5 or 5,6), isomerism around C-3 (the sulfur or the nitrogen is in the alpha position), as these are determining factors in the mechanism of hydrolysis, binding and final release of the active species, as illustrated by the effect of the location of the double bond:

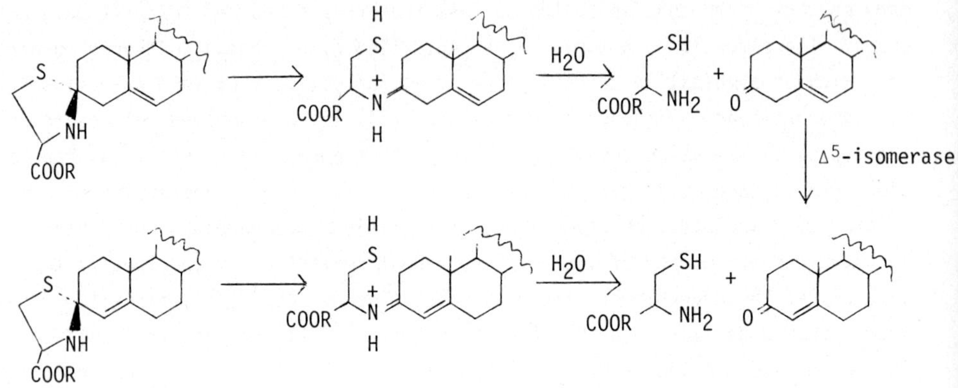

TABLE 12

Relative antiinflammatory activity[a] of selected cysteine based 3-spirothiazolidine derivatives of hydrocortisone

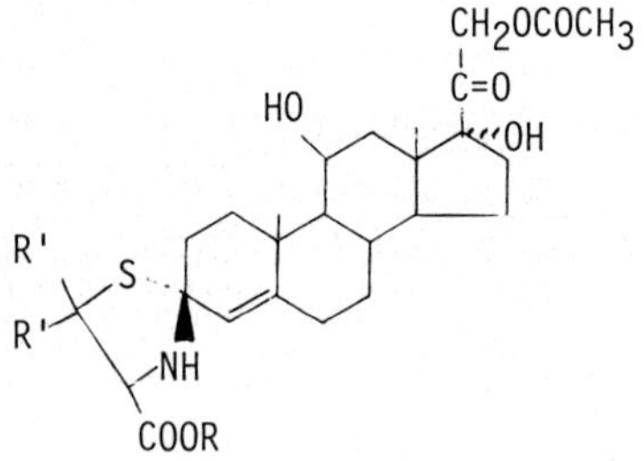

| Nr | Compound R | R' | $ED_{50}$ (M)[b] | Relative potency to hydrocortisone |
|---|---|---|---|---|
| 56 | $CH_3$ | H | 0.0035 | 3.1 |
| 57 | $C_2H_5$ | H | 0.0033 | 3.2 |
| 58 | $C_4H_9$ | H | 0.0027 | 4.0 |
| 59 | $C_6H_{13}$ | H | 0.0039 | 2.7 |
| 60 | $C_{10}H_{21}$ | H | 0.0036 | 3.0 |
| 61 | $C_2H_5$ | $CH_3$ | 0.0055 | 1.9 |
| 54 | Hydrocortisone | | 0.0107 | 1.0 |
| 55 | Hydrocortisone 21-acetate | | 0.0203 | 0.5 |
| 62 | Hydrocortisone 17α-butyrate | | 0.0011 | 10.0 |

[a]The test compounds were applied in acetone solution containing 2% croton oil on each the anterior and posterior surface of the right ear. Three hours later, the mice (male DDY) were sacrificed and both ears were removed. Circular sections were punched out and drug effect expressed as percent inhibition of inflammation compared to the control.

[b]Linear regression analysis of data obtained at $3x10^{-5}$, $3x10^{-4}$, $3x10^{-3}$ and $3x10^{-2}$ M

If the double bond (as usual for tetrahedral C-3- derivatives) would migrate to the 5,6- position, the $\Delta^5$-3-ketosteroid isomerase would be required for the release of the active hydrocortisone. Detailed $^{13}C$ NMR and other studies have established (refs. 34, 35) that in this specific case of 54 or 55, under certain conditions, the only isolable isomer is the one with the unchanged 4,5- double bond and the sulfur in the $\alpha$ position.

A series of the spirothiazolidines were then tested (ref. 33) for their topical antiinflammatory activity using the mouse ear assay. The results are given in Table 12.

It is evident that the 3-spirothiazolidines based on cysteine (56-60) provide a 3-4 fold improvement over hydrocortisone (54) and a 6-8 fold one over the corresponding hydrocortisone acetate. Hydrocortisone-17$\alpha$-butyrate, 62, was included to confirm the known relative potencies. Note, that 62 is not a prodrug of hydrocortisone. It is interesting to note that 3-spirothiazolidines of the 17$\alpha$-butyrate did not show improvement over 62.

The effect of the topically applied steroids on the thymus involution was also assessed, using weanling rats (45-50 g). As shown in Table 13, the 3-spirothiazolidine 57 had significantly lower systemic side effects than even hydrocortisone (54) or hydrocortisone acetate (55).

TABLE 13

Thymus involution[a] in rats after topical application of steroids

| Compound | mg of thymus / 100 g of rat ± S.D. | % reduction in thymus[b] |
|---|---|---|
| Blank[c] | 268 ± 25 | |
| Vehicle | 257 ± 59 | |
| 54 | 168 ± 30 | 35 |
| 55 | 167 ± 18 | 35 |
| 57 | 204 ± 25 | 21 |
| 62 | 206 ± 20 | 20 |

[a]All compounds were administered in a total of 50 µl as a 0.03 M acetone/IPM (90:10) solution to 10 rats, each.

[b]Compared to vehicle.

[c]Untreated rats.

A logical explanation for the better separation of activity-toxicity after local topical application of the 3-spirothiazolidine 57 as compared to 55 would be a lower amount of systemic delivery of hydrocortisone when using 57, but a higher amount bound locally in the skin, allowing a more sustained release of the active component at the site of the inflammation. Indeed, diffusion studies through freshly excised hairless mice skin have shown that only about half as much hydrocortisone (and only hydrocortisone, indicating total skin metabolism of 57) appeared in the receptor phase when 57 was applied compared to the case in which hydrocortisone was used. The hydrocortisone acetate delivered substantially higher amounts. The results are given in Table 14.

TABLE 14

Steroid diffusion[a] through fresh hairless mouse skin

| Compound | Mole % hydrocortisone[b] diffused ± S.D.[c] (hours after application) | | | | |
|---|---|---|---|---|---|
| Hydrocortisone 54 | | 2.1±0.8(4) | 4.1±1.3(9) | 7.5±1.8(18) | 8.4±3.0(24) |
| Hydrocortisone acetate 55 | | 1.7±0.6(4) | 3.5±1.3(9) | 5.2±1.3(18) | 14.1±5.9(24) |
| Thiazolidine 57 | 0.1±0.05(2) | 0.6±0.1(4) | 1.2±0.2(7.4) | 1.8±0.3(12) | 3.2±0.7(24) |

[a]50 μl of 0.03 M acetone:IPM (90:10) was applied to the whole skin placed over a reservoir with the epidermal side up. The reservoir contained 44 ml of normal saline with 0.01% gentamycin. The cells were kept stirred at 32°C. HPLC was used for the analysis.

[b]Only hydrocortisone was found in the receptor side.

[c]Triplicate experiments.

Based on these results, it was assumed that the thiazolidines undergo ring opening to the intermediate 63 which then binds as indicated by structure 64 followed by sustained release of hydrocortisone:

This theory is supported by *in vivo* studies on analogous thiazolidine derivatives of progesterone (65), which were synthesized to provide sustained progesterone release in the skin for the treatment of acne (ref. 36). Thus, when radiolabelled 65 and 66 were applied topically to hairless mice (ref. 37), more than twice of the activity was found in the skin when 66 was given than when progesterone, 65, was given indicating a more sustained source for local progesterone release.

## THE INACTIVE METABOLITE APPROACH

The inactive metabolite approach is one of the most promising and most versatile methods for developing safe, soft drugs. The principles of the inactive metabolite approaches are: 1) start the design with a known inactive metabolite of a drug, 2) perform chemical modifications on the metabolite to obtain a structure which resembles (isosteric and/or isoelectronic) the starting or an analogous drug, 3) design the structure and the metabolism of the new, soft compound in such a way as to yield the starting inactive metabolite in one step and without going through toxic intermediates, 4) control transport and binding properties, as well as the rate of metabolism and pharmacokinetics by molecular manipulations in the activation stage.

The easiest way to get a feeling of this approach is by analyzing the data in Table 15, which gives some toxicity data of known, structurally related pesticides.

TABLE 15

Toxicity of some pesticides

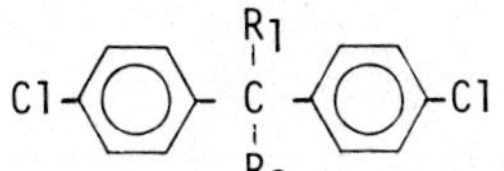

Cl–C(R1)(R2)–Cl

| | $R_1$ | $R_2$ | Name | $LD_{50}$ (mg/kg) oral | Carcinogen Conc. (ppm) |
|---|---|---|---|---|---|
| 65 | -H | $-CCl_3$ | DDT | 120 | 300 |
| 66 | -OH | $-CCl_3$ | Kelthane | 800 | 300 |
| 67 | -OH | $-COOC_2H_5$ | Chlorobenzylate | 1500 | 6000 |

The two major common metabolites for each of these pesticides are the acids 68 and the ketone 69.

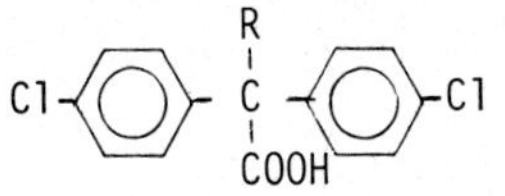

Cl–C(R)(COOH)–Cl

68 R = H, OH

Cl–C(=O)–Cl

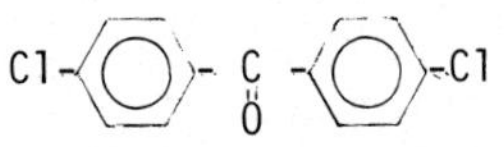

69

It is easy to recognize that the reason for the significantly lower toxicity for 67 is due to the fact that it is a simple ester of the common metabolite 69 which is inactive and is excreted. The deactivation of 67 requires only a simple ester hydrolysis, contrary to the metabolism of 65 and 66. As all three are good pesticides of comparable activity, one should obviously use 67. From the point of view of the design of soft compounds, 67 is formally derived from

References p. 163

the inactive metabolite 68, by masking the polar acid function. The metabolism-deactivation is in one hydrolytic step, predictable and it could further be controlled by introducing other alcohol functions instead of the ethoxy group.

On a more general basis, the metabolism of a large number of drugs were analyzed by us and many useful inactive metabolites were found. For example, major antiinflammatory steroidal agents undergo among others, oxidative metabolic degradation of the dihydroxyacetone side chain. Thus, the prototype hydrocortisone (55) will get oxidized stepwise to the ketoaldehyde 70, the 20-oxo-21-oic acid, 71 and cortienic acid, 72, in addition to the various A ring reduced products,

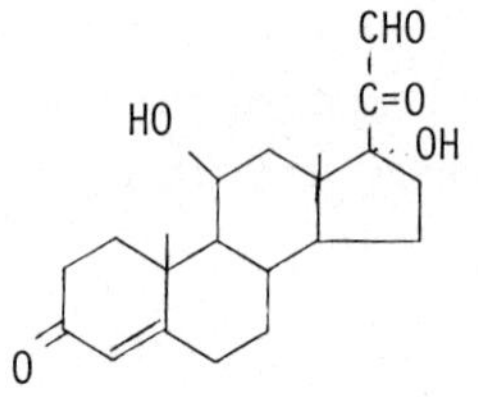

70 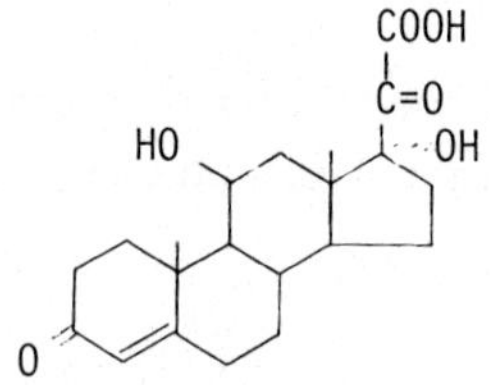 71 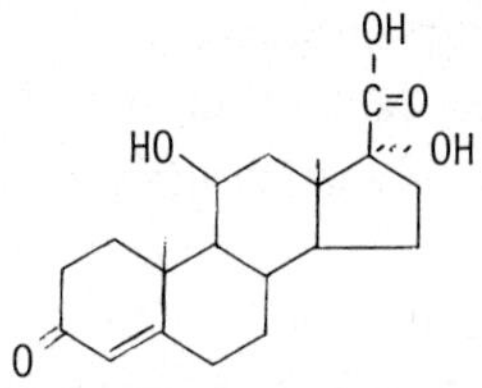 72

which, however, are of no interest to us at this stage. The acids 71 and 72 are inactive and can be used as lead compounds to design isosteric and/or isoelectronic analogs of the 17α- and 21- substituted hydrocortisone represented by the general formula 73 (ref. 38). The corresponding 74 and 75, if judiciously chosen, will have good local activity, but will be void of any systemic acitivity-toxicity, such as thymus and adrenal suppression and others.

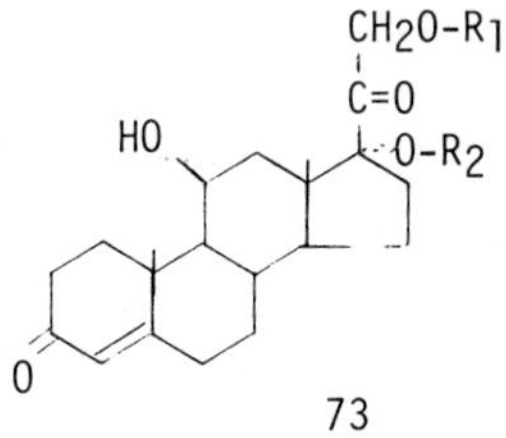

73 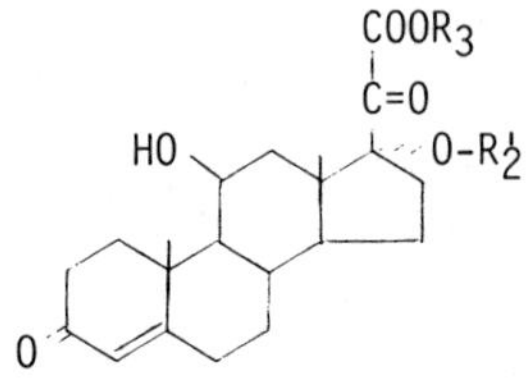 74 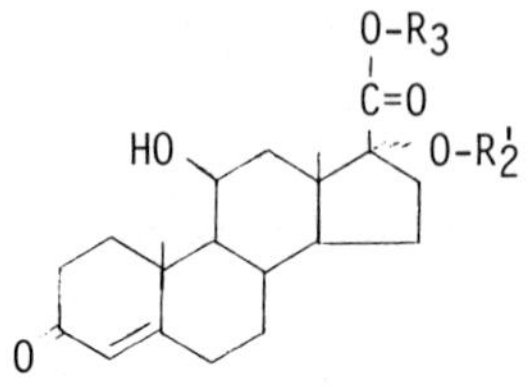 75

$R_1$ = $CH_3CO$-, $(CH_3)_3CCO$-, ...
$R_2$ = H, $C_3H_7CO$-, $C_2H_5CO$-, ...

$R_2'$ = $R_2$ or others
$R_3$ = $C_1$-$C_6$ alkyl
-$CH_2OCR_5$ (C=O)
-$CH_2$-X-$CH_3$, etc.

For example, using the known McKenzie-Stoughton human blanching test, some of the cortienic acid derivatives, such as 76 and 77 showed good activity, while the fluorinated derivatives 79 and 80 were more potent than hydrocortisone 17α-valerate (81) (Table 16).

TABLE 16

Human blanching activities of selected soft steroids

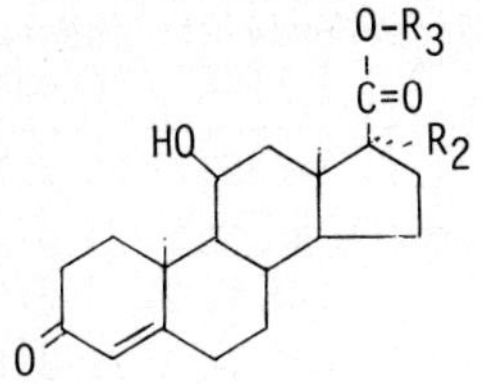

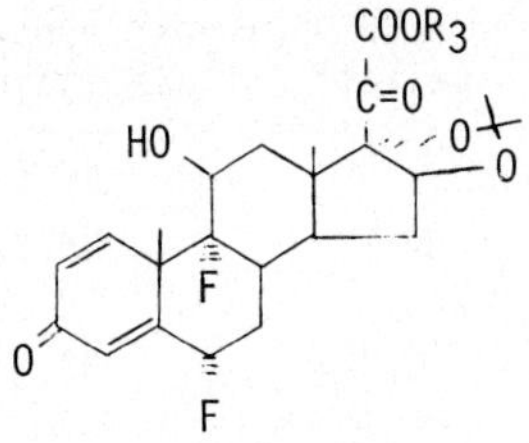

| Nr. | $R_2$ | $R_3$ | Relative Blanching[a]: Conditions (occlusion time, conc. in vehicle[b]), activity |
|---|---|---|---|
| 76 | $C_4H_9CO$- | $-CH_2-O-C(=O)CH_3$ | 6h; 1% EtOH/IPM; 1.5 vs. 2.5 (81) |
| 77 | $C_4H_9CO$- | $-CH_2COOC_2H_5$ | 6h; 1% EtOH/IPM; 1 vs. 2.5 (81) |
| 78 | $C_4H_9CO$- | H | 6h; 1% EtOH/IPM; inactive |
| 79 | -- | $-CH_2SCH_3$ | 6h; 1% EtOH/IPM; 2.5 ≃ 2.5 (81) |
| 80 | -- | $-CH_2OC(=O)CH_3$ | 6h; 1% EtOH/IPM; 3 > 2.5 (81) |

[a]Direct comparison to 1% 81.

[b]Ethanol:isopropylmyristate = 70:30.

The corresponding 17α-substituted cortienic acid 78 was inactive. One of the analogs of 73, compound 82, was studied in detail simultaneously for its in vivo local activity using the rat granuloma test and for its systemic activity-toxicity, compared to hydrocortisone 17α-butyrate (62) and betamethasone valerate (83). The results are given in Table 17 and are self-explanatory.

The inactive metabolite approach was successfully applied more recently to a variety of cardiovascular drugs (ref. 39).

It should be mentioned that one does not have to wait for an inactive metabolite to be isolated. The inactive metabolite can be designed during the general drug design process, based on our knowledge of structural requirements for activity, as well as, elimination and enzymatic cleavage.

TABLE 17

Relative activity[a] and toxicity of the soft steroid 82 as compared to 62 and 83

| Test Compound | Dose (mg/ pellet) | Number of test Animals | Body wt. gain (g) | Granulation Tissue Dry wt. (mg/100g body wt.) | Granulation Tissue Inhibition % | Relative organ wt. mg/100 g Body wt. (decrease %) Thymus | Relative organ wt. mg/100 g Body wt. (decrease %) Adrenals |
|---|---|---|---|---|---|---|---|
| None (control) | | 10 | 40.5±0.8 | 43.7±4.2 | | 326±22 | 23.7±1.1 |
| 82 | 0.1 | 8 | 36.0±2.8 | 34.7±4.3 | 20.6 | 282±13 (13.5) | 22.9±2.6 (3.4) |
| | 0.3 | 8 | 33.0±1.3*** | 25.3±2.3** | 42.1 | 298±16 (8.6) | 22.8±1.0 (3.8) |
| | 1 | 8 | 32.8±0.9*** | 14.0±1.8*** | 68.0 | 304±10 (6.7) | 21.8±1.3 (8.0) |
| | 3 | 7 | 30.7±1.5*** | 18.7±2.3*** | 57.2 | 278±21 (14.7) | 19.6±1.1* (17.3) |
| Hydrocortisone 17-butyrate 62 | 1 | 8 | 33.4±1.4*** | 32.2±5.0 | 26.3 | 73±5*** (77.6) | 27.1±1.4 (-14.3) |
| | 3 | 8 | 15.9±1.4*** | 21.6±2.2** | 50.6 | 47±3*** (85.6) | 16.5±1.2*** (30.4) |
| | 10 | 8 | 4.9±1.0*** | 29.2±3.1* | 33.2 | 32±3*** (90.2) | 16.8±1.2*** (29.1) |
| Betamethasone valerate 83 | 1 | 8 | 16.6±1.9*** | 35.4±7.3 | 19.0 | 47±2*** (85.6) | 15.5±1.3*** (34.6) |
| | 3 | 8 | 14.9±1.7*** | 31.6±2.1 | 27.7 | 38±3*** (88.3) | 13.6±0.9*** (42.6) |
| | 10 | 8 | 17.0±2.1 | 40.7±2.6 | 6.9 | 43±4*** (86.8) | 12.6±0.9*** (46.8) |

*$p < 0.5$ **$p < 0.01$ ***$p < 0.001$ (mean s.e.)

[a]The compound was injected in acetonic solution into the pellet which then was implanted subcutaneously and left there for 6 days. After the rats were sacrificed and removal of the pellet, the dry pellet weight, the thymus and adrenal glands were analyzed, together with the relative body weight gain.

## CONCLUSIONS

The field of design of safer drugs based on the soft drug approach has opened a number of general ways leading to very successful separation of drug activity and toxicity, in other words, to significant improvement in therapeutic index. This highly logical approach has just started to gain recognition as one of the most important and integral parts of the drug design process. The methods of applying the basic concept can differ and can involve the usual basic structure-activity relationships or using computer optimized structures, etc. The main point is that in order to avoid many toxic effects of drugs, the design of drug metabolism should be involved at a very early stage of the drug design process.

ACKNOWLEDGEMENTS

I am truly indebted to my very able former and present co-workers who helped me to develop many of the soft drug ideas. These include among others, Drs. J. Kaminski, R. Woods, K. Sloan, Y. Oshiro, H. Farag, C. Raper, T. Loftsson, N. Kuo, as well as, R. Little, S. Selk, K. Knutson, P. Kearney, N. Gildersleeve and L. Caldwell. Encouraging discussions with Drs. T. Higuchi and W. Morozowitch are also acknowledged. Financial support by Otsuka Pharmaceutical Co., the National Institute of Health, Key Pharmaceutical Co., and $Inter_X$ Research Corp. are gratefully acknowledged.

REFERENCES

1 E.J. Ariëns, in E.J. Ariëns (Ed.), Drug Design, Vol. 1, Academic Press, New York and London, 1971, p. 1-270.
2 E.J. Ariëns, in E.J. Ariëns (Ed.), Drug Design, Vol. 2, Academic Press, New York and London, 1971, p. 1-127.
3 A. Albert, Selective Toxicity, 6th edn., Wiley, New York, 1974.
4 A.A. Sinkula and S.H. Yalkowsky, J. Pharm. Sci., 64 (1975) 181-210.
5 E.B. Roche (Ed.), Design of Biopharmaceutical Properties through Prodrugs and Analogs, Academy of Pharmaceutical Sciences, Washington, D.C., 1977.
6 N. Bodor, Drugs of the Future, 6 (1981) 165-182.
7 B.N. Ames, Science, 204 (1979) 587-589 and ref. cited.
8 S.D. Nelson, M.R. Boyd and J.R. Mitchell in P.M. Jerina (Ed.), Drug Metabolism Concepts, Am. Chem. Soc., 1977, 155-185.
9 G.T. Miwa and A.Y.H. Lu, Ann. Reports Med. Chem., 13 (1978) 206-218.
10 W.A. Mahon, T. Ihaba and R.M. Stone, Clin. Pharmacol. Ther., 22 (1977) 228-233.
11 F. Oesch, Biochem. Pharmacol., 25 (1976) 1935-1937.
12 H.R. Glatt, M. Metzler, H.G. Neumann and F. Oesch, Biochem. Biophys. Res. Comm., 73 (1976) 1025-1029.
13 B.H. Migdalof, Ann. Reports Med. Chem., 13 (1978) 196-205.
14 E.J. Ariëns, Pharmacochemistry Library, 2 (1977) 1-27 and ref. cited.
15 E.J. Ariëns and A.M. Simonis, in Drug Design and Adverse Reactions, Alfred Benzon Symposium X, Munksgaard, 1977, 317-330.
16 N. Bodor, in E.B. Roche (Ed.), Design of Biopharmaceutical Properties through Prodrugs and Analogs, Acad. Pharm. Sci., Washington, D.C., 1977, 98-135.
17 N. Bodor, U.S. Patent 4,061,722, Dec. 6, 1977.
18 N. Bodor and L. Freiberg, U.S. Patent 4,264,765, April 28, 1981.
19 N. Bodor, J. Kaminski and S.H. Selk, J. Med. Chem., 23 (1980) 469-474.
20 F.S. Kilmer McMillan, H.M. Reller and F.H. Snyder, J. Invest. Dermatol., 43 (1964) 363-377.
21 N. Bodor, R. Woods, C. Raper, P. Kearney and J.J. Kaminski, J. Med. Chem., 23 (1980) 474-480.
22 W.B. Geiger and H. Alpers, Arch. Int. Pharmacodyn., 148 (1964) 352-358.
23 N. Bodor and Y. Oshiro, unpublished results.
24 N. Bodor, J.J. Kaminski, S.D. Worley, R.J. Colton, T.H. Lee and J.W. Rabalais, J. Pharm. Sci., 63 (1974) 1387-1391.
25 J.J. Kaminski, N. Bodor and T. Higuchi, J. Pharm. Sci., 65 (1976) 553-557.
26 J.J. Kaminski, N. Bodor and T. Higuchi, J. Pharm. Sci., 65 (1976) 1733-1737.
27 J.J. Kaminski, M.M. Huycke, S.H. Selk, N. Bodor and T. Higuchi, J. Pharm. Sci., 65 (1976) 1737-1742.
28 M. Kosugi, J.J. Kaminski, S.H. Selk, I.H. Pitman, N. Bodor and T. Higuchi, J. Pharm. Sci., 65 (1976) 1743-1746.
29 H.H. Kohl, W.B. Wheatley, S.D. Worley and N. Bodor, J. Pharm. Sci., 69 (1980) 1292-1295.
30 N. Bodor and J.J. Kaminski, J. Med. Chem., 23 (1980) 566-569.

31 R.J. Francis, P.B. East, S.J. McLaren and J. Larman, Biomed. Mass Spectrometry, 3 (1976) 281-285.
32 W.M. Schubert and Y. Motoyama, J. Am. Chem. Soc., 87 (1965) 5507-5508.
33 N. Bodor, K.B. Sloan, R.J. Little, S.H. Selk and L. Caldwell, in print.
34 K.B. Sloan, N. Bodor and R.J. Little, Tetrahedron, in print.
35 K.B. Sloan, N. Bodor and J. Zupan, Tetrahedron, in print.
36 N. Bodor and K.B. Sloan, U.S. Patents 4,069,322, Jan. 17, 1978 and 4,239,757, Dec. 16, 1980.
37 N. Bodor and K.B. Sloan, J. Pharm. Sci., in print.
38 N. Bodor and R.J. Little, unpublished results.
39 N. Bodor and Y. Oshiro, unpublished results.

J.A. Keverling Buisman (Editor), *Strategy in Drug Research*



# OPTIMALIZATION OF PHARMACOKINETICS - AN ESSENTIAL ASPECT OF DRUG DEVELOPMENT - BY "METABOLIC STABILIZATION"

E.J. ARIËNS and A.M. SIMONIS
Institute of Pharmacology and Toxicology, University of Nijmegen, the Netherlands

## 1) INTRODUCTION

Generally speaking, the chemical properties and hence the chemical structure of a compound definitely determine the way in which it participates in the various part-processes involved in biological action. A structure-action relationship (SAR), therefore, has to be a fundamental characteristic of bioactive agents. The apparent absence of such a relationship can only be due to deficient methods of investigation and to the multiplicity and complexity of the process as a whole. Although the various part-processes are biochemical and physicochemical in nature, they differ greatly. Totally different SAR patterns may be expected for, for instance, the rate of absorption, the mode of distribution, the renal excretion, the various types of metabolic conversion, and the capacity of the agent to activate the molecular sites of action (the receptors) in the target tissue - the structure-action relationship in a strict sense. Absorption, distribution and excretion, which are mainly based on passive diffusion processes, will largely depend on partition coefficients. Metabolic conversion will depend mainly on the presence in the molecule of particular groups that are open to attack by enzymes. These groups as a rule have little or nothing to do with the chemical characteristics which are essential for the induction of the effect. Whether an agent is hydrolysed by esterases, for instance, depends mainly on the presence of a suitable ester group in the molecule. The ester group, however, has little or nothing to do with the question whether the agent has a curariform, an anticholinergic, a local anesthetic action, is an insecticide, a herbicide, a plasticizer, or some toxon. Whether an agent is capable of inducing a particular type of biological effect is usually dependent on various specific chemical characteristics in the molecule.

SAR will emerge most clearly if it is studied for particular part-processes such as those involved in absorption, distribution or excretion, where passage of membranes is essential, those involved in drug metabolism, where SAR will depend on the particular enzyme, and SAR for the final step of action, the induction of the effect. In a comparison of the quantitative dose-effect relationship for a

*References p. 178*

group of compounds the in vivo-SAR is the resultant of the integrated contribution of SAR for the various part-processes.

2) THE MAIN PHASES IN BIOLOGICAL ACTION

The complex of processes involved in biological action can be split up in three phases (Fig. 1) (ref. 1, 2).

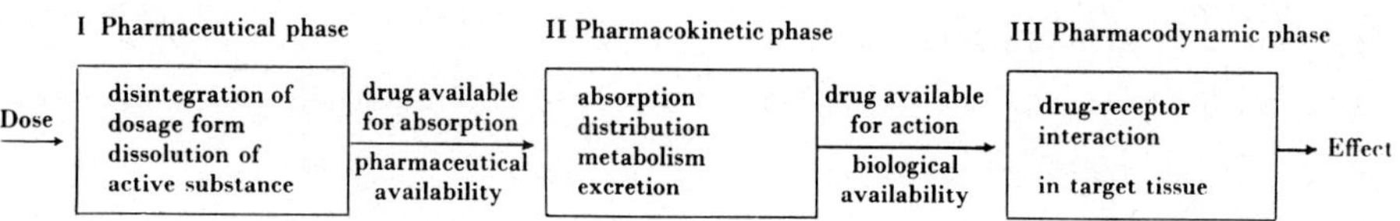


Fig. 1.

I. The pharmaceutical phase

This phase comprises the processes that are determinant for the efficacy of the application. Here the disintegration of the dosage form, tablets, capsules, etc., in such a way that the active agent becomes available in a molecular dispersed form suitable for absorption, and avoidance of chemical or enzymatic activation of the active agent before absorption, e.g. in the intestinal tract, count. In general, for the absorption - which implies passage of biological membranes - the lipid/water solubility and therewith the partition coefficient is determinant. For weak bases and acids also the degree of ionization and therewith the $pK_A$ of the compound and the pH at the site of absorption count. The fraction of the dose available for absorption is indicated as the "pharmaceutical availability". The time course of the events has to be taken into account, too, and results in the "pharmaceutical availability profile".

II. The pharmacokinetic phase

This phase comprises the processes involved in absorption, distribution, excretion and metabolic conversion of the agent after absorption. The fraction of the dose that reaches the general circulation is indicated as the "biological (systemic) availability". Also here the time course represented in the "biological availability profile" is of particular significance. The concentration of the active agent in the target tissue as a function of time is represented by the "pharmacological availability profile". In the pharmacokinetic phase, besides the lipid/water solubility and degree of ionization of the agent, particularly its sensitivity to various enzymes counts. The presence in the molecule of vulnerable moieties accessible to enzymatic attack plays a predominant role. In this respect, like in the case of active, carrier-related transport, the charge distribution of the agent and its steric properties are determinant factors. The metabolic conversion of the agent applied may result in its bioinactivation (biodetoxification) or bioactivation (biotoxification).

The involvement of various metabolites greatly complicates pharmacokinetics. Metabolic conversion usually increases hydrophilicity thus facilitating renal excretion.

III. The pharmacodynamic phase

This phase comprises the processes involved in the interaction between the bioactive compounds and their molecular sites of action, receptors, enzymes, etc. Pharmacon-receptor interaction results in the induction of a stimulus which initiates a sequence of biochemical and biophysical events which finally lead to the effect observed.

3) PHARMACON METABOLISM, A NATURAL DEFENCE AGAINST INTRUSION OF CHEMICALS (XENOBIOTICS), INCLUDING DRUGS

Although one might get the impression that the toxicological risks involved in the exposure to chemicals, including drugs, are generated by the evolvement of chemical and pharmaceutical industries and thus are of recent origin, this is definitely not the case. Already since the very beginning of evolution living systems have been exposed to chemicals. This especially holds true for the heterotrophic organisms (in general, animal life) which are to a large extent dependent on the consumption of autotrophic organisms (mainly plant material) and are exposed, therefore, to a great variety of potentially toxic chemicals of plant origin. These plant products are xenobiotic to the animal concerned. The term "biogenic xenobiotics" is appropriate here.

As long as life was limited to the oceans, the problems were relatively small, since there was a tremendous water compartment available for the disposal of undesired body-foreign chemicals, even if these were rather lipid-soluble. The "affinity" thereof for the relatively lipophilic biomass was counterbalanced by the tremendous volume of the disposal compartment. Photodegradation and oxidation in the surface layers of the waters largely took care of chemical degradation. By the time animal life switched from water to land, this opportunity got lost. Water became relatively scarce and only a small volume became available for disposal (for man about 1 liter a day). This increased the danger of accumulation of lipophilic, poorly water-soluble agents in the biomass. In the line of evolution an answer was found in the development of enzyme systems which take care of the conversion of relatively lipophilic compounds into highly water soluble end-products suitable for renal excretion (table 1). This conversion occurs in two steps: a first predominantly oxidative step and a second predominantly conjugational step (Fig. 2). Simultaneously, a strong increase in the concentration of plasma albumin took place (table 1), important for osmotic regulation but serving as well as a temporary sink, a kind of parking lot, for lipophilic xenobiotics. Such agents would easily pass the various membranes in the body and so enter tissues and cells where damage

TABLE 1. EVOLUTIONARY ASPECTS OF PLASMA PROTEIN AND DRUG METABOLISM (ref. 3).

| *Species* | *Plasma protein* % | *Oxidative N-demethylation*[c] | *Phenol glucuronidation*[d] | *Species* |
|---|---|---|---|---|
| man | 6.5 | 19 ± 2 | 21 ± 3 | mouse |
| dog | 6.1–6.7 | 15 ± 2 | 46 ± 13 | rat |
| turtle | 4.8 | 26 ± 8 | 85 ± 22 | pigeon |
| crocodile | 3.69 | 4 ± 0.6 | 8.9 ± 2.3 | lizard |
| frog | 1.5–4.3 | 1.6 ± 0.45 | 1.26 ± 0.47 | frog |
| skate | 2.4–3.1 | 1.1 ± 0.30 | 1.72 ± 0.25 | trout |
| menhaden | 0.72–2.9 | 0.71 ± 0.28 | 1.9 ± 0.33 | goldenorfe |
| goosefish | 1.4–2.2 | 0.86 ± 0.23 | 2.68 ± 0.65 | carp |

[c] µmoles formaldehyde formed per gram fresh liver tissue/hour.
[d] µmoles p-nitrophenol glucuronidation per gram fresh liver tissue/hour.

Note the increases at the switch from water to land animals.

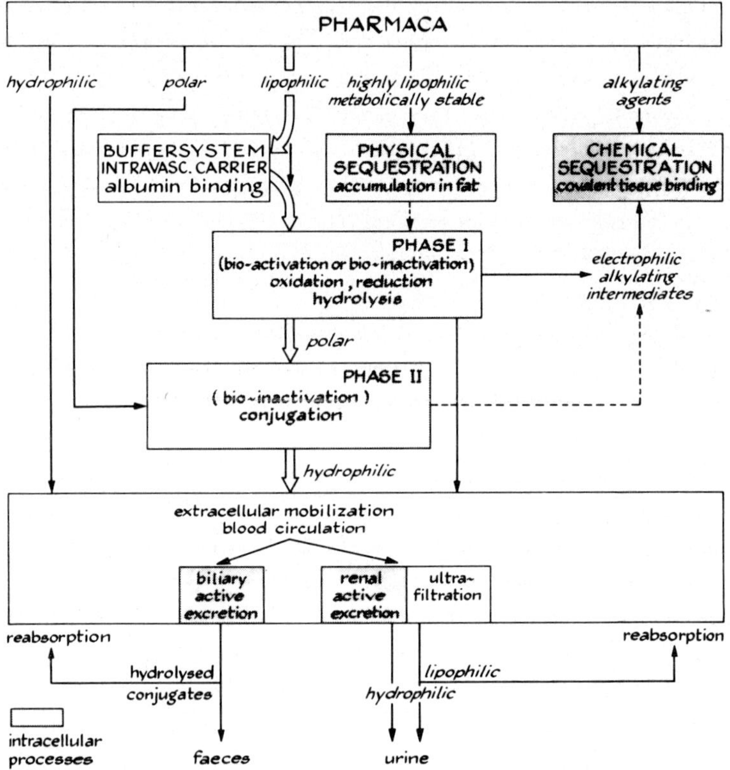


Fig. 2. Schematic representation of the main steps in drug metabolism and elimination.

might be done. Binding to albumin implies lowering of the free concentration in plasma and therewith lowering of the effective concentration to which cells and tissues are exposed. The agents involved are temporarily stored on the albumin in the circulation, where they are available for the enzymes, particularly in the liver, that especially take care of biochemical conversion to products that are suitable for renal excretion (ref. 3).

In short, by the time chemical and pharmaceutical industry came to development, animal and man were more or less prepared for dealing with - in fact for defence against - exposure to the products of these industries, "synthetic xenobiotics", including drugs, thanks to their experience with "biogenic xenobiotics".

## 4) DRUG METABOLISM - DETOXIFICATION AND TOXIFICATION

In the early days of studies on this subject, drug metabolism was put more or less synonymous with detoxification as indicated, for instance, by the classic book entitled "Detoxication Mechanisms" by R.T. Williams, 1959 (ref. 4). In the case the metabolic elimination of xenobiotics concerns the application of drugs as therapeutics, the action is considered, at least by the prescribing physician, as desirable, although some components in the action still may count as undesirable, i.e. as side-effects. In fact in drug metabolism two classes of undesirable aspects can be distinguished:

1) the generation of toxic metabolites, still xenobiotic in nature, biotoxification;
2) the untimely elimination of the drug and complication of pharmacokinetics with as a consequence blurring of the dose-effect relationship due to drug metabolism.

## 5) BIOTOXIFICATION

Drug metabolites may be biologically active and in some cases are fully responsible for the action of the drug, which then in fact must be considered as a prodrug. With regard to the bioactive metabolites, distinctions can be made between:

a) Stable metabolites, active in a pharmacological sense, producing effects mostly related to that of the mother compound. This type of bioactivation which depending on the circumstances may be considered positive or negative will not be discussed in further detail here.

b) Chemically highly reactive, electrophilic, biologically alkylating intermediate products with a very short half-life time, formed in the course of the metabolic conversion - particularly oxidation, but also conjugation reactions. These intermediates act under covalent binding with nucleophilic groups on biological macromolecules such as nucleic acids and proteins. The resulting "chemical lesions" may have serious consequences such as:

a) carcinogenesis, involving chemical lesions in chromosomal DNA
b) mutagenesis, also involving chemical lesions in chromosomal DNA
c) possibly accelerated aging, caused by an increase in the error frequency in-

duced in chromosomal DNA,

d) teratogenesis, caused by disturbed cell proliferation due to chemical lesions during embryogenesis,

e) allergic sensitization, due to chemical lesions in proteins that cause them to act as allergens,

f) cell degeneration and necrosis, due to chemical damage to the membranes of lysosomes or to essential enzymes,

g) photosensitization, involving formation of reactive products by radiation of the drug or its metabolite(s), thus causing local chemical lesions, or formation of allergens.

As a matter of fact, toxic effects such as the ones just mentioned may also be induced by directly alkylating agents, such as some cytostatics used in the chemotherapy of cancer. Particularly troublesome with regard to the carcinogenesis and mutagenesis is the latency, the long lag-time between exposure to the agent and the appearance of the effect. This is partly due to the irreversible nature of the chemical lesions, which implies an accumulation of the effect. Like in the case of exposure to ionizing radiation, in fact each dose, how small it may be, counts and contributes to the effect. The total lifetime exposure constitutes the dose. Further, especially for lesions in chromosomal DNA, "syncarcinogenesis" due to various agents has to be taken into account. The chemical lesions in proteins are reversible to a certain extent on the basis of de novo synthesis of proteins. If the damage is limited, it may be largely reversible. This is not the case for protein damage resulting in allergic sensitization where the immunological memory of the lymphocytes is involved. In the case of damage to DNA, to a certain extent, especially short term, repair mechanisms may eliminate part of the chemical lesions.

## Metabolic systems protecting against biochemical lesions

In the line of evolution, nature not only developed biochemical clearance systems for xenobiotics, but also systems to control the risks thereof, namely those involved in the formation of reactive intermediate metabolites. The major protecting systems are: the glutathione transferase system, coupling glutathione to the chemically reactive, biologically alkylating metabolic intermediate, under the formation of conjugation products that appear in the urine as water soluble mercapturic acid derivatives (Fig. 3) and methylthiolation which implies the coupling of a methylthio ($-SCH_3$) group to the chemically reactive, electrophilic group in the alkylating metabolic intermediate, which thus is detoxicated. Further there is the epoxide hydratase system taking care of the hydrolysis of alkylating epoxides under the formation of diols which appear in the urine mostly as water-soluble phenol sulphate conjugates (Fig. 3) (ref. 1, 2, 5, 6).

Conjugation products such as those formed by acetylation or sulphate conjugation

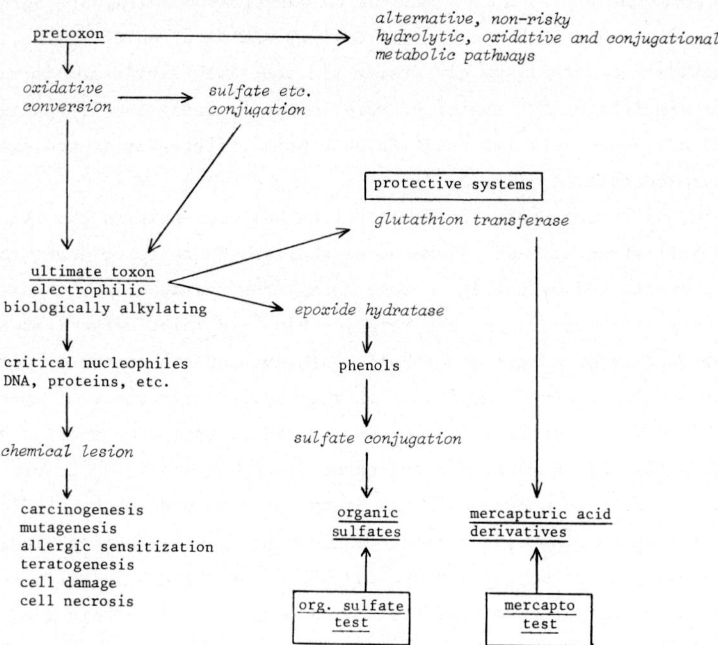


Fig. 3.

a rule are considered as harmless final detoxification products. However, although exceptionally, also such conjugation products, may be chemically reactive, biologically alkylating, and thus toxic. Also here the glutathione transferase system has a protective function.

Oxidation products formed in the course of drug metabolism may also lead to peroxides and oxidation products with a toxic character with regard to redox systems. An example of the damage caused is the formation of methemoglobin from hemoglobin. The latter type of action is well known for aniline derivatives. Again, glutathione has a protecting action since it contributes to the regeneration of hemoglobin from methemoglobin.

## Early detection of biotoxification

It will be clear from the foregoing that considerations on drug metabolism and its consequences such as biotoxification are essential already in an early phase, if possible on the drawing table, of drug design. Reasoning on the relationship between chemical structure and action in this respect implies recognition in the

*References p. 178*

structures of chemical groups potentially open to metabolic conversion. One has to differentiate between moieties leading to non-risky conversion - being particularly significant for the bioavailability and duration of action, i.e. the pharmacokinetics - and to risky conversion via reactive, alkylating intermediates particularly significant for toxicity. Moieties determining the lipophilicity of the compound are especially important in absorption, distribution and excretion and thus for pharmacokinetics (ref. 1, 2).

Remarkably, up to now, very little attention has been paid to the relationship between chemical structure and pharmacon metabolism. There is no doubt that such a relationship exists and even that in many cases, for instance in the case of particular enzymatic conversion, the relationships are relatively clear and simple. In vivo, however, often multiple metabolic pathways and a sequence of different metabolic steps are involved. Avoidance in the chemical structure of moieties potentially involved in biotoxification is advisable. Once compounds have been synthesized, a testing on mutagenic and carcinogenic action is advisable, in order to select or at least incorporate in the groups of compounds to be studied, the agents with a reduced risk with respect to the causation of chemical lesions. The use of the Ames-test, or better a properly chosen set of such in vitro tests, gives a reasonable indication of the risk for a mutagenic and carcinogenic action (ref. 7, 8, 9). By the way, one has to be well aware that even, although there is not a 100% correlation between mutagenic action as detected by such in vitro tests and the carcinogenic action in vivo, mutagenesis as such - for which the bill will be paid by future generations - , should be taken at least as serious as carcinogenesis.

A covalent binding of the toxon to biopolymers has as a consequence that the toxon cannot be extracted from the tissues anymore with hydrophilic or lipophilic solvents. A chemical sequestration is involved, to be distinguished from a physical sequestration where the compound, due to its metabolic stability combined with high lipophilicity, is kept back in the organism, predominantly by dissolution in the body fat. In balance studies, relating the dose to the quantity of the agent excreted, the fraction missing in that balance is important, even if it may be small, especially if chemical sequestration is involved (ref. 10).

The final inevitable step in the testing of a new drug, before its release for practical use, is the study of its carcinogenic potential in animal species. This still does not present a 100% safeguarding. Even after the agent has been released for application to the patient it has to be monitored in a toxicological sense. Introduction in a number of steps, comprising larger and larger groups of individuals, for drugs widely used for minor ailments numbering many thousands of individuals, is advisable.

## 6) BLURRING OF PHARMACOKINETICS AND THUS OF THE DOSE-EFFECT RELATIONSHIP BY DRUG METABOLISM

Therapeuticals usually are metabolized and eliminated at the time that the action is still wanted; thus sequential dosages have to be supplied. This in fact means a drug waste. Also other aspects of drug metabolism count as negative, e.g. the first-pass losses, due to metabolic conversion in the intestinal wall and the liver, the patient-to-patient and intra-patient variations in metabolic capacity with as a result a highly variable bioavailability, and the drug interactions related to drug metabolism. A highly variable relationship between dose and plasma level due to drug metabolism makes expensive therapeutic monitoring on basis of plasma level measurements, especially of drugs with a small therapeutic margin, necessary. Species differences, mostly related to differences in drug metabolism make extrapolation of animal data to the human situation difficult. An answer to the problems inherent in drug metabolism may be the development of drugs resisting drug metabolism, metabolic stabilization (ref. 1, 2, 11).

If short or ultrashort action is required or at local application, systemic action has to be avoided, introduction of suitable, safe, vulnerable moieties may be required. The same holds true in the case that the prodrug principle is to be applied. In general, however, avoidance of drug metabolism or reduction of it to the possible minimum will be advantageous.

For metabolically stable agents pharmacokinetics (absorption, distribution and excretion) are mainly determined by the balance between lipid and water solubility as expressed by the partition coefficient which in its turn is related to the $pK_A$-value. An exception has to be made for active transport processes. A modulation of pharmacokinetics on the basis of adaptation in the partition coefficient will usually be much simpler than adaptation in the metabolic pathways and the rates of conversion. Often various metabolic pathways and a sequence of different metabolic conversions are involved in the processing of one drug.

With regard to metabolic stabilization two aspects have to be taken into account:
1) Metabolic stabilization in general, predominantly aimed at the simplification and control of pharmacokinetics. In this case a reduction of the fraction of the dose metabolized counts.
2) Metabolic stabilization, particularly concerned with those moieties in the molecule that can be converted to electrophilic, alkylating groups. The aim is to control biotoxification. In this case a reduction in the absolute quantity of reactive intermediates counts.

## 7) METABOLIC STABILIZATION TO CONTROL PHARMACOKINETICS

Metabolic stabilization implies a longer half-life time and therewith less drug waste, less exposure to unnecessary quantities of the drug in repeated application, and simpler dosage regimens and therewith a better patient compliance.

Metabolic stabilization contributes to a reduction in drug interactions which in many cases are generated on the drug metabolic level.

Metabolic stabilization reduces the patient-to-patient and the intra-patient variability in the relationship between dose and effect, since this variability is largely based on differences and variations in the drug metabolic capacity.

Metabolic stabilization will reduce the variability in the relationship between dose and plasma concentration. This will reduce or eliminate the need for expensive therapeutic monitoring via plasma drug concentration measurements for drugs with a relatively small therapeutic margin. The uncertainty in the dose-effect relationship which enforces plasma level monitoring is largely related to the variability in drug metabolism. Therapeutics that require therapeutic monitoring should be replaced as soon as possible by analogously acting new drugs which are pharmacokinetically better controlled, an aim which may be realized by metabolic stabilization. Such new drugs definitely cannot be regarded as "me-too" drugs, but in fact are badly needed revisions in the therapeutic arsenal (ref. 12, 13, 14).

Metabolic stabilization implies a reduction in species differences which are largely related to species differences in metabolic capacities. It will make the now highly uncertain transfer of animal data to man more reliable.

Metabolic stabilization will greatly reduce the number and significance of possibly active metabolites, which implies a fargoing reduction of elaborate and expensive studies on drug metabolites on both the preclinical and clinical level.

Metabolic stabilization will reduce the chance that the drug applied in fact is a prodrug or the situation that, besides the active agent applied, a number of more or less similarly active, but pharmacokinetically different metabolites complicate the picture. These situations which occur incidentally should in no way be regarded as advantageous. In the given circumstances it is advisable to consider (one of) the active metabolite(s) as a potential drug. Clearcut examples of this situation are found among the benzodiazepines (table 2). Various benzodiazepines on the market are in fact benzodiazepine metabolites. The use of the therapeutically active metabolites as such, especially the ones in the most advanced oxidized state, will automatically reduce the impact of metabolic conversion and thus reduce both the metabolic toxicological risks and the complexity of pharmacokinetics. If so required , the metabolite can be presented as a prodrug - e.g. to enhance absorption of the usually more hydrophilic metabolite. This has as a matter of fact to be based on a safe metabolic handle for bioactivation. As such,hydrolytic cleavage is to be preferred,but also oxidation of a saturated alkyl side-chain may be considered. Unsaturated alkyl side-chains may lead to risky epoxides. Similar reasonings hold true if a vulnerable moiety has to be introduced into the molecule in order to obtain an ultrashort or short action or to avoid systemic action after local application.

TABLE 2

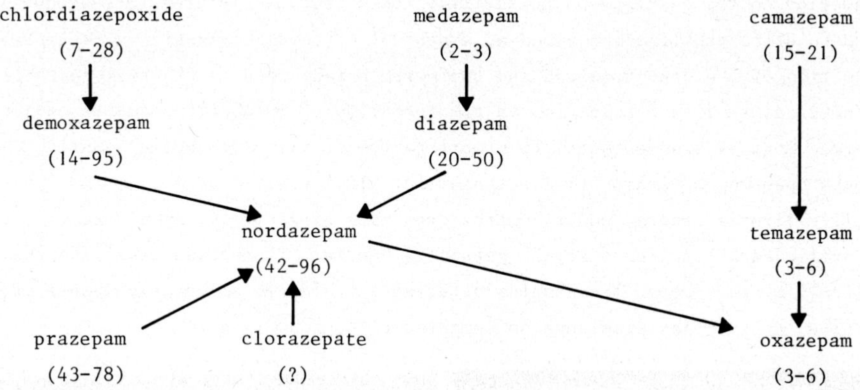


Flow scheme of benzodiazepine metabolism.
All substances (half-life in hours) are in use as drugs.

8) METABOLIC STABILIZATION AND CONTROL OF BIOTOXIFICATION

The aim is a reduction in the absolute quantity of reactive intermediates formed. There are two approaches here:

a) reduction in the dose of the drug required;

b) metabolic stabilization.

A reduction in the quantity of reactive, potentially carcinogenic, mutagenic, etc. intermediate products is to a certain extent a natural consequence of the development of highly potent agents. Only low dosages are required then, which implies the reduction of the quantity of metabolites anyway and therewith a reduction in the risk of induction of chemical lesions.

An increase in potency, as far as related to the process in the pharmacodynamic phase - that is to the induction of the effect on specific sites of action, and not to, for instance,reduction in first pass loss - implies that lower plasma and tissue concentrations are needed for the induction of the effect desired. If the therapeutic effect and side-effect are induced on different target molecules (receptors, enzymes, etc.), an increase in the affinity to the sites involved in the therapeutic action only under particular circumstances will go hand in hand with a comparable increase in the affinity to the sites on which the side-effects are induced. An exception has to be made for those cases in which the higher therapeutic potency is related to accumulation of the agent in a phase (e.g. a lipophilic phase), in which both the sites for therapeutic effect and side-effect are located. In those cases that the increase in therapeutic potency is related to a higher degree of complementarity of the active agent to the molecular sites for therapeutic action, as a rule, this tends to enhance selectivity and thus to reduce side-effects. Besides this the lowering of the dose required also implies a smaller metabolic turnover and thus a reduction in the quantity of potentially toxic reactive intermediate products.

Metabolic stabilization aimed at a control of pharmacokinetics also implies a reduction of the dose required and therewith a reduction in the risky metabolic turnover as well as a reduction in the formation of metabolic products causing pharmacological side-effects. If stabilization of risky metabolic handles, chemical groups open to conversion to electrophilic, alkylating moieties, is involved, biotoxification is brought under control even more effectively. An alternative to metabolic stabilization of risky metabolic handles, is introduction into the molecule of safe metabolic handles offering a preferred alternative route of conversion. An example is toluene as compared to benzene (see fig. 4).

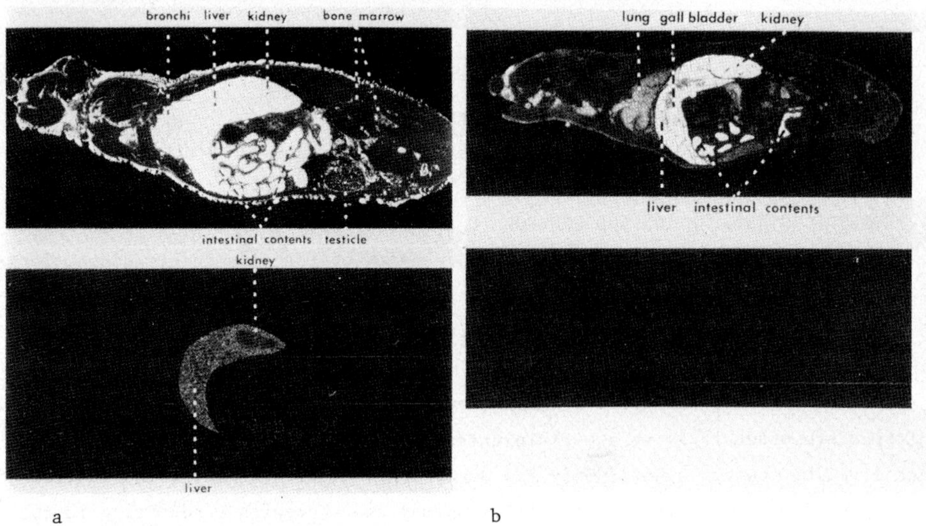


Fig. 4 a-b. Autoradiograms of mice 1 h after inhalation for 10 minutes of 5 µl $^{14}C$-benzene (a) and 10 µl $^{14}C$-toluene (b). Preparation: dried and evaporated (upper), additionally extracted (lower). Note: benzene metabolites are irreversibly bound in kidney cortex and liver (a); all toluene metabolites are completely extractable (b). After Bergman (ref.10).

The oxidative attack on the benzene ring leads to the formation of an epoxide as toxic reactive intermediate. In toluene the methyl group serves as a safe metabolic handle preferably attacked by the mixed function oxidases leading to benzoic acid as an end product. This principle is further elucidated in fig. 5.

The objection that metabolically stable agents, lipophilic enough to penetrate the central nervous system, would not be eliminated by renal excretion can be rejected for a number of reasons. Centrally active compounds excreted to a large extent unmetabolized exist. Examples are anorectic agents, such as phentermine and derivatives and phenphluramine, which still have relatively short half-life times

Fig. 5. AVOIDANCE OF RISKY AROMATIC RING OXIDATION (PHENOL FORMATION) BY INTRODUCTION OF ALTERNATIVE SAFER METABOLIC HANDLES.

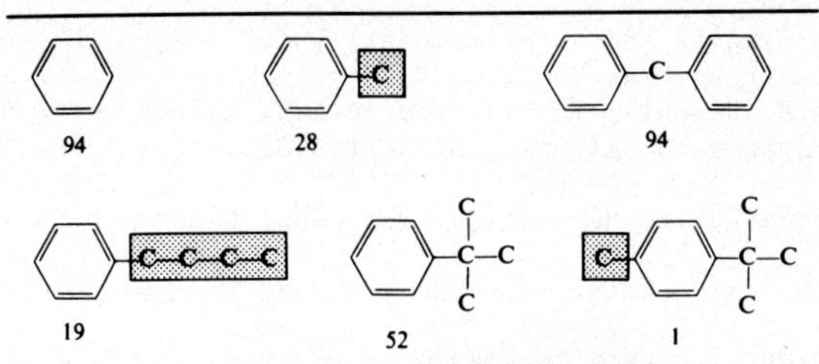


The figures indicate the organic (phenolic) sulphate as a fraction of the total sulphate excretion in the urine (rat). High values imply ring oxidation, low values imply attack along safer metabolic pathway. The low value 1 for the last compound - which implies nearly complete ring oxidation - results from the combination of blockade in the ring (tertiary butyl group) and alternative pathway (methyl group). Based on data from H.W. Gerarde. "Toxicology and Biochemistry of Aromatic Hydrocarbons." Elsevier, Amsterdam 1960 (ref. 15).

in the order of 10 to 30 hours (ref. 16). Metabolically stable agents are not necessarily highly lipophilic. On the other hand, prolonged half-life times in the order of 48 hours or even longer may allow for simple dosage regimens. If so required, the drugs, as far as tertiary amines, mostly weak bases, or weak acids are involved, - many centrally acting drugs belong to these categories - can be driven out by acidifying or alkalinizing the urine by means of, for instance, ammonium chloride or sodium bicarbonate, respectively.

Although our insight in the relationship between structure and metabolic conversion is still scanty, a number of principles applicable in metabolic stabilization or, if required so, metabolic destabilization, have been worked out and proven effective. As such can be mentioned the principle of "packing" of the vulnerable moiety thus sterically or otherwise hindering the enzymatic attack on the group concerned and blocking of vulnerable positions in the drug molecule, for instance by substitution of hydrogen by fluorine or possibly deuterium. For examples the reader is referred to various reviews in the literature (1, 2, 11, 21, 22).

In conclusion, drug metabolism should be regarded as acceptable only if it has a particular, well defined purpose, such as: realization of short or ultrashort action; solely local action under the avoidance of systemic action; prodrug formation aimed at, for instance, facilitation of absorption; avoidance of local irritation; protection against first-pass loss; selective bioactivation, e.g. in the target tissue; increase in water solubility for intravenous application; increase in lipophilicity to obtain depot preparations, etc. These are areas for the "soft drug approach" (ref. 17, 18, 19, 20).

REFERENCES

1 E.J. Ariëns, in E.J. Ariëns (Ed.), Drug Design, Vol. IX, Academic Press, New York, 1980, pp. 1-46.
2 E.J. Ariëns, A.M. Simonis and J. Offermeier, Introduction to General Toxicology, 2nd edn., Academic Press, New York, 1978.
3 E.J. Ariëns and A.M. Simonis, in S.H. Yap, C.L.H. Majoor and J.H.M. van Tongeren (Eds.), Clinical Aspects of Albumin, Nijhoff Medical Division, The Hague, 1978, pp. 149-171.
4 R.T. Williams. Detoxication Mechanisms, 2nd edn., Chapman & Hall Ltd., London, 1959.
5 R. van Doorn, Ch.M. Leijdekkers, R.P. Bos, R.M.E. Brouns and P.Th. Henderson, Ann. occup. Hyg., 24 (1981) 77-92.
6 W.G. Stillwell, TIPS, 2 (1981) 250-252.
7 V.A. Ray, Pharm. Rev.,30 (1978) 537-546.
8 F.A. de la Iglesia, R.S. Lake and J.E. Fitzgerald, Drug Metab. Revs.,11 (1980) 103-146.
9 T. Sugimura, S. Sato, M. Nagao, T. Yahagi, T. Matsushima, Y. Seino, M. Takeuchi and T. Kawachi, in P.N. Magee, S. Takayama, T. Sugimura and T. Matsushima (Eds.), Fundamentals in Cancer Prevention, Univ. of Tokio Press, Tokyo/Univ. Park Press, Baltimore, 1976, pp. 191-215.
10 K. Bergman, Scand. J. Work Environm. and Health, 5 (1979) suppl. 1, 5-263.
11 E.J. Ariëns and A.M. Simonis, in D.D. Breimer (Ed.), Towards Better Safety of Drugs and Pharmaceutical Products, Elsevier/North-Holland Biomedical Press, Amsterdam, 1980, pp. 3-29.
12 F.A. de Wolff, H. Mattie and D.D. Breimer (Eds.), Therapeutic Relevance of Drug Assays, Leiden University Press, Leiden, 1979.
13 L.F. Prescott, P. Roscoe and J.A.H. Forrest, in D.S. Davies and B.N.C. Prichard (Eds.), Biological Effects of Drugs in Relation to their Plasma Concentrations, MacMillan Press Ltd., London, 1973, pp. 51-81.
14 R. Sommer (Ed.), Kontrolle der Plasmaspiegel von Pharmaka, Georg Thieme Verlag, Stuttgart, 1980.
15 H.W. Gerarde, Toxicology and Biochemistry of Aromatic Hydrocarbons, Elsevier, Amsterdam, 1960.
16 H.A.J. Struyker-Boudier, in L. Szekeres (Ed.), Handb. exp. Pharmacol. 54/II, Adrenergic Activators and Inhibitors, Springer Verlag, Berlin, 1981, pp. 386-416.
17 E.J. Ariëns, in E.J. Ariëns (Ed.), Drug Design, Vol. II, Academic Press, New York, 1971, pp. 1-127.
18 S.H. Yalkowsky and W. Morozowich, in E.J. Ariëns (Ed.), Drug Design, Vol. IX, Academic Press, New York, 1980, pp. 121-185.
19 T. Higuchi and V. Stella (Eds.), Pro-drugs as Novel Drug Delivery Systems, ACS Symposium Series 14, American Chemical Society, Washington D.C., 1975.
20 N. Bodor, The Soft Drug Approach: Strategies for Design of Safer Drugs, 2nd Noordwijkerhout IUPAC-IUPHAR Symposium 1981, this volume.
21 J.F. Thomson, Biological Effects of Deuterium, Pergamon Press, Oxford, 1963.
22 T.A. Baillie (Ed.), Stable Isotopes, MacMillan Press Ltd., London, 1978.

J.A. Keverling Buisman (Editor), *Strategy in Drug Research* 


# STRUCTURE-PHARMACOKINETICS RELATIONSHIPS IN DRUG DESIGN

J.K.SEYDEL
Borstel Research Institute, Biochem.Dept., D-2061 Borstel (G.F.R.)


## ABSTRACT

Using linear or nonlinear models, quantitative structure-pharmacokinetics relationships are presented for different classes of drugs in various biological systems.

Pharmacokinetic parameters as rate constants for absorption, metabolism, and elimination, protein binding constant and volume of distribution and their variation as a function of structural modifications have been quantitatively explained by the variation in the lipophilic, steric, and electronic properties of the substituents or whole molecules. From the results presented the important role of overall lipophilicity of the drug molecule becomes obvious. The estimation of drug concentration profiles in plasma within homologous series of compounds knowing the relevant physicochemical properties is demonstrated. As pharmacodynamic effects are in most cases depending on more specific structural and physicochemical properties of the drug molecule, a more rational design of active drugs with special pharmacokinetic properties seems feasible.


---

## INTRODUCTION

The final aim in "rational drug design" is to predict or estimate pharmacodynamic, pharmacokinetic, and toxic properties before synthesis. Besides a scientific interest there are strong economic considerations behind these efforts.

The statement may be valid that considerable progress has been achieved in the understanding of drug action and in drug development during the last decades. This process was essentially stimulated by the methods applied in the analysis of structure-activity relationships. The development of high performance computer technology was the necessary precondition to change from qualitative (SAR) to quantitative

*References p. 199*

structure-activity relationship (QSAR) analysis during the last 20 years. These computerized statistical methods try to explain on a quantitative basis the observed variation in biological effects caused by the variation of substituents within certain classes of compounds. The variation in biological response as a reflection of the molecular changes in a series of drug molecules makes it feasible to interpret quantitatively the functional interdependence of both changes. In other words: the quantitative and qualitative influence of chemical and physicochemical properties of the drug molecule on the release of a biological response is recognized by such an analysis.

These methods can be a great help in guiding synthesis of more suitable derivatives and especially in gaining a better understanding of factors and processes important in drug action and in estimating the height of a biological effect, thus enabling a more rational design and development of drugs. In addition QSAR analyses enable the investigator to find exceptions within a data set which may allow the generation of a new lead.

The major problem in QSAR analysis is the ignorance about the molecular organization of the biological receptors and especially the complexity of the biological system. Drug action is proceeding in several branched or consecutive reaction steps. Each of these steps can be rate-determining. Due to these complex events the derivation of significant and meaningful QSAR is often difficult. Even if a statistically sound equation is obtained by regression analysis or other approaches it might still be difficult to interpret the results by physicochemical or biochemical reasoning.

These difficulties can be reduced if more simple biological models are selected, that means if the biological activity data are not determined in whole animals but in isolated systems, thus excluding the influence of pharmacokinetic properties in the first step. It is therefore not surprising that QSAR techniques have mainly successfully been applied to describe biological activities in isolated systems, especially in enzyme preparations. The results and the applied QSAR methods are discussed and summarized in several review articles and books (refs.1-5). In contrast published results on qualitative and especially quantitative structure-pharmacokinetics relationships are still rare. One of the reasons is the complexity of the pharmacokinetic processes. It is obvious, however, that the optimization of drug action under in vitro conditions does not guarantee a sufficient efficacy in vivo. The reason for this are the pharmacokinetic properties of a certain drug molecule, i.e. the lack of desirable therapeutic activity may not be due to inadequate drug-receptor interaction but rather to an inappropriate concentration and/or time course of drug presence at the specific receptor. Because of the complexity of biotransformation, metabolism, excretion, and unspecific binding one is inclined to deny the existence of straight forward relations between pharmacokinetic behaviour and molecular structure of the drug molecules. The derivation of such relations and their quantitative aspects is, however, a necessary precondition for a more rational drug design. The interest of this contribution is therefore focused on pharmacokinetic processes and parameters and to the demonstration of their qualitative and quantitative dependence on variations in molecular properties of drug molecules. The aim is to enable the drug designer to modify the chemical structure of a pharmacodynamically active drug in such a way that mainly the pharmacokinetic properties and not its pharmacodynamic action is changed. This implies restriction of the modifications to certain groups or moieties of the molecule. It requires information about the relationship between structure and activity especially with regard to the pharmacodynamic action. To achieve a more rational design of drugs our interest has to be to answer the question: how can pharmacokinetic properties and thereby the therapeutic effects be altered by structural modifications?

In general the degree of freedom for structural manipulations will be large with respect to pharmacokinetic behaviour as it depends mainly on overall properties of the molecule as for instance drug distribution and partitioning between lipid/water phases. The reason for this is the more or less uniform construction of biological membranes (ref. 6). This paper attempts to highlight the significance of pharmacokinetics in drug design and to discuss the most important factors on examples selected partly from the literature. It is obvious that most of the examples are derived from chemotherapeutics (antibacterials) where one of the important preconditions for the application of quantitative structure-pharmacokinetics relationships (QSPR) analysis is fullfilled, i.e. homologous series are available and have been tested.

## RESULTS

### Structure-pharmacokinetics relationships - general remarks

It is the object of pharmacokinetics to describe the change in drug and drug metabolite concentrations in various body fluids and tissues as a function of time. Mathematical equations and models are derived to describe the experimental data and to derive pharmacokinetic parameters as rate constant of absorption, $k_a$, of metabolism, $k_m$, of elimination, $k_{el}$, the volume of distribution, $V_d$, the degree of binding to serum proteins, $K_A$ (refs. 7-9). Pharmacokinetics describe the action of the macroorganism on the drug molecules. The knowledge of pharmacokinetic parameters has been used and is essential for:

- calculation of dose and dose interval
- estimation of bioavailability
- correlation of pharmacokinetic properties to pharmacodynamic effects
- use of pharmacokinetic information as diagnostic tool for detection of disturbance of the metabolic system and/or kidney functions

The possible quantitative relations between structure and pharmacokinetic parameters has, however, not been considered so far. The action of the macroorganism on the drug molecules can be summarized as follows: absorption, distribution, metabolism, binding to biopolymers (serum proteins), and elimination. The macroorganism acts differently on the molecules of different classes of drugs, however, in the same way on identical molecules. This is reflected in the pharmacokinetic parameters. These parameters are characteristic for a certain drug molecule similarly as its melting point, solubility, pKa, etc. though we have to admit that the determination is less accurate and the observed variation is larger because of the influence of the biological system.

As already pointed out at least 5 pharmacokinetic consequences can be expected as a result of structural changes in the drug molecule. These are changes in the:

1) rate and order of absorption, $k_a$
2) volume of distribution, $V_d$
3) rate and type of metabolism, $k_m$
4) affinity constant for "unspecific" binding to serum proteins and other biopolymers, $K_A$,(dissociation constant $K_D$)
5) rate and type of elimination, $k_{el}$ (clearance, Cl)

To estimate correctly the influence of small structural changes on the pharmacokinetics of a drug all 5 aspects have to be considered simultaneously. It is possible that the variation in structure is also changing the pharmacodynamic (or antibacterial) activity of the molecule.

In a homologous series of compounds the observed variation for the above pharmacokinetic parameters should show a structural dependence, i.e. the variation in the physicochemical parameters of the drug molecules should be reflected in a variation in their pharmacokinetic behaviour. This functional relation can be expressed by:

$$\Delta k_{el} = f(\Delta EL; \Delta Li/Hy; \Delta E_{St} \text{ etc.}) \quad (1)$$

where for example $\Delta k_{el}$ is the observed difference in the elimination rate constant comparing two members in a homologous series of compounds. The change in electron density of certain substructures in molecule A compared to B is expressed by ΔEL, the change in lipophilic/hydrophilic properties by ΔLi/Hy and the change in steric influence of a substituent by $\Delta E_{St}$. Electronic influences can be expressed for example by the dissociation constant (pKa), spectroscopic data (UV, NMR, IR) or σ-Hammett constants, lipophilic properties by the partition coefficient log P, $R_m$ values (ref.5) or retention times from high pressure liquid chromatography (ref.69) and steric influences by the molar volume or by other steric parameters like $E_s$-Taft. A more detailed description of this approach which is generally called the Linear Free Energy (LFE) approach or Hansch method and of other approaches are reviewed by Martin, Hansch and Seydel and Schaper (refs. 3-5). The basis of the Hansch approach is the assumption that different biological responses of the members of a homologous series correspond to changes of the free energy ΔG of the compounds occurring at their interaction with receptors or in biochemical reactions. Both gradations (of activity and ΔG) are supposed to be linearly related. Constants like rate constants, equilibrium constants and derived parameters like partition coefficients are also linearly related to free energy. For this reason the above function (eq 1) and the dependent variable (biological parameters) are expressed in the logarithmic form:

$$\log k_{el} = a \log P + b\, pKa + c\, E_{St} + k' \quad (2)$$

By computerized multiregression analysis the regression (a, b, c etc.) coefficients and the significance of their contribution are determined.

## Linear and nonlinear models

The following equations have proven to be suitable for the description of the observed variation in pharmacokinetic parameters or biological effects (BE) as a function of structural changes (lipophilicity, log P) of drug molecules. For a review see refs. 4-5 and 10-12.

$$\log BE = b \log P + x \qquad \text{linear} \quad (3)$$

$\log BE = -a(\log P)^2 + b \log P + c$ parabolic (4)

$\log BE = a \log P - b(\log P + 1) + c'$ linear ascending and descending; parabolic (5)

$\log BE = a \log P - \log(b P^d + 1) + c'$ nonlinear (6)

$\log BE = \log(a + b P^c)$ nonlinear (7)

The time dependence of such relations was stressed in papers of Penniston and Dearden (refs. 13-15). The transport phenomena were studied again by Kubinyi (refs. 16-17) using a 3-compartment model. The following bilinear equation was derived:

$\log BE = a \log P - b \log (\beta P + 1) + c'$ (8)

If P values are assumed to be different in biological systems compared to the P values measured in the system octanol/water this is accounted for by eq 8a introduced by Kubinyi (ref.10).

$\log BE = a \log P - b \log (\beta P^{\alpha} + 1) + c$ (8a)

If partly ionized drugs are considered this can be accounted for by

$\log BE - \log(1+10^{pH-pKa}) = -a(\log P)^2 + b \log P + c$ (4a)

This correction can also be applied to eq 8.

## Absorption and transport

One of the major demands for a drug to be used therapeutically is its bioavailability. Not only the fraction absorbed of a given dose but also its time course is of great importance for its therapeutic usefulness.The overall physicochemical character of a molecule should be decisive for its rate of absorption if distribution and transport of drug within a biological system are based on free diffusion through hydrophilic and lipophilic membranes. The absorption as determined by the diffusion coefficient, $k_d$ (Fick's law), depends on molecular properties as hydrophilicity, lipophilicity, polarity, degree of ionization, and molecular size. Strong acids or bases will not permeate lipophilic membranes or only to a small degree. A general equation 9 for the absorption of acids was derived from an aqueous/ lipid 2-compartment model with perfect sink on the second side of the lipid barrier (refs. 11, 18-19). If the rate constants for absorption of the ionized ($k_i$) and unionized ($k_{ui}$) forms are described by the corresponding partition coefficient $P_i$ and $P_{ui}$, eq 9 is obtained where $c\, P_{ui}{}^d$ and $g\, P_i{}^h$ are describing the influence of the unstirred layer on partitioning.

$$k_a = \frac{k_{ui}}{1 + 10^{pH-pKa}} + \frac{k_i}{1 + 10^{pKa-pH}} \qquad (9)$$

homologous series $\log P_i$ is linearly related to $\log P_{ui}$. Considering this the following general equation was derived for absorption of homologous acids and bases:

$$k_a = \frac{a\,P_{ui}^{\,b}}{c\,P_{ui}^{\,d} + 1 + 10^{pH-pKa}} + \frac{e\,P_i^{\,f}}{g\,P_i^{\,h} + 1 + 10^{pKa-pH}} \qquad (9a)$$

For acids the first term of eq 9 is an expression for pH dependent absorption of the unionized fraction and the second one for the ionized fraction whereas for bases the sequence is reversed. Both parts of eq 9a show a "nonlinear" dependence of absorption rate $\log k_a$ (undissociated or dissociated) on log P (see eq 4 - 8a). The terms reflecting the influence of the unstirred diffusion layer are important mainly for compounds of high lipophilicity. For this reason the term $g\,P_i^{\,h}$ in the equation for transport of acids probably can be neglected so that in practice eq 9b might be more realistic. In addition it can be assumed that in homologous series $\log P_i$ is linearly related to $\log P_{ui}$. This is described by eq 9b:

$$k_a = \frac{a\,P_{ui}^{\,b}}{c\,P_{ui}^{\,d} + 1 + 10^{pH-pKa}} + \frac{e\,P_{ui}^{\,f}}{1 + 10^{pKa-pH}} \qquad (9b)$$

This equation was applied to the data for buccal absorption of alkyl carboxylic acids (ref.20) and the values of a to f were determined by nonlinear regression analysis (ref. 11).

$a = 0.0527;\ b = 0.500;\ c = 0.0706;\ d = 0.564;\ e = 3.31\cdot10^{-4};\ f = 0.467$

$n = 71;\ r = 0.967;\ s = 0.119,\ k_a$ in $\min^{-1}$ (10)

The absorption data (rate of absorption $k_a$) for a series of sulfonamides (SA) (ref. 21) can be fitted to nonlinear models using eq 8:

$$\log k_a = 0.5 \log P - 0.61 \log(0.07P + 1) - 0.39 \qquad (11)$$

$n = 12,\ r = 0.89,\ s = 0.18$

or eq 4:

$$\log k_a = 0.44 \log P - 0.09 \log P^2 - 0.396 \qquad (12)$$

$n = 12,\ r = 0.89,\ s = 0.16$

i.e. the rate of absorption depends nonlinearly on the lipophilicity of the drug molecules.

It is interesting to note that similar results were obtained for SA from in vivo studies using a Satorius absorption simulator ($k_D$) (ref. 22) and in vivo data ($k_a$)

$$k_D \times 10^{-3} = 5.74\, k_a + 0.61 \qquad (13)$$

$n = 15,\ r = 0.93,\ s = 0.43$

Binding to serum proteins

Protein binding which decreases the free fraction which can diffuse to the receptor site can influence the following parameters:

1) the necessary therapeutic dose
2) the volume of distribution
3) the degree of metabolism
4) the rate and type of elimination (only the unbound fraction is glomerularly filtered)
5) the serum protein binding of other drugs administered simultaneously

It is not accidental that especially for the relation between degree of protein binding of drugs and their physicochemical properties many quantitative examples have been published (see ref. 11). The reason for this is that the protein binding can be determined separately from other influences of the macroorganism in in vitro experiments. Again most of the examples are derived from antibacterial drugs because long homologous series are available and the influence of protein binding on antibacterial effects is important. It has been shown that only the free not protein bound fraction of chemotherapeutics can diffuse to the locus of infection. Arguments concerning the contribution of ionic or lipophilic forces on protein binding have often been described in the literature. From the many published results it becomes obvious, however, that in most of the given examples both forces are operative if ionizable compounds are involved. Opposite results are explainable by the characteristics of the series studied. As long as the pKa is kept almost constant, a discriminating role in the determination of the degree of protein binding cannot be expected. Increasing degree of binding of SA to albumin with increasing fractions of ionized drug has for example clearly been demonstrated (refs. 21, 23-25) by studying the protein binding of SA as a function of pH.

Binding of homologous series of various drugs has been determined by Scholtan (refs. 26-27). Some of these quantitative relationships are given in the following equations:

| | | n | r | s | |
|---|---|---|---|---|---|
| Penicillins: | $\log K = 1.32 \log P + 0.37$ | 8 | 0.97 | 0.14 | (14) |
| SA: | $\log K = 1.15 \log P + 1.23$ | 8 | 0.97 | 0.17 | (15) |
| Steroidbisguanylhydrazones: | $\log K = 1.23 \log P - 0.05$ | 15 | 0.97 | 0.11 | (16) |
| Steroid-hormones: | $\log K = 1.65 \log P - 2.57$ | 4 | 0.99 | 0.06 | (17) |

The binding constant K as defined by Scholtan is not identical with

$K_A$ obtained from a Scatchard plot. If the binding data derived by Singhvi et al. (ref. 28) are analyzed where percent binding (%) is given, the following correlation equation is obtained for penicillins:

$$\log\left(1 - \frac{\%}{100}\right) = -1.12 \log P + 1.01 \qquad (18)$$

$n = 7, \quad r = 0.98, \quad s = 0.15$

It is remarkable that the influence of lipophilicity on the protein binding of these very different classes (eq 14-18) of compounds is very similar (similar regression coeff.). Only the intercept differs indicating the contribution of the parent molecule. The influence of the parent molecule can also be demonstrated on two closely related series of SA, i.e. sulfapyrimidines and sulfapyridines which per se show highly significant correlations between their protein binding (dissociation constant, $K_D$) and lipophilicity (ref. 29) (Fig. 1) (eq 19-20).

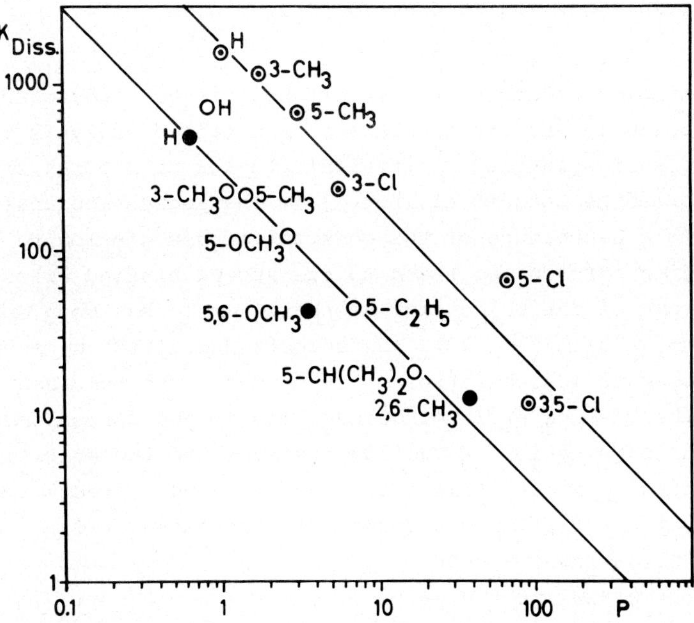


Fig. 1. Correlation between log $K_D$ (dissociation constant of the drug albumin complex) and log P (partition coefficient, octanol/water) for a series of sulfapyridines (⊙) and 2- and 4-sulfapyrimidines (o, •).

In combination (eq 21), however, a remarkable drop in the significance of the correlation is observed. If the difference in the contribution of the parent molecule is considered with an indicator variable I (I = 1 for sulfapyrimidines and I = 0 for sulfapyridines) a highly significant correlation for the combined data set is observed (eq 22):

| | | n | r | s | |
|---|---|---|---|---|---|
| Sulfapyridines: | $\log K_D = -0.97 \log P + 3.24$ | 6 | 0.96 | 0.24 | (19) |
| Sulfapyrimidines: | $\log K_D = -0.99 \log P + 2.49$ | 9 | 0.96 | 0.17 | (20) |
| in combination: | $\log K_D = -0.85 \log P + 2.73$ | 15 | 0.84 | 0.39 | (21) |
| | $\log K_D = -0.97 \log P - 0.70\, I + 3.24$ | 15 | 0.97 | 0.169 | (22) |

The protein binding increases with increasing lipophilicity. If in addition the ionization varies (different pKa of the SA) and substituents are in o-position ($I_o$) eq 23 is obtained for a set of sulfapyridines and their binding ($K_A$) to rat serum (ref. 30), where $I_o$ is an indicator variable which is equal to 1 for o-substituted derivative and 0 for other derivatives.

$$\log K_A = 0.20 \log P - 0.13\, pKa - 0.47\, I_0 - 4.96 \qquad (23)$$

$n = 19, \quad r = 0.92, \quad s = 0.20$

The last examples underline the importance of the study of closely related series in the first data set. A detailed analysis of the binding of sulfonylureas to different classes of binding sites has been performed by Goto et al.(ref. 31). The regression analysis resulted in a dependence of the constant of association to the first binding site on log P and to the second binding class on log P and pKa of the molecules. Another example has been described by Lüllmann et al. (ref. 32). The authors described the accumulation (T/M = tissue to medium ratio) of 16 neutral, cationic and anionic drugs in the resting atria of guinea pigs by the corresponding log P or a linear combination of the log P values and the ability of the drugs to bind to atrial homogenate (log % bound/% free = log B/F). An identical correlation was found for stimulated atria.

$$\log T/M = 0.446 \log P - 0.06 \qquad (24a)$$

$n = 16, \quad r = 0.928, \quad s = 0.44$

$$\log T/M = 0.247 \log P + 0.464 \log B/F + 0.729 \qquad (24b)$$

$n = 16, \quad r = 0.978, \quad s = 0.25$

It seems necessary to remark that there is a significant intercorrelation between log P and log B/F (r = 0.80).

Volume of distribution

The apparent volume of distribution of a drug ($V_D = D/c_0$) where D is the administered dose and $c_0$ is the plasma concentration at t = 0 after i.v. injection, cannot be smaller than the volume of the blood plasma. It can become larger if the drug can pass biological membranes such as the capillary membranes or the blood-brain barrier, or if the degree of distribution in certain tissues increases. The degree of distribution therefore depends on the following factors:

1) Lipophilicity of the drug molecule and lipophilicity of the tissue
2) Degree of ionization of the drug molecules
3) Degree of binding to serum proteins and tissue constituents

Kjaer et al. (ref. 33) have reported that the administration of the more lipophilic methoxymethylester of hetacillin resulted in a more extensive distribution into tissue compared to ampicillin. By esterification the distribution increases from 3 % of body volume to 85 %. Even if most of the examples describing the relation between physicochemical structure and the degree of distribution are still of qualitative or semiquantitative nature, it is obvious that structural modifications for a specific drug distribution can become of great importance in drug design. Especially antimicrobial drugs are most suitable for this type of research, as structural influences on pharmacokinetic behaviour and on pharmacodynamic effect (antibacterial effect) can separately be studied. Because many of these drugs as antibiotics like penicillins, cephalosporins, but also sulfonamides, are very often highly protein bound, this must be considered to understand their distribution pattern. As these drugs show large variation in protein binding and in lipid solubility they have also varying degrees of distribution into tissues and therefore different $V_d$ values. The characteristics of penetration to the locus of infection in various tissues is a selection criterion in therapy and thus important for drug design.

The relationship for a nonhomologous series of 15 basic drugs between $V_d$ and partition coefficients and degree of ionization has been studied by Watanabe and Kozaki (refs.34-35) and a mathematical expression has been derived to estimate $V_d$ based on this relationship. This expression can be simplified by combining constants to give:

$$\log V_d = \log (a + b P^c) \qquad (25)$$

Applied to the data of Watanabe and Kozaki (refs. 34-35) the following values for the constants are obtained (ref. 11):

$$a = 1.325;\ b = 0.19;\ c = 0.83;\ n = 15;\ r = 0.91;\ s = 0.281 \qquad (26)$$

There are two mechanisms for penetration of capillary membranes: transcapillary diffusion for lipid soluble drugs and passage via water channels for strongly hydrophilic drugs. Distribution from the capillary system has been quantitatively correlated with the lipophilicity of penicillins and cephalosporins (ref. 36). For characterization of lipophilicity $R_m$ values have been used. The regression equation obtained was:

$$\log V_{d_u} = 0.629\, R_m + 1.48 \qquad (27)$$

$n = 7, \quad r = 0.986, \quad s = 0.09$

In this correlation $V_{d_u}$, the volume of distribution of the unbound fraction, has been used to eliminate the influence of protein binding on the relationship. The volume of distribution is linearly increasing with increasing lipophilicity ($R_m$ value) of the penicillins.

Another example can be derived from SA. The volume of distribution for the free unbound drug (SA) depends on lipophilicity of the neutral form and ionization of the SA as well as on o-substitution ($I_0$).

$$\log V_{d_u} = 0.30 \log P_{ui} - 0.04\, pKa - 0.39\, I_o + 2.99 \qquad (28)$$

$n = 18, \quad r = 0.92, \quad s = 0.14$

This can reasonably be expected because more lipophilic drugs can leave the capillary system more easily and they may also be bound to lipid and tissue, thus decreasing the concentration in the central compartment. These examples are a special case of the more general preceding equation (eq 25). It is limited to its linear ascending part.

It is well known from practice that hydrophilic and ionized drugs can only with difficulty pass the blood brain barrier due to the very special construction of this membrane (ref. 37). This has been used to prevent side effects of the central type without losing the wanted peripheral action. One example is atropine which can penetrate the brain barrier whereas methylatropine cannot because of its quaternary structure. Another example is the neurotoxic effect of penicillins which is clearly related to their lipophilicity (ref. 38). This information can serve for the estimation of the neurotoxicity of penicillins. Using the nonlinear model of eq 25 this relationship has been quantified (ref. 11) (Fig. 2) (eq 29).

$$\log \text{neurotox.index} = \log (11.38 + 14.2P^{2.2}) \qquad (29)$$

$n = 8, \quad r = 0.997, \quad s = 0.005$

Other interesting results on the permeation of the brain barrier have also been obtained (see refs. 39-41). In these studies the analgesic activity (ED) of 11 morphine-like compounds after intravenous (iv) and intraventricular (iventr.) application has been measured and compared. A dramatic difference in analgesic activity was observed.

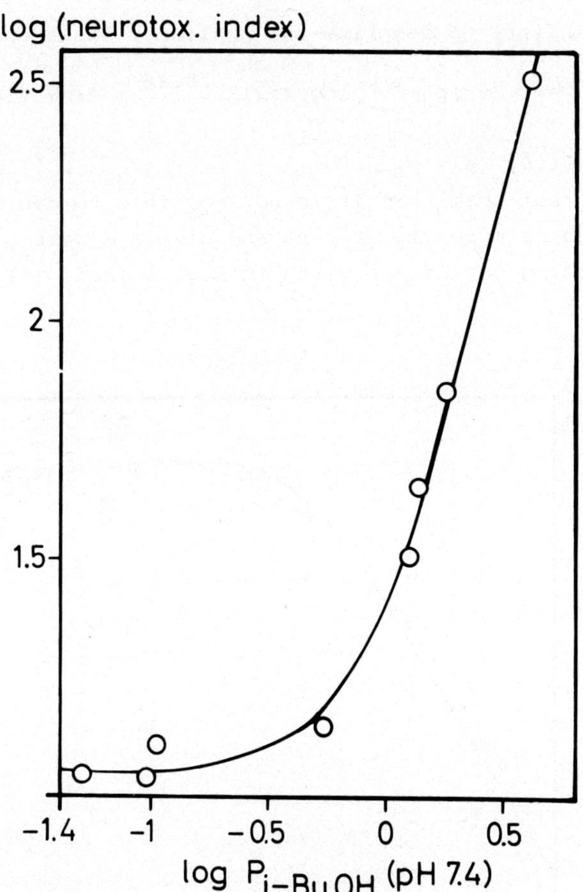


Fig. 2. Nonlinear dependence of the neurotoxic index of penicillins on their lipophilicity (ref. 11, 38).

After intraventricular administration ($c_{iventr.}$) the effect of the different derivatives was 3-3000 times stronger than if they were injected ($c_{iv}$) outside the brain compartment. There was a nonlinear dependence of the logarithm of the ratio $c_{iventr.}/c_{iv}$ on the lipophilicity of the derivatives. The lipophilic character was expressed by the partition coefficient P, determined in the system heptane/ phosphate buffer pH 4.7. The following equation was obtained by regression analysis:

$$\log \frac{c_{iventr.}}{c_{iv}} = 0.036 \log P - 0.09 (\log P)^2 - 0.673 \qquad (30)$$

$$n = 11, \quad r = 0.97, \quad s = 0.297$$

Another possibility to describe the nonlinear dependence is eq 31:

$$\frac{\log c_{iventr.}}{\log c_{iv}} = 0.79 \log P - \log (32.2 P^{0.86} + 1) + 0.82 \qquad (31)$$

n = 11, r = 0.99, s = 0.35

With the data set available it is not possible to decide unequivocally which equation is more significant and allows a more precise predictio The corresponding curves are given in Fig. 3 (ref. 11).

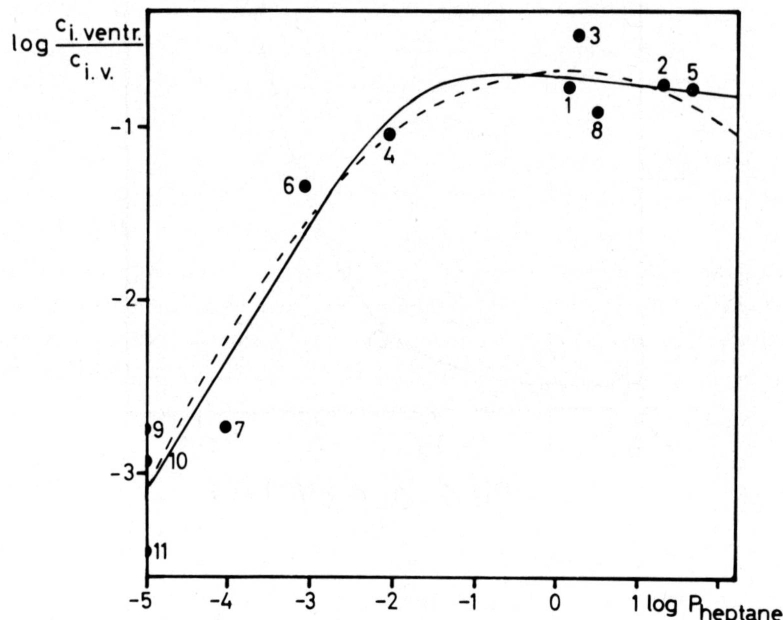


Fig. 3. Dependence of the logarithm of $c_{iventr.}/c_{iv}$ on log P parabolic (ref. 39)(---), bilinear (ref.19)(——).

The dependence of distribution into the brain on lipophilicity has been described also for barbiturates (ref. 42).

$$\log V_d = 0.17 \log P + 1.74 \qquad (32)$$

n = 7, r = 0.84, s = 0.06

Ritschel and Hammer (ref. 43) found that the dependence of the volume of distribution for 123 different drugs on their partition coefficient could be described by a single equation of high statistical significance.

$$\Delta'_{extrap.(f)} = 0.156\ P + 0.86 \qquad (33)$$

$n = 123,\ r = 0.94$

where $\Delta'_{extrap.(f)}$ is the volume of distribution, corrected for protein binding and extrapolated using a 2-compartment open model. The dependent and the independent variable are used in the non-logarithmic form. We can conclude that this pharmacokinetic parameter again depends mainly on the lipophilicity of the drug molecule (further examples are given in ref. 11).

Metabolism (biotransformation)

Variation in effectivity within a series of chemically related compounds is related to intrinsic potency at the specific receptor site, pharmacokinetic behaviour and biotransformation properties of the drug molecules. Metabolism studies are therefore an important part in drug development programs. The study of the pharmacokinetics and metabolic properties of drugs has essentially contributed to the safety of new drugs. Therefore drug design must consider the influence of metabolism.

Only few quantitative SAR studies are available in the literature. The reason is the lack of homologous series studied and the complexity of the biological system and biological pathway. Quantitative and semiquantitative aspects of structure-metabolism correlations have been reviewed in refs. 12 and 44-49. Depending on route of administration, drug, structure, and distribution, metabolism can take place in different organs. Again a separate study on isolated biological systems is indicated. Even in such isolated systems at least 2 processes may become rate determining:

1) diffusion to and binding at the metabolizing enzyme
2) biochemical reaction at the receptor site and/or release of the products formed

An example is given from studies of the $N^4$-acetylation of SA in vitro on crude microsomal preparations of rat liver (ref. 30). The observed variation of acetylation can be described by eq 34:

$$\log k_m = -0.21 \log P + 0.13\ pKa - 1.29 \qquad (34)$$

$n = 10,\quad r = 0.90,\quad s = 0.18$

The rate of acetylation decreases with increasing lipophilicity and decreasing ionization. This is opposite to the results obtained for protein binding (eq 23) and opposite to the general opinion that more lipophilic drugs are metabolized to a greater extent.

An excellent support for these results given in eq 34 was obtained by the analysis of in vivo data of the $N^4$-acetylation of SA in human (data from ref. 50). The following regression equation was achieved:

$$\log k_m = -0.42 \log P + 0.14 \, pKa - 2.89 \tag{35}$$

$n = 11, \quad r = 0.84, \quad s = 0.34$

Both regression equations (34-35) show a striking similarity. The larger regression coefficient with log P in eq. 35 is easily explained by the larger amount of protein available in vivo for binding of SA.

The results are in agreement with the assumption that only the not protein bound fraction of SA is accessible to metabolism by the liver microsomes. This is underlined by the highly significant dependence of $k_m$ on the percentage unbound and unionized drug as described for the data of Wiseman and Nelson (ref. 50) by eq 36:

$$\log k_m = 0.44 \log (\% \text{ unbound, unionized}) - 2.05 \tag{36}$$

$n = 11, \quad r = 0.90, \quad s = 0.25$

The rate determining step seems to be the diffusion of SA from the SA protein complex to the microsomes during liver passage. The variation in rate of N-dealkylation (DEA) of 15 N-alkylsubstituted amphetamines in humans has been quantitatively described as a function of lipophilicity and volume of the substituent (ref. 51).

$$\log DEA = 0.28 \log P - 0.015 \, V_R \tag{37}$$

$n = 16, \quad r = 0.93, \quad s = 0.142$

This equation indicates that dealkylation increases with increasing lipophilicity of the molecule and decreases with the volume of the substituent ($V_R$) which is eliminated. According to the authors this might be due to two factors:

1. High lipophilicity favours the affinity to the cytochrome P-450 and hence a fast reaction
2. The more bulky the split off substituents are, the slower the initial $C_\alpha$-hydroxylation ultimately leading to N-dealkylation appears to be.

Other examples where the relationship between rate of metabolism of compounds by various microsomal preparations and physicochemical properties are discussed are given in refs. 52-57.

Elimination

Drug elimination from the various body compartments occurs via excretion of unmetabolized and metabolized drugs. The main routes are renal and biliary excretion. Renal excretion occurs normally by first order processes (c = drug concentration).

$$dc/dt = k_{el}\ c \qquad (38)$$

Besides the elimination rate constant the clearance concept is used in pharmacokinetics to characterize the decrease in concentration of a drug in plasma. Clearance is defined as the volume of plasma which is cleared from the drug per unit of time by the clearing organ. It is related to the physiological organ perfusion rate and extraction efficacy. In case of monoexponential decay clearance is expressed by

$$Cl = k_{el}V_d \qquad (39)$$

If more than one route of elimination exists, total clearance is the sum of the individual clearances.

$$Cl_{tot} = Cl_{metabolic} + Cl_{renal} + Cl_{hepatic} \text{ etc.} \qquad (40)$$

The renal excretion of a drug may involve 3 processes: glomerular filtration, tubular secretion and tubular reabsorption (refs. 58-59). As glomerular filtration is a physicochemical filtration process with a filtration rate of approximately 125 ml/min for human, no influence of structure and molecular size can be observed. It is important to recognize that only the unbound fraction of a drug is filtered by the glomeruli. The degree of binding, however, is depending on certain physicochemical properties of the drug molecule. The remaining 82 % of the renal plasma flow can deliver drug that may be secreted directly into the tubule. Tubular secretion is generally considered as an "active" or carrier mediated process and the number of receptor sites is necessarily limited. Therefore other drugs may compete with certain types of drugs for binding sites and inhibit their tubular secretion. A classical example is the inhibition of the tubular secretion of penicillin by probenecid. Again there will be a structural precondition for this type of interaction. No first order elimination is possible in case of saturation, i.e. the tubular excretion must be described by Michaelis-Menten kinetics. Probenecid itself is also tubularly secreted. The relative clearance for a homologous series of probenecid analogs has been evaluated (ref. 60) and correlated with log P ($CHCl_3$) (ref. 61). Omitting two derivatives the following regression equation was obtained:

$$\log Cl_R = -0.242 (\log P)^2 - 0.035 \log P + 0.578 \quad (41)$$

$n = 5, \quad r = 0.98, \quad s = 0.16$

Using the whole data set of Beyer (ref. 60) and estimating two log P values (-3.0 and + 3.5) nonlinear regression was performed to give eq 42:

$$\log Cl_R = -\log (0.35 + 0.013\, P^{1.12}) \quad (42)$$

$n = 7, \quad r = 0.99, \quad s = 0.14$

Tubular reabsorption of the drug from the tubule is caused by increasing concentrations in the tubular lumen. This return into the circulating plasma can be an "actively" or "passively" controlled process. The interest is focussed on the passive process because it is diffusion controlled. This type of reabsorption occurs in the distal portion of the tubule and requires uncharged drug molecules to permeate the lipid barrier of the renal tubular epithelium and to diffuse back into the circulating plasma. Thus the combination of the pH of the urine, the pKa of the drug molecule and its lipophilicit can determine the extent and rate of the reabsorption process as a function of the concentration of the effectively diffusable uncharged species. The influence of urinary pH on the rate of elimination has been shown and studied by many authors for several types of drugs. As an example the change in biological half life of SA with different pKa at various urinary pH values is given in Table 1 (ref. 62).

TABLE 1

The influence of the urine pH and of the state of wakefulness on the renal excretion of acidic drugs. Biological half lives, $t_{50\%}$ (hr), of 12 sulfonamides with different pKa' values (ref. 62).

| Compound | pKa' | pH 5 $t_{50\%}$ | pH 8 $t_{50\%}$ | $Q_{pH}$ | night $t_{50\%}$ | day $t_{50\%}$ | $Q_{n/d}$ |
|---|---|---|---|---|---|---|---|
| Sulfisoxazole | 4.9 | 9.5 | 4.7 | 2.0 | - | - | - |
| Sulfaethidole | 5.1 | 11.4 | 4.2 | 2.7 | - | - | - |
| Sulfasymazine | 5.5 | 17.8 | 7.3 | 2.4 | 35.0 | 13.5 | 2.9 |
| Sulfamethoxazole | 5.7 | 10.7 | 7.0 | 1.5 | 37.9* | 23.4* | 1.6 |
| Sulfadimethoxine | 5.9 | - | - | - | 38.7 | 26.3 | 1.5 |
| Sulfamethoxypyrazine | 6.1 | - | - | - | 110.6 | 49.1 | 2.3 |
| Sulfadiazine | 6.4 | - | - | - | 13.9 | 9.7 | 1.4 |
| Sulfamethoxine | 6.5 | - | - | - | 91.5 | 27.3 | 3.6 |
| 2-Sulfa-5-ethylpyrimidine | 6.9 | | | | 67.8 | 27.3 | 2.5 |
| Sulfadimethyloxazole | 7.2 | 8.0 | 6.7 | 1.2 | - | - | - |
| Sulfasomidine | 7.4 | 8.9 | 7.3 | 1.2 | 10.9 | 7.6 | 1.4 |
| Sulfanilamide | 10.5 | 9.6 | 9.6 | 1.0 | 12.7 | 11.1 | 1.1 |

* Values obtained from 3 patients with renal insufficiency

Only sulfanilamide with a pKa of 10.5 shows - as expected - no dependence of the biological half life on urinary pH. Another interesting example is the rate of renal excretion of amphetamines at different pH values of the urine (refs. 63-64). The reabsorption rate of only 4 SA has been studied by Owada et al. (ref. 65). From a regression analysis performed (ref. 11) the following equation was obtained:

$$\log k_{reabs.} = 0.39 \log P_{oct.(pH\ 7.4)} - 0.10 \qquad (43)$$

$n = 4, \quad r = 0.73, \quad s = 0.20$

The interrelation between reabsorption rate and biological half life $t_{50\%}$ is given in eq 44:

$$\log t_{50\%} = 1.93 \log k_{reabs.} + 1.54 \qquad (44)$$

$n = 4, \quad r = 0.97, \quad s = 0.15$

The rate of elimination is a very important factor in drug design. A too rapid or too slow excretion may exclude an active drug from therapeutic use. In combined therapy it might be desirable to have comparable excretion rates for two different drugs for a more convenient regimen. For a series of sulfapyrimidines with very similar pKa and some o-substituted derivatives studied in human the following equation was obtained:

$$\log k_{el} = -0.24 \log P_{ui} + 0.36\ I_o - 1.35 \qquad (45)$$

$n = 7, r = 0.90, \quad s = 0.15$

For a series of sulfapyridines with large variation in pKa studied in rats (ref. 30) the regression equation is:

$$\log k_{el} = -0.43 \log P_{ui} + 0.28\ I_o + 0.22\ pKa - 2.21 \qquad (46)$$

$n = 19, \quad r = 0.94, \quad s = 0.19$

The rate of elimination decreases with increasing lipophilicity and increasing ionization. The biliary excretion of penicillin seems to depend nonlinearly on their lipophilicity (refs. 61, 66).

$$\log \%_{excret.} = 0.13 (\log P)^2 - 0.79 \log P + 2.27 \qquad (47)$$

$n = 9, \quad r = 0.93, \quad s = 0.08$

in case of sulfathiazole an additional contribution of pKa is observed.

$$\log \%_{excret.} = -0.72 (\log P)^2 + 0.86 \log P - 0.40\ pKa + 3.2 \qquad (48)$$

$n = 9, \quad r = 0.94, \quad s = 0.242$

As pointed out in the general discussion of the processes in renal clearance we can expect rather simple relations between excretion rates and physicochemical properties of drug molecules as far as glomerular filtration and reabsorption rates are concerned. Yet there are only very few successful quantitative relationships cited in the literature. The main reason is the lack of data from homologous series of compounds where no change in the type of elimination and metabolism may occur and which are therefore suitable for a quantitative analysis of structure-pharmacokinetic relationships. Most of the data can only qualitatively be discussed. Some of these qualitative examples are reviewed by Fung et al. (ref. 67).

Finally an example is given, where the correlation equations derived between lipophilicity and degree of ionization and $V_d$ and $k_{el}$ (eq 28, 46) have been used to estimate a blood concentration curve after iv injection of SA to rats. In Fig. 4 the experimental curve obtained and the curve predicted from knowing the lipophilicity and ionization constant are compared using eq 49 and inserting eq 28 and 46 for $V_{d_u}$ and $k_{el}$.

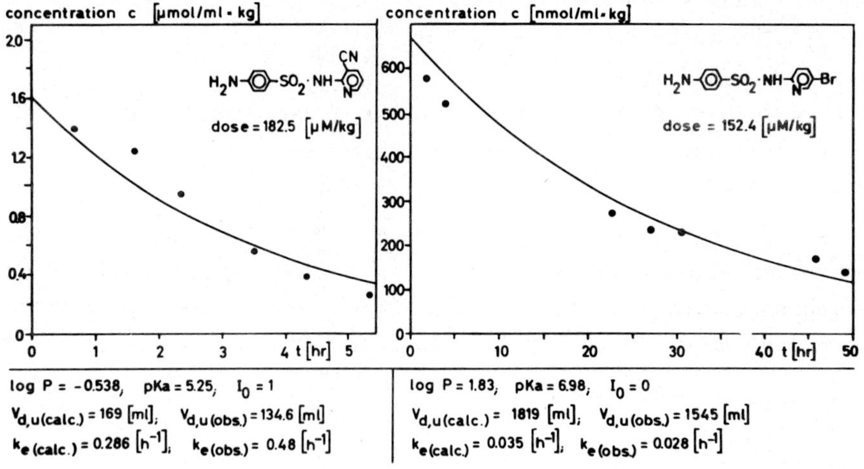


Fig. 4. Plasma concentration curve of sulfonamides after iv injection into rats; (●) measured values, solid line simulated according to equations 28, 46, 49. (ref. 70).

$$c_p = \frac{D}{V_{d_u}(1 - p)\,G}\, e^{-k_{el}\, t} \qquad (49)$$

where $c_p$ is the plasma concentration, D means dose, $V_d$ volume of distribution, G body weight, (1 - p) correction for protein binding $k_{el}$ elimination rate constant and t time. Such calculations have also been published by Ritschel and Hammer (ref. 43).

## Concluding remarks

Despite the interrelationship of pharmacokinetic parameters the analysis of quantitative structure-pharmacokinetics relationships seems to be feasible. Because of the discussed limitation one should not always expect correlation equations with high statistical significance. If it can be assumed from additional information and knowledge that the correlation is biologically meaningful this information can be of great help in further development of the studied series. Another important tool in QSPR analysis is the detection of outliers, i.e. the detection of derivatives which deviate significantly from the regression found. They may lead to the detection of unexpected metabolic or excretion patterns.

The scale up of information from separately performed QSAR and QSPR analyses can become a decisive instrument for a rational drug design (refs. 30, 68).

## REFERENCES


1 W.P.Purcell, G.E.Bass and J.M.Clayton, Strategy of Drug Design: a Molecular Guide to Biological Activity, Wiley, New York, 1973.

2 C.Hansch, Relations structure-activité, Societe de Chimie Therapeutique, Paris, 1975.

3 C.Hansch in N.B.Chapman and J.Shorter (Ed.),Correlation Analysis in Chemistry: Recent Advances, Plenum, New York, 1978, pp397-438.

4 Y.C.Martin, Quantitative Drug Design, Marcel Dekker, New York, 1978.

5 J.K.Seydel and K.-J.Schaper, Chemische Struktur und biologische Aktivität von Wirkstoffen. Methoden der Quantitativen Struktur-Wirkung-Analyse, Verlag Chemie, Weinheim, 1979.

6 E.D.Korn, Annu.Rev.Biochem., 38(1969)263-288.

7 R.E.Notari, Biopharmaceutics and Pharmacokinetics, Marcel Dekker, New York, 1975.

8 E.Gladtke and H.M.von Hattingberg, Pharmacokinetics, Springer, Berlin, 1979.

9 W.A.Ritschel, Angewandte Biopharmazie, Wissenschaftliche Verlagsgesellschaft, Stuttgart, 1973.

10 H.Kubinyi, in E.Jucker (Ed.), Progress in Drug Research, Vol. 23, Birkhäuser Verlag, Basel, 1979

11 J.K.Seydel and K.-J.Schaper, in M.Rowland and G.Tucker (Eds.), Pharmacology and Therapeutics, Pergamon Press, Oxford, 1982.
12 Y.C.Martin, J.Med.Chem., 24(1981)229-237.
13 J.T.Penniston, L.Beckett, D.L.Bentley and C.Hansch, Mol.Pharmacol., 5(1969)333-341.
14 J.C.Dearden and M.S.Townend, J.Pharm.Pharmacol., 28(1976)13P.
15 J.C.Dearden and M.S.Townend, Pestic.Sci., 10(1979)87-89.
16 H.Kubinyi, J.Med.Chem., 20(1977)625-629.
17 H.Kubinyi, J.Pharm.Sci., 67(1978)262-263.
18 K.-J.Schaper, J.Chem.Res., (1979)S,357.
19 K.-J.Schaper, unpublished results.
20 A.H.Beckett and A.C.Moffat, J.Pharm.Pharmacol. 20(1968)239S-247S.
21 K.Kitao, K.Kubo, T.Morishita, N.Yata and A.Kamada, Chem.Pharm.Bull., 21(1973)2417-2426.
22 M.Yamazaki, Y.Ito, J.Iwane and N.Yata, Yakuzaigaku,37(1977)1-7.
23 R.Elofsson, S.O.Nilsson and A.Agren, Acta Pharm.Suecica, 7(1970) 473-482.
24 R.Elofsson, S.O.Nilsson and B.Kluczykowska, Acta Pharm.Suecica, 8(1971)465-474.
25 A.Agren, R.Elofsson and S.O.Nilsson, Acta Pharm.Suecica, 8(1971). 475-484.
26 W.Scholtan, Arzneim.-Forsch., 18(1968)505-517.
27 W.Scholtan, Arzneim.-Forsch., 28(1978)1037-1047.
28 S.M.Singhvi, A.F.Heald and E.C.Schreiber, Chemotherapy, 24(1978) 121-133.
29 J.K.Seydel, G.Miller and P.H.Doukas, in P.Pratesi (Ed.), Medicinal Chemistry, Butterworths, London, 1973, pp.139-151.
30 J.K.Seydel, D.Trettin, H.P.Cordes, O.Wassermann and M.Malyusz, J.Med.Chem., 23(1980)607-613.
31 S.Goto, H.Yoshimoto and M.Nakase, Chem.Pharm.Bull., 26(1978)472-480.
32 H.Lüllmann, P.B.M.W.M.Timmermans, G.M.Weikert and A.Ziegler, J.Med.Chem., 23(1980)560-565.
33 T.B.Kjaer, P.G.Welling and P.O.Madison, J.Pharm.Sci., 66(1977) 345-347.
34 J.Watanabe and A.Kozaki, Chem.Pharm.Bull., 26(1978)3463-3470.
35 J.Watanabe and A.Kozaki, Chem.Pharm.Bull., 26(1978)665-667.
36 W.A.Craig and P.G.Welling, Clin.Pharmacol. 2(1977)252-268.
37 T.S.Reese and M.J.Karnovsky, J.Cell Biol. 34(1967)207-217.
38 T.R.Weihrauch, Naunyn Schmiedebergs Arch.Pharmakol. 289(1975) 55-64.
39 E.Kutter, A.Herz, H.Teschemacher and R.Hess, J.Med.Chem. 13(1970) 801-805.
40 E.Kutter, Arzneimittelentwicklung. Grundlagen - Strategien - Perspektiven, Georg Thieme, Stuttgart, 1978.
41 B.Von Cube, H.Teschemacher, A.Herz and R.Hess, Naunyn-Schmiedebergs Arch.Pharmakol. 265(1970)455-473.
42 Y.J.Lin, S.Awazu, M.Hanano and H.Nogami, Chem.Pharm.Bull. 21 (1973)2749.
43 W.A.Ritschel and G.V.Hammer, Int.J.Clin.Pharmacol.Therapy, Toxicol., 18(1980)298-316.
44 F.J.Di Carlo, Drug Metabolism Reviews, Vol.1, Marcel Dekker, New York, 1973.
45 D.C.Hobbs and H.M.McIlhenny, Ann.Rep.Med.Chem., 11(1976)190-199.
46 J.W.Bridges and L.F.Chasseaud, Progress in Drug Metabolism, Vol. 1, John Wiley and Sons, London, 1976.
47 B.H.Migdalof, in F.J.Di Carlo (Ed.), Drug Metabolism Reviews, Vol. 13, Marcel Dekker, New York, 1978, pp. 196-205.
48 G.T.Tucker, Br.J.Anaesth., 51(1979)641-648.
49 C.Hansch, in F.J.Di Carlo (Ed.), Drug Metabolism Reviews, Vol. 1, Marcel Dekker, New York,1973, pp. 1-14.

50 E.H.Wiseman and E.Nelson, J.Med.Chem. 53(1964)992.
51 B.Testa and B.Salvesen, J.Pharm.Sci., 69(1980)497-501.
52 T.D.Yih, J.M. van Rossum, Biochem.Pharm., 26(1977)2117.
53 Y.C.Martin and C.Hansch, J.Med.Chem., 14(1971)777-779.
54 R.E.Gammans, R.D.Sehon, M.W.Anders and P.E.Hanna, Drug Metab. Disposition, 5(1977)310.
55 I.M.Kapetanovic, J.M.Strong and J.J.Mieyal, J.Pharm.Exper.Ther., 209(1979)20.
56 T.D.Yih and J.M. van Rossum, J.Pharm.Exper.Ther., 203(1977)184.
57 M.Tichy, Ergeb.Exp.Med. 29(1978)17-28.
58 P.Brazeau, in L.S.Goodman and A.Gilman (Eds.), The Pharmacological Basis of Therapeutics, 5th ed., Macmillan, New York, 1975, pp. 848-859.
59 P.Brazeau in ref.58, pp. 860-866.
60 K.H.Beyer, Arch.Int.Pharmacodyn., 98(1954)97-117.
61 E.J.Lien, in E.J.Ariens (Ed.), Drug Design, Vol. 5, Academic Press, New York, 1975, pp. 81-132.
62 L.Dettli and P.Spring, Proc.3rd Internat.Pharmacol.Meeting 1966, 7(1968)5-32.
63 A.H.Beckett, R.N.Boyes and G.Tucker, J.Pharm.Pharmacol., 20(1968) 277-282.
64 P.Turner, J.H.Young and J.Paterson, Nature 215,(1967)881-882.
65 E.Owada, K.Takahashi, R.Hori and T.Arita, Chem.Pharm.Bull., 22 (1974)594-600.
66 A.Ryrfeldt, J.Pharm.Pharmacol., 23(1971)463-464.
67 H.-L.Fung, B.J.Aungst and R.A.Morrison, Ann.Rep.Med.Chem., 14 (1979)309-320.
68 J.K.Seydel, Int.J.Quantum Chem., in press.
69 B.-K.Chen and C.Horvath, J.Chromatogr., 17(1979)15-28.
70 J.K.Seydel and K.Visser, unpublished results.

J.A. Keverling Buisman (Editor), *Strategy in Drug Research*



# DRUG BIOTRANSFORMATION AS A SOURCE OF DRUG DEVELOPMENT

H. OELSCHLÄGER
Institut für Pharmazeutische Chemie der Universität Frankfurt,
Frankfurt am Main (G.F.R.)

## ABSTRACT

The knowledge of pharmacokinetics is attaining increasing importance for the planning and the synthesis of new drugs. In particular research related to biotransformation contributes essential facts. Not only are the enzymes of the endoplasmatic reticulum (especially those of the liver and the cytosol) able to metabolize drugs but the enzymes of the mitochondria (Oelschläger and Blume 1975) have this ability, as well. In regard to phase I and phase II reactions significant differences of the latter have sometimes been observed when compared with the enzymatic reactions catalyzed by microsomes. The influence of biotransformation on the pharmacodynamics of drugs can be classified according to the following mechanisms:

1) transformation of drugs into nearly inactive metabolites
2) transformation of drugs into metabolites with similar activity
3) formation of active metabolites from inactive preliminary forms (prodrugs)
4) transformation of drugs into toxic metabolites.

Examples of these mechanisms will be presented. Very often pharmacological and clinical trials of promising metabolites have been very advantageous, because drugs of improved properties resulted. Structural changes providing favourable pharmacokinetic properties are results of biotransformation research too.

---

## INTRODUCTION

There should be an ideal method for the synthesis of causal acting drugs: elucidation of the pathophysiology of a disease, discovery of the pathobiochemical aspects and after a study of the receptor site situation, the synthesis of the pharmacon molecule, which was formulated in advance while sitting at the desk. This intelligent procedure, avoiding

*References p. 222*

the detours of empirism, would definitely lower the high costs and shorten the large amounts of time necessary for the development of new drugs.

However, up to now this route could hardly be used, simply because the pathophysiology and pathobiochemistry of most diseases are unknown.

Therefore drug research is dominated by the following traditional disposition: thousands of substances have to be synthesized and submitted to screening using animal models. Only a very small selection of substances with superior pharmacodynamic activity and promising therapeutic index can be made available for clinical trials. The concepts for drug synthesis are derived from different areas. Native substances are often used as leads. The a priori synthesis, independent of natural substances but using certain hypothetical routes, has up to now yielded the best results. Naturally this procedure is expensive and uneconomical. Most of the drugs used today were created this way. Very often good fortune has been the companion of success. This was perfectly expressed by the Nobel prize winner (1979) in biochemistry, Christia de Duve:

" ... however rationally we may try to design a drug, we should always allow for serendipity and welcome it gratefully when it comes our way."

## IMPORTANCE OF BIOTRANSFORMATION

Since pharmacokinetic parameters have been recognized to influence the pharmacodynamic activity, biotransformation (defined as the enzymatic transformation of drugs in the animal and human organism) has increasingly become a matter of interest in drug research. By biotransformation the lipophilicity of a drug is decreased, thus enlarging the possibility of renal elimination, due to the extended solubility in water. Therefore lipophilic pharmaca, mostly being weak acids or bases are metabolized to various extents, whereas hydrophilic drugs are hardly subject to biotransformation. On principle every living cell is able to undergo biotransformation. The main enzymes are localized in th endoplasmatic reticulum (e.r.) and bound to membranes. Nevertheless, some of the enzymes are found in the cytosol.

During the last years at our Institute (ref. 1) highly purified mitochondria derived from rat liver have been tested for their potency in drug metabolism. The investigation of 60 drugs of known microsomal metabolism (i.e. chlorpromazin, fomocain, imipramin, methamphetamin, nitrazepam, paracetamol, phenacetin, procain, tolbutamid) has surprisingly revealed that mitochondria are able to cause oxidative, reductive a hydrolytic reactions (phase I) as well as conjugation (phase II) reactions.

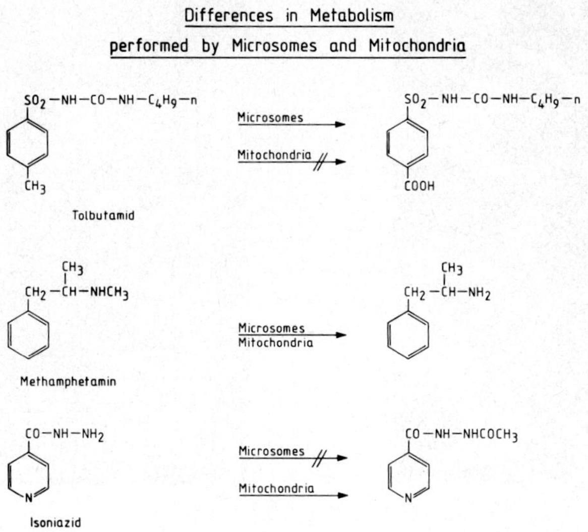

Differences in Metabolism
performed by Microsomes and Mitochondria

$SO_2-NH-CO-NH-C_4H_9-n$ (Tolbutamid, $CH_3$) — Microsomes → ; Mitochondria ↛ — $SO_2-NH-CO-NH-C_4H_9-n$ ($COOH$)

$CH_2-CH(CH_3)-NHCH_3$ (Methamphetamin) — Microsomes, Mitochondria → — $CH_2-CH(CH_3)-NH_2$

$CO-NH-NH_2$ (Isoniazid) — Microsomes ↛ ; Mitochondria → — $CO-NH-NHCOCH_3$

Figure 1

The main difference between metabolism caused by microsomal or mitochondrial enzymes is the fact that $sp^2$- and $sp^3$-hybrid carbon atoms cannot be hydroxylated by the latter enzymes. Thus neither from hexobarbital nor from the local anaesthetic fomocain can a hydroxylation product be found. This means the cytochrome P-450 of the mitochondria is more specific than the cytochrome P-450 of the e.r. (Fig. 1).

Also with regard to phase II reactions important differences exist. Whereas the main reactions performed by the microsomal enzymes are methylation and formation of glucuronides, the mitochondrial enzymes are able to synthesize acetyl- and hippuric acid derivatives as well as glutathion conjugates. Sulfate esters are only formed by the soluble enzymes of the cytosol.

The validity of all experiments with mitochondria is strongly dependent upon their purity and integrity. For that purpose a special procedure based on density gradient centrifugation with Percoll™ as a new medium was developed by Blume (ref. 2). Percoll is colloidal silica coated with polyvinylpyrrolidone. Fig. 2a shows highly purified and integral mitochondria and Fig. 2b destroyed mitochondria, caused by a two weeks storage at -18°C.

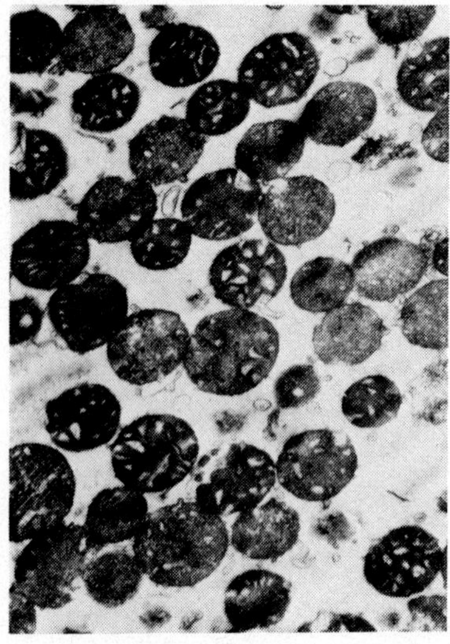

Fig. 2a. Integral Mitochondria
(Magnification 10 000 : 1)

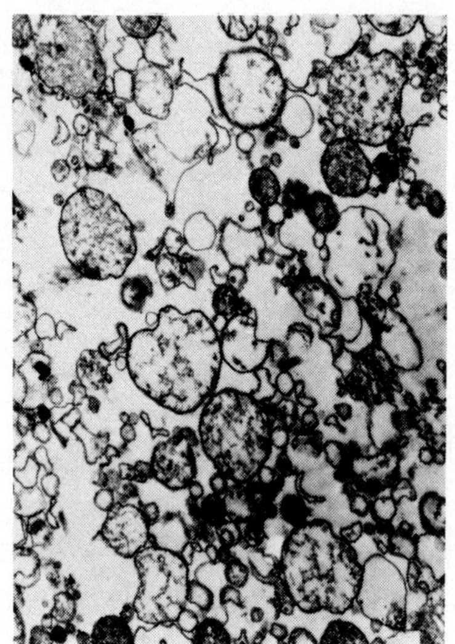

Fig. 2b. Destroyed Mitochondria
(Magnification 10 000 : 1)

With regard to changes in the velocity of the drug-elimination and thereby in the plasma concentration when constant doses are administered we raised the question of possible stimulation of the mitochondrial enzymes by phenobarbital. Our experiments did not reveal any enzyme induction. This is most probably due to the fact that phenobarbital cannot pass the double layer of the mitochondrial membrane and thus does not stimulate protein synthesis. Generally the turnover rates caused by mitochondria are lower than those of microsomes (roughly 10 - 40%). This can be attributed to the limited capacity of the membrane transport processes. If the permeability barrier is removed, using ultrasonics or detergents, drastically enlarged turnover rates result in most cases (latency phenomenon).

Because of its size and large supply of blood the liver is highly suitable for biotransformation. The numerous pores of the loose endothelium of the sinusoids and the special membrane of the parenchyma make an intensive exchange of substances possible. When oral administered drugs are considered the liver together with the intestinal mucosa may cause a first enzymatic attack (first pass effect) inactivating in some cases up to 50% of the absorbed drug (examples: lidocain, propranolol, nitroglycerin, morphin, diphenhydramin, etc.).

There is no doubt that frequently observed differences in drug activity in man are partly due to interindividual differences in the capability of drug metabolism. Results obtained with twins revealed a genetic origin. There are epidemologic references indicating genetic defects in the cytochrome P-450 dependent hydroxylation in about 5% of our population. Though no differences in biotransformation between males and females have been observed in human beings, there are differences in laboratory animals.

To an increasing extent a certain regio- and stereoselectivity in drug metabolism in view of the substrate has been noticed. Thus conjugation of 4-nitrophenol with glucuronic acid is much faster than the corresponding conjugation of 2-nitrophenol (regio selectivity). When R(-)-amphetamin is incubated separately its deamination and N-oxidation occurs more rapidly than observed with the S(+)-amphetamin (stereo selectivity). However, if both enantiomers are incubated simultaneously S(+)-amphetamin is metabolized more rapidly, due to its higher affinity to the enzyme system.

An experienced therapy is impossible without paying attention to the age dependence of biotransformation. The fetal liver is already equipped with the fully developed microsomal monooxygenases 6 to 8 weeks after conception. However, contrary to the adult liver the fetal liver is not able to execute conjugation reactions like glucuronidation and,therefore,is unprotected against active metabolites formed by hydroxylation. Consequently these metabolites might react with biopolymers which are important for further evolution of the organism and homeostasis. This possible detrimental potency of xenobiotica has not yet been investigated. The biotransformation rate slowly decreases with age. Estimation of the extent is problematic due to the restriction of the kidney function of the elderly.

Up to now only few reliable facts about the influence of liver and renal dysfunctions on biotransformation are known. As a rule the enzyme capacity even of an affected liver will not be exhausted by the low doses of drugs commonly administered. Only those drugs needing a high dosage or showing a tendency to cumulate due to their long half-life (i.e. phenobarbital, diphenylhydantoin, phenylbutazon, rifampicin, and acetylsalicylic acid) have to be administered carefully if the kidney is affected. Drugs undergoing extensive metabolism are to be preferred in cases of renal dysfunction. For example propranolol, which is extensively metabolized, should be used as ß-blocker instead of pindolol, which is metabolized only to about 40% (Fig. 3).

*References p. 222*

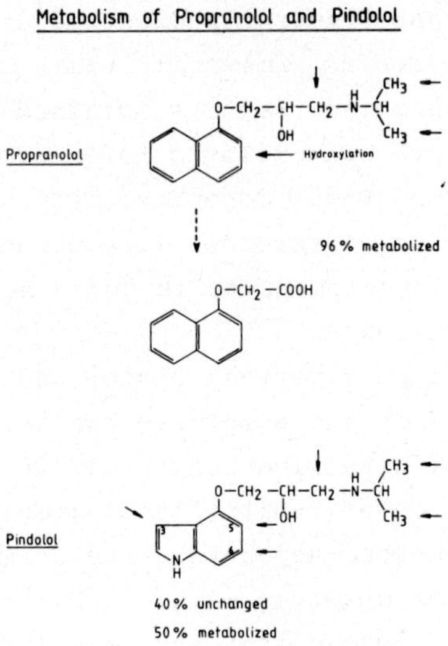

Metabolism of Propranolol and Pindolol

Propranolol

$O-CH_2-CH(OH)-CH_2-NH-CH(CH_3)_2$

Hydroxylation

96 % metabolized

$O-CH_2-COOH$

Pindolol

$O-CH_2-CH(OH)-CH_2-NH-CH(CH_3)_2$

40 % unchanged

50 % metabolized

Figure 3[+]

The most important exogen factor influencing biotransformation of drugs is ethanol, which is metabolized to acetic acid via acetic aldehyde in the liver. The activity of the alcohol dehydrogenase remains constant but ethanol shows some affinity to the monooxygenases, too, and therefore catabolism of drugs (i.e. aminophenazone) might be inhibited. In 1979 Oelschläger and Ueberall (ref. 3) demonstrated that via interference between drugs and ethanol, unexpected biosynthetics are formed in man and rats. When for example N-[N-methylnorleucyl]-2,6-dimethylaniline (O/G 10), a local anaesthetic, or other anilides with a secondary amine residue are administered to rat and man simultaneously with ethanol, substituted imidazolidinones result (Fig. 4).

[+]The arrows in the figures are pointing to atoms which are sites of further metabolic attack.

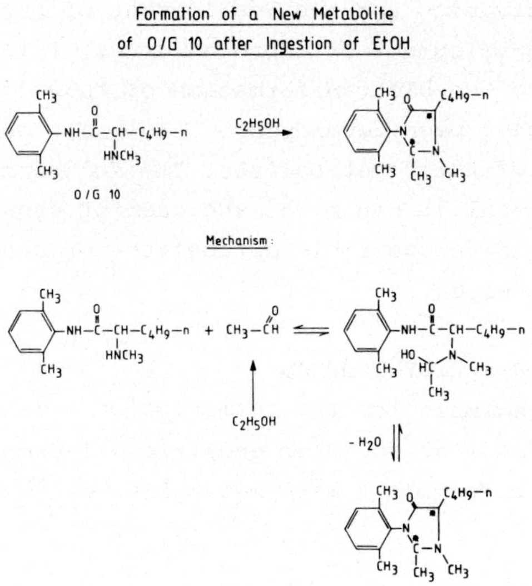

Formation of a New Metabolite
of O/G 10 after Ingestion of EtOH

$C_2H_5OH$

O/G 10

Mechanism:

$C_2H_5OH$

$-H_2O$

Figure 4

This formation can only be explained considering a reaction of acetic aldehyde, an ethanol metabolite, with the secondary N-atom forming a carbinol amine as an intermediate before cyclization. Following the reaction scheme, the compounds were also synthesized in the laboratory. Presently these substances are under pharmacological evaluation. Their toxicity is lower than those of the parent compounds. Our observations may lead to an understanding of unexpected reactions in man, which have been noticed when alcohol and drugs are administered simultaneously and which so far cannot be explained. Trager et al. (ref. 4) have expressed considerations in the same direction.

Just some decades ago only a few scientists were concerned with the biotransformation of drugs. Today the pharmaceutical industry has to consider biotransformation of drugs in order to obey drug legislation and to ensure drug safety. The enzymes which perform drug metabolism cannot of course distinguish between products useful or detrimental to the organism. They alter the structure of the substrates along their mechanistic schemes and by doing so often modify the activity of the substrates. This may cause different consequences. Four different mechanisms influencing pharmacodynamics have to be considered:

1. Transformation of a drug into metabolites without activity.
2. Transformation of a drug into metabolites with similar activity.
3. Formation of active metabolites from inactive preliminary forms.
4. Transformation of a drug into toxic metabolites.

Today the bioactivation and the development of prodrugs are important factors in the development of improved drugs. This will be so in the future too. Since the biotransformation of known drugs was elucidated, many new drugs have been developed on the basis of pharmacological and clinical trials of their metabolites. The following examples will demonstrate how useful it can be to the chemist engaged in synthesizing new drugs, to consider possible metabolites of a drug in advance when planning new syntheses.

## METABOLITES AS INDEPENDENT DRUGS

A well-known example for the formation of a metabolite into an independent drug, showing superior qualities if compared to the parent compound, is paracetamol, a main metabolite of the analgesic phenacetin (Fig. 5).

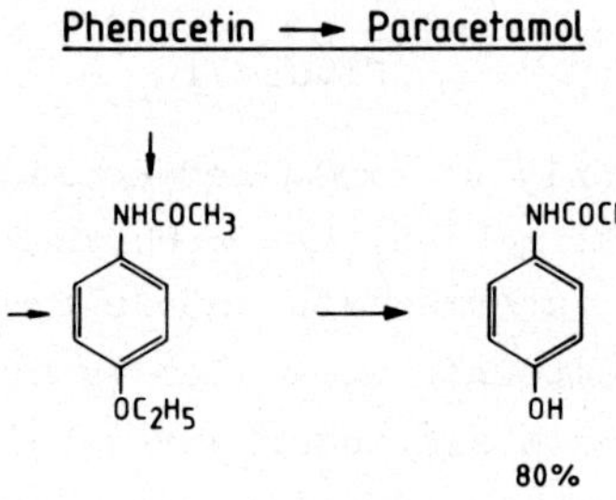

**Phenacetin → Paracetamol**

$NHCOCH_3$ / $OC_2H_5$ → $NHCOCH_3$ / OH

80%

Figure 5

The main advantage of paracetamol is the fact that it does not produce methemoglobinemia in children and that it does not cause drug addiction. Renal dysfunctions, which were found after longterm administration of phenacetin have not been noticed with paracetamol.

Oxyphenbutazon is a minor metabolite of phenylbutazone (Fig. 6).

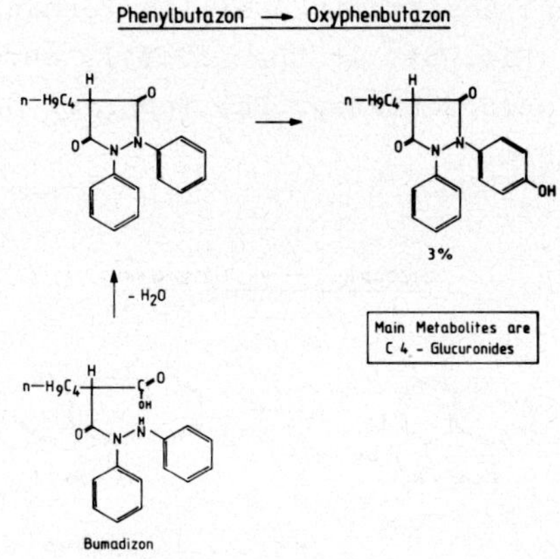

Phenylbutazon → Oxyphenbutazon

3%

Main Metabolites are C 4 - Glucuronides

Bumadizon

Figure 6

Its antiphlogistic activity should be superior to that of phenylbutazon, therefore it is used in the therapy of inflammations and non-rheumatic oedema. Comparing oxyphenbutazon to phenylbutazon side effects are less frequent. The development of bumadizon is unnecessary because it is cyclized to phenylbutazon in the organism.

The secretolytic bromhexin is to a small extent subject to N-demethylation and hydroxylation. One product of biotransformation (Fig. 7), ambroxol, shows stronger secretolytic activity whereas the weak bronchoconstriction caused by bromhexin has disappeared.

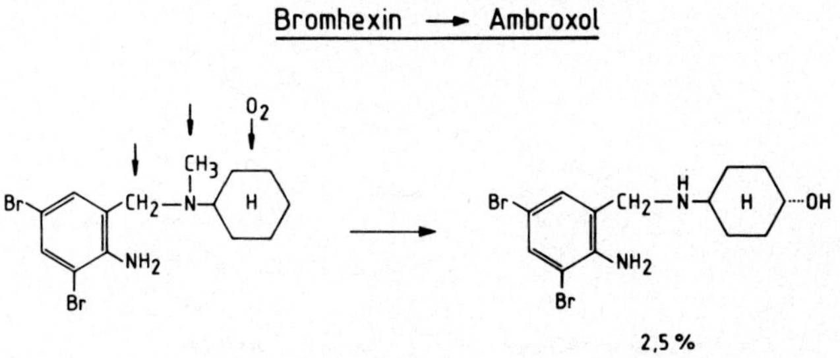

Bromhexin → Ambroxol

2,5 %

Figure 7

The antidepressant desipramin owes its formation to the N-demethylation of imipramin (Fig. 8). It specifically cures depressions with decreased psychomotoric activity. The superior bioavailibility of desipramine is noticeable.

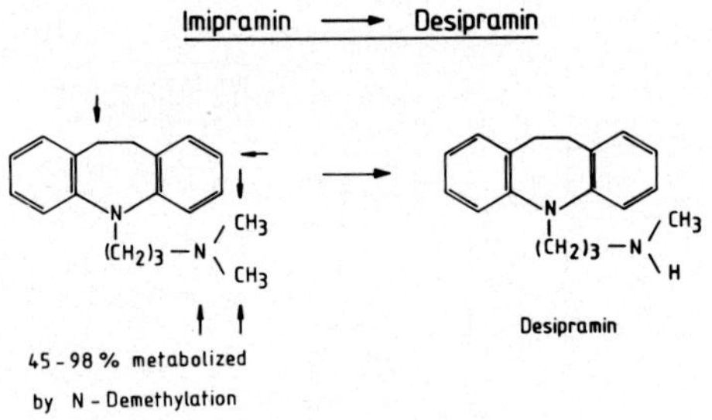

Imipramin → Desipramin

N

$(CH_2)_3-N(CH_3)_2$

45 - 98 % metabolized by N - Demethylation

$(CH_2)_3-N(CH_3)H$

Desipramin

Figure 8

An excellent illustration of the potentialities of biotransformation research in therapeutic as well as in economical respect is represented by the biotransformation of the tranquilizer chlordiazepoxid to the corresponding lactam demoxepam (Fig. 9).

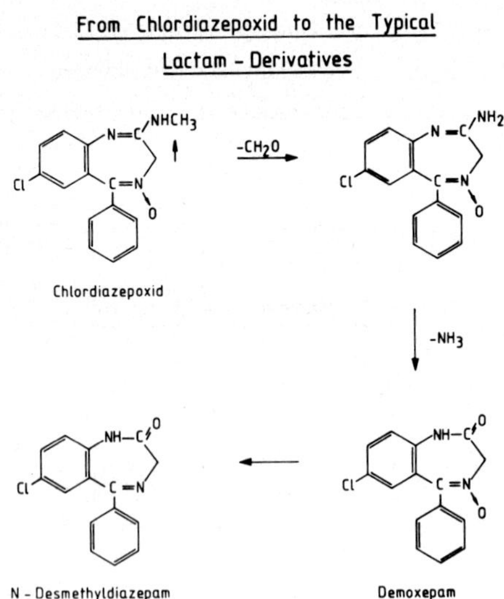


Figure 9

Demoxepam was not put on the market; but its product of reduction, the long acting N-desmethyldiazepam, also a metabolite of the older diazepam, is in therapeutic use. The C-3-hydroxylation noticed in the organism with both lactams led to the independent tranquilizers temazepam and oxazepam. Both are less anxiolytic (Fig. 10).

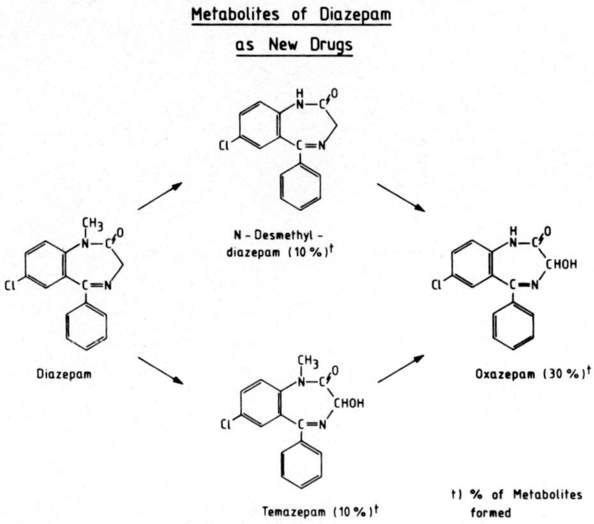

Metabolites of Diazepam as New Drugs

Diazepam

N - Desmethyl - diazepam (10 %)†

Oxazepam (30 %)†

Temazepam (10 %)†

†) % of Metabolites formed

Figure 10

From an analytical point of view the fact that 1,5-benzodiazepines (i.e. clobazepam) are not hydroxylated at C-3 but show C-4'-hydroxylation is very significant. A second main metabolite is the N-desmethyl-derivative (Fig. 11).

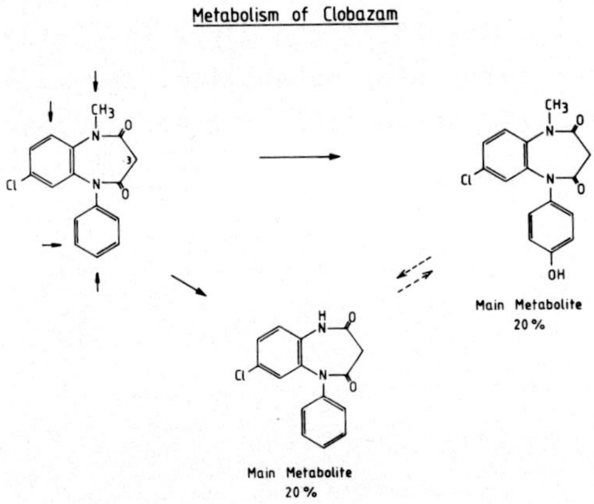

Metabolism of Clobazam

Main Metabolite 20 %

Main Metabolite 20 %

Figure 11

*References p. 222*

Thioridazin, which was put on the market in 1973, is oxidized to the sulfoxide and consecutively to the sulfone (Fig. 12).

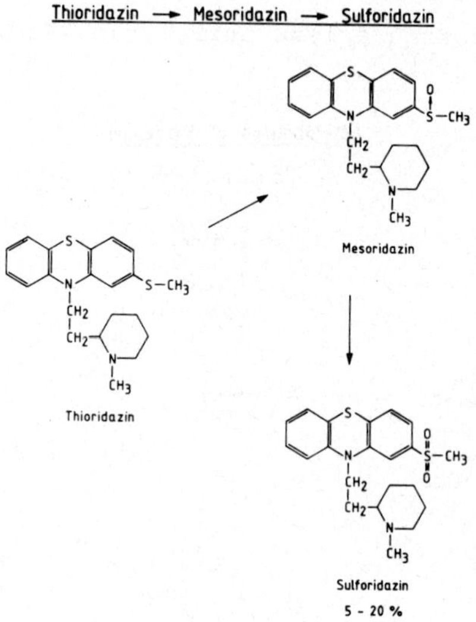

Thioridazin → Mesoridazin → Sulforidazin

Mesoridazin

Thioridazin

Sulforidazin
5 - 20 %

Figure 12

There are important differences in the pharmacodynamic pattern of sulforidazin compared to the parent compound. Above all the depression of the psychomotor system is about 2-3 times stronger and there is a pronounced cataleptic effect.

Another interesting example, showing the relevance of biotransformation research, is the activation of vitamine $D_3$. Cholecalciferol is hydroxylated in position 25 in the liver resulting in a small increase in activity of the first step metabolite. The main activation occurs in the renal mitochondria where it is further hydroxylated to form $1,25\text{-}(OH)_2\text{-}D_3$ (Fig. 13).

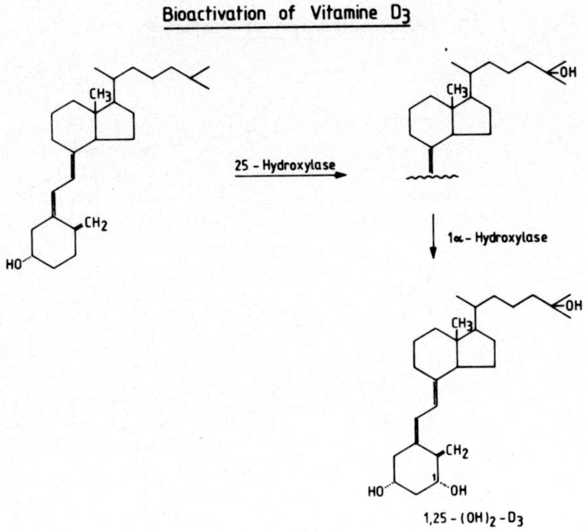

**Bioactivation of Vitamine $D_3$**

25 - Hydroxylase

1α - Hydroxylase

1,25 - $(OH)_2$ - $D_3$

Figure 13

The latter is classified as a hormone, as its mechanism of action is identical to that of the steroid hormones. 1,25-$(OH)_2D_3$ (Calcitriol) enlarges the calcium- and phosphate uptake from the intestine and increases the rate of syntheses of membrane proteins. 1,25-$(OH)_2$-$D_3$ as well as 1α-(OH)-$D_3$ are already therapeutically used.

Looking at such impressive results one may ask why the knowledge of biotransformation is not used to a greater extent. Why, for example, is trichlorethanole, the active principle of chloralhydrate, not used as an agent? Could it be due to decreased absorption or faster metabolism via glucuronidation? Why have neither the active principle of the analgesic dextro-propoxyphen, the N-desmethylderivative, nor the active principle of the saluretic mefruside, the lactone, formed by biotransformation, yet been registered as drugs? Are there perhaps no pharmacokinetic reasons but simply economic considerations the decisive factors? The answers to such questions may only be guessed at.

When considering the XOD-blocker allopurinol the reason is obvious. The half-life of allopurinol has been estimated to be about only 40 minutes. It is rapidly transformed into the main metabolite oxipurinol, which possesses a half-life of 14 h after oral administration (Fig. 14).

*References p. 222*

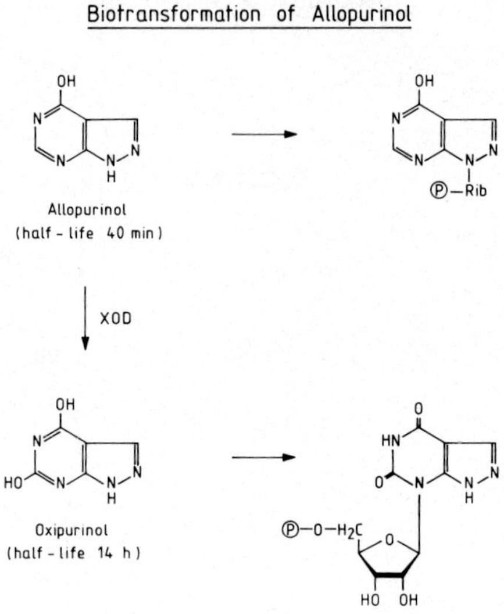

Biotransformation of Allopurinol

Allopurinol
(half - life 40 min)

XOD

Oxipurinol
(half - life 14 h)

Figure 14

Oxipurinol itself inhibits the xanthine oxidase. Nevertheless, oxipurinol could not become an independent drug as its absorption from the intestine is negligible.

## THE NECESSITIES OF PRODRUGS

In rational drug design prodrugs demand significant interest (Fig. 15).

Necessities for Prodrugs

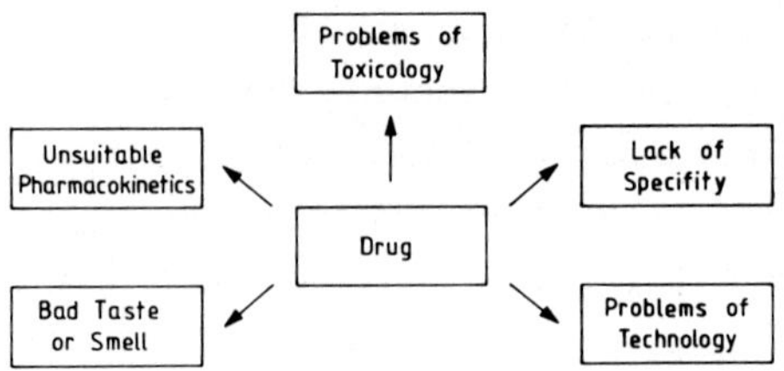


Figure 15

Figure 15 shows the potentialities of prodrugs. Most important is the possible manipulation of pharmacokinetics. As examples, let us consider a substance too polar to pass the blood-brain barrier and a substance subjected extensively to a first pass effect. In both cases low plasma levels may cause ineffectivness. The prodrug principle was confirmed in an impressive manner in the therapy of Parkinson's disease, which is caused by a lack of dopamine in certain areas of the brain. Theoretically, administration of dopamine should be a possible form of therapy. Unfortunately, this is not possible in practice as dopamine (pKa 8.93) is highly ionized at physiological pH and thus cannot pass the blood-brain barrier. When the natural precursor of dopamine, the amino acid L-dopa is used, the blood-brain barrier is overcome by means of an active carrier system. L-dopa then is metabolized to dopamine by the dopa-decarboxylase in the gangliocytes of the brain (Fig. 16).

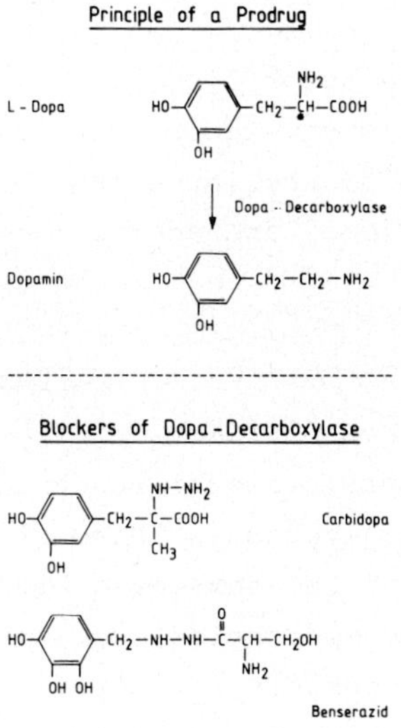

Figure 16

As L-dopa is decarboxylated into dopamine in the periphery, too, causing side effects of the autonomic nervous system, a blocker of the peripheral decarboxylase, i.e., carbidopa or benserazid, which itself is unable to pass the blood-brain barrier, is administered simultaneously. This allows an essential reduction of the dosage of L-dopa.

Among plant derived drugs the anthraglycoside cathartics are important natural prodrugs. Because of their hydrophilic sugar component, absorption in the small intestine is prevented. Moreover, the sugar moiety protects the emodines from metabolic attacks in the small intestine. After microbial removal of the sugar moiety (Fig. 17),

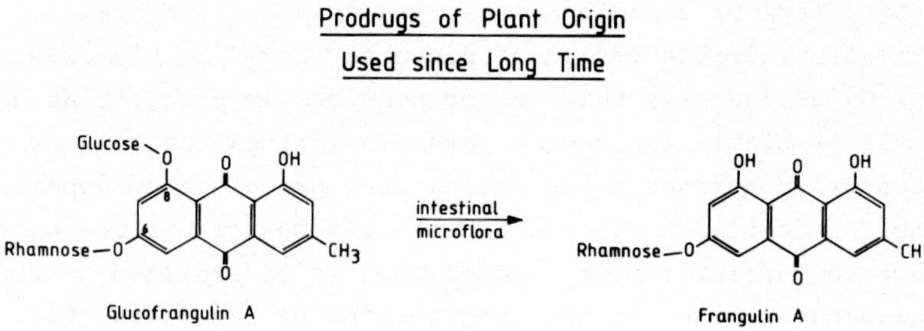


Figure 17

the emodines inhibit the absorption of sodium ions and water from the intestine resulting in doughy feces. The voluminous filling of the gut causes a stretching of the intestinal wall leading to a reflectory defecation. If the aglycones are administered then they are absorbed and metabolized.

## BIOTRANSFORMATION AND DRUG DESIGN

The results of biotransformation research are increasingly taken into consideration in drug synthesis. More stable connecting links are used in the molecules and the enzymatic transformation of the parent compound is regulated by appropriate substituents. Thus the plasma concentration which is responsible for the interaction with the receptor can be modified as necessary for a superior therapeutic effect.

Three examples will demonstrate this situation. Procaine shows, as all local anaesthetics do, an antiarrhythmic activity due to its influence on the saltatoric excitation. This activity cannot be used therapeutically, since the procaine molecule is rapidly hydrolyzed by plasma esterases. When the ester group is substituted by an amide group, which is stable against the esterases, but can be hydrolyzed by the liver amidases, the stability of the molecule is increased and a longer half-life results (Fig. 18).

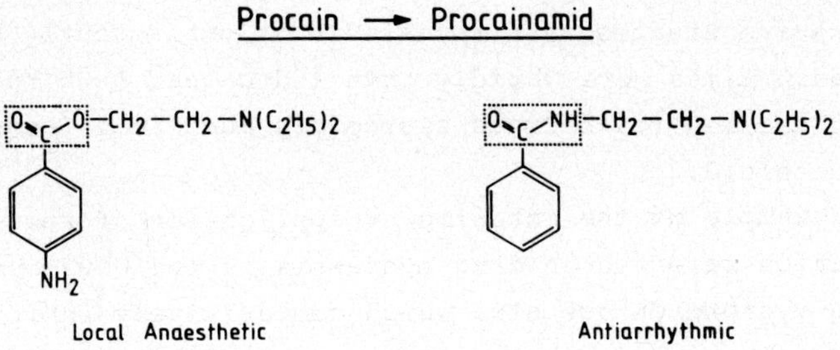

Figure 18

This is also proved by the investigation of the elimination-process for up to 70% of the administered dose is found unchanged in the urine. Besides, due to the amide bond, toxicity is lowered to at least 50%.

The chemically very stable local anaesthetic lidocaine has a half-life of 100 minutes. The catabolism of lidocaine in man is initiated by an oxidative N-dealkylation, followed by the hydrolysis of the amide bond (Fig. 19).

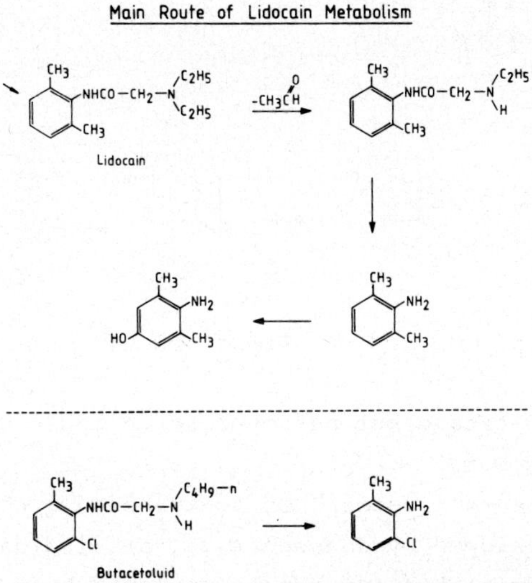

Figure 19

*References p. 222*

Butacetoluid contains in its molecular structure a secondary amine, therefore, the first step of biotransformation is already completed, and comparative studies have revealed that consequently butacetoluid is metabolized 5 times more rapidly than lidocaine. As a result side effects in the central nervous system are much less frequently observed with butacetoluid.

A fine example of the intelligent application of results from biotransformation research in drug synthesis is the development of the antiandrogen cyproteron acetate, which competitively inhibits the testosterone effect by competing for the cytoplasmatic dihydrotestosterone receptor. When orally administered, the cyproterone C-20-keto-function is rapidly reduced and a C-17-ketosteroid metabolite is produced after removal of the C-17-side chain. Acetylation of the C-17-hydroxy group significantly hinders the reduction process on account of a steric effect. The tertiary C-17-acetoxygroup is removed in vitro and in vivo only to a very small extent (Fig. 20).

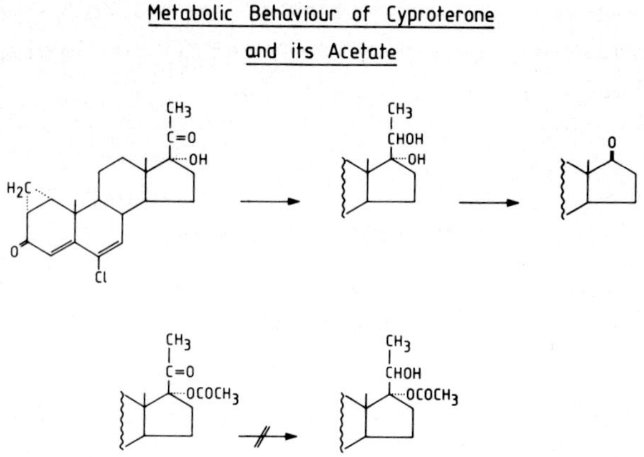

Metabolic Behaviour of Cyproterone and its Acetate



Figure 20

Only cyproteron acetate but not cyproteron could be detected in the plasma of volunteers.

For the long term treatment of schizophrenia the new fluorodiphenylbutylamines, developed by Janssen c.s., are indicative of great progress because daily administration can be replaced by i.m. injection or oral administration once a week. This has been demonstrated using fluspirilen with a half-life of 7 days. There is no doubt that the properties of the fluorobutyrophenones (e.g., haloperidol) namely extreme lipophilicity, biliary excretion with consecutive reabsorption from the feces and slow biotransformation have contributed to a great extent to the development of this new group of drugs.

The plasma half-life of haloperidol is 12 - 38 h after ingestion. The fluorinated phenylring is not hydroxylated. Introduction of a second fluorophenyl substituent into the haloperidol molecule yielded a steady long lasting therapeutic activity of about 6 - 12 days (Fig. 21).

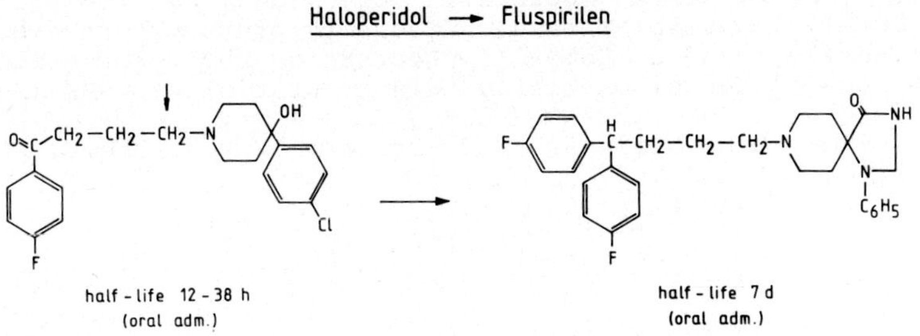

Haloperidol → Fluspirilen

half-life 12 - 38 h (oral adm.)

half-life 7 d (oral adm.)

Figure 21

There are many more examples, which have not been mentioned in this lecture. All of them demonstrate the growing influence of biotransformation research. It has resulted in metabolites becoming independent drugs, as well as in drugs with improved pharmacokinetic properties. Our own experiments using mitochondria reveal a significant contribution to the biotransformation of many drugs. This contribution could have a beneficial influence on drug toxicity. To sum it up in one sentence: For the development of new drugs the results of biotransformation research can profitably be used.

ACKNOWLEDGEMENTS

I am obliged to all pharmaceutical firms which supported me with details on their mentioned drugs.

*References p. 222*

REFERENCES


1 H. Oelschläger, Lecture on the 4th Xenobiotica-Symposium held at Pezinok/CSSR (May 7th, 1975).
H. Oelschläger, Lecture on the Symposium on Drug Metabolism held at Guildford/U.K. (April 6th, 1976).
H. Oelschläger, Discussion on the 2nd International Symposium on The Biological Oxidation of Nitrogen in Organic Molecules held at Chelse College, London (September 20th - 23rd, 1977).
H. Blume and H. Oelschläger, Arzneim.-Forsch./Drug Res., 28, 956 (1978).
H. Blume, Arzneim.-Forsch./Drug Res., 30, 1566 (1980).
H. Blume, Arzneim.-Forsch./Drug Res., 31, 805 (1981).
H. Blume, Arzneim.-Forsch./Drug Res., 31, 994 (1981).
H. Blume and H. Oelschläger, Arzneim.-Forsch./Drug Res. (in press)
H. Blume, Pharmazie (in press)

2 H. Blume, Arch. Pharm. (Weinheim, Ger.), 312, 561 (1979).

3 S. Ueberall, Doctoral-Thesis, University of Frankfurt a.M. (1979).
H. Oelschläger and S. Ueberall, Lecture on the International Conference on Xenobiochemistry held at Bratislava/CSSR (June 10th, 1980).

4 S.D. Nelson, G.D. Breck and W.F. Trager, J. Med. Chem., 16, 1106 (1973).

J.A. Keverling Buisman (Editor), *Strategy in Drug Research* 


# THE QUANTITATIVE MEASUREMENT OF BIOLOGICAL EFFECTS

P. J. GOODFORD
Biochemistry Division, Wellcome Research Laboratories, Langley Court, Beckenham, Kent, BR3 3BS, England.

"Seek and ye shall find, Knock and it shall be opened unto you"

Luke, Chapter 11, Verse 9.

## ABSTRACT

Good drugs are, generally speaking, both potent and specific in their biological effects. In order to ensure adequate potency and specificity, a drug molecule must have the right combination of properties. Thus one might be seeking a compound which reacts specifically with the relevant receptor; which is concentrated near that receptor; which has low concentrations elsewhere in the body; and which is metabolised and excreted at appropriate rates. A good drug-design strategy is an attempt to optimise as many of these properties as possible in order to give the desired clinical effect. Two general requirements must therefore be satisfied. First, one must have a clear understanding of the different factors which need to be considered. This can only come from an adequate comprehension of the biological processes which are to be influenced, and from a careful study of the properties of the chosen compounds. Second, one must have good methods for measuring the properties of the compounds and the biophase. These general requirements will be illustrated by recent work on diseases of the blood. The haemoglobin molecule itself is the primary receptor target for therapy, but a wide range of inter-related experimental approaches will be described covering the whole spectrum of investigation from receptor to patient.

## INTRODUCTION

There are many different reasons why attempts to discover new therapeutic agents may fail. The first requirement for success is superabundant good luck, and many a worthwhile investigation has drawn a blank because luck was against it. On the other hand a seemingly coincidental run of bad luck may turn out, after more thorough analysis, to have been caused by inappropriate decisions. If these happen early in an investigation, and appropriate corrective action is not taken in time, a great deal of money and effort can be wasted. In order to find new therapeutic agents, one must seek for them in the right way.

*References p. 249*

The character of the overall approach may often be determined at a very early stage, long before any detailed research has taken place. For example a "management" decision might be taken to discover compounds which should fill a previously unexplored gap in a market, say for antiallergics. However, certain fundamental requirements must be satisfied if such a decision is to be implemented in an effective way leading to worthwhile novel therapeutic agents. The exact scientific target must be explicitly defined in scientific as well as marketing terms. Appropriate experimental methods must be established in the laboratory, and it must be unequivocally demonstrated that these test systems are appropriate and relevant models of the chosen disease in man. Additional laboratory tests may be required in order to demonstrate the selectivity or, on the other hand, the breadth of the biological spectrum covered by any novel compounds. Then, finally, the response characteristics of each test must be established so that genuine responses can be unambiguously detected and, if possible, quantified. **The initial decision to discover a novel type of therapeutic agent cannot be implemented reliably, unless the above criteria for the biological tests are fully satisfied.**

An alternative approach might stem from prior scientific knowledge, such as a chemical appreciation of some class of compounds or functional groups or reaction mechanisms. For example prior knowledge of the penicillins and penicillin chemistry would naturally provide an impetus in the direction of novel antibiotics, and antibiotic screening is a good example of a biological test system which is both relevant to the chosen disease and easily quantified. On the other hand an expertise in peptide chemistry would not lead to such a narrow and well-defined field of biological testing. Peptides can show such diverse biological effects that particular care would be needed in devising relevant, accurate and precise biological tests to support a chemical initiative in this area. Clearly, any chemically-based strategy will have profound effects on the necessary biological tests, and this interaction must be borne in mind from the outset if the desired therapeutic research objective is to be effectively achieved.

Only one more overall research philosophy need be considered. The innovatory approach may stem neither from management nor from chemical considerations, but from an investigation of the biological system itself. For example, studying the physiology of heart muscle or the detailed mechanisms of an enzyme pathway might be the primary research approach, in the belief that a better understanding of the biology and biochemistry should provide a basis for improved therapy. Once again, however, the same requirement holds good. **The relevance of the biological tests to the human disease must be demonstrated unequivocally, and their selectivity, accuracy and reproducibility must be adequate.**

## THE OVERALL APPROACH

Although a line of research may be initiated by a marketing, or a chemical or a biological concept, it is necessary for all three aspects to be thoroughly assessed at the outset. It is wishful thinking to start with a good idea and assume that one can muddle through any unexpected difficulties which may arise later. On the contrary, **the greatest difficulties should be identified as early as possible, so that appropriate measures can be taken well in advance.**

The need for an all-embracing strategy will now be illustrated by considering one example in some detail. The Wellcome Foundation has a long research tradition in the area of tropical medicine, and this has led to some notable therapeutic advances especially in the area of parasitology. There has been a simultaneous improvement in controlling the vectors which transmit parasitic infections, but although this progress has been spectacular, it has not helped those patients in the tropics who suffer from non-parasitic diseases. It was natural for an organization like Wellcome to consider these patients as well, and so the possibility of drug therapy for Sickle Cell Disease came up for assessment.

Sickle Cell Disease is an anaemia which almost exclusively occurs in people of negro descent. It presents as a disease of the young, and the infant mortality rate is extremely high. Even under good economic conditions with adequate clinical care as many as 10% of patients die in the first year of life, and the proportion may well be much higher in less favourable environments. Irreversible changes have occurred in the patient's spleen by the age of 4 or 5, and further characteristic developments present throughout childhood and in the young adult. The chronic advance of the disease is interrupted from time to time by acute painful attacks, and many patients die before middle age from cardio-vascular or kidney damage. On the other hand some patients have a much less traumatic life, and many people with Sickle Cell Disease may be completely free of symptoms. To demonstrate the clinical efficacy of any new therapeutic agent in such a variable disease cannot be easy.

One therapeutic approach might be to administer the potential new drug chronically, in order to prevent the slow progression of the disease and eliminate the acute painful crises. Even with carefully selected patients and matched controls, however, a large and long trial would be needed before the efficacy of such chronic administration could be clearly demonstrated in man, and so alternative approaches have to be considered. One possibility might be to treat neonatal patients alone and to measure the reduction in infant mortality, but the chronic treatment of newborn babies with a novel compound would raise ethical questions and might not be acceptable to many parents. Another possibility might be to study only those patients who claim they can anticipate the onset of a painful crisis, and then use the compound to prevent its predicted onset. However this approach would be critically dependent upon the patient's initial subjective assess-

*References p. 249*

ment, and in order to avoid any subjective influence it might be preferable to concentrate on those times when no crisis was anticipated and the patients were apparently in a steady state. Some parameter might be chosen, perhaps the severity of the anaemia, and this would be monitored regularly to find out whether drug treatment produced a more favourable blood picture. Nevertheless, it might still be an open question whether the proposed therapy would confer real clinical benefit to the patient by extending his life or reducing the incidence of painful crises, even if a drug were efficacious in such a steady state blood test. In fact, the requirement for a worthwhile clinical assessment of potential therapeutic agents for Sickle Cell Disease is not easily met, and the obvious difficulties argue strongly against even making the attempt to find new drugs. The effort can only be justified because the disease is life threatening, and because no effective therapy is available.

It is in precisely these circumstances that there is the greatest requirement for relevant biological tests. **If the laboratory tests are well-conceived and sufficiently broad-ranging, it should be possible to select a compound with a relatively high probability of success on clinical evaluation. Initially, as a first step in the choice of good test systems, it is necessary to study the target disease in significantly more detail.**

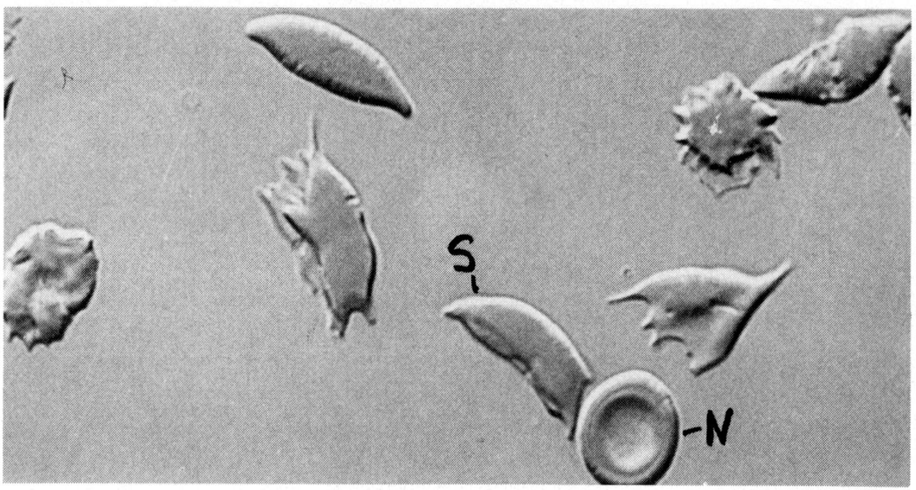


Fig 1. Photomicrograph of sickle cells viewed under Nomarski Optics. Homozygous sickle blood was incubated at $37^{\circ}$C under a reduced oxygen tension, and samples of cells were fixed in formal phosphate-buffered saline. The field reveals cells at various stages of sickling from an unchanged normal discoid erythrocyte (N) through to a fully sickled cell (S) with the characteristic crescent-shaped appearance. Note also the "pitted" appearance of some of the cells, due to the presence of membrane vesicles which are characteristic of the splenic dysfunction in Sickle Cell Disease (photomicrograph provided by Mr. K. D. Patel).

## SICKLE CELL DISEASE

In 1915 Cook and Meyer (ref 2) described a patient suffering from "severe anaemia with remarkable elongated and sickle-shaped red blood cells", and two years later Emmel (ref 3) detected the presence of sickle cells (Fig 1) in the father of this patient. This suggested that there might be a genetic basis for sickling, and by 1923 Taliaferro and Huck (ref 8) showed that the disease was inherited. Patients with the heterozygous form of the disease show few if any symptoms, but those who have inherited it from both parents in the homozygous form can suffer from the full range of symptoms (ref 5). The former asymptomatic condition is called "Sickle Cell Trait", to distinguish it from the disease proper which is known as "Sickle Cell Anaemia".

At almost exactly the same time biochemical investigations demonstrated (ref 6) that the haemoglobin from a patient with Sickle Cell Anaemia was different from a normal person's haemoglobin, and that someone with Sickle Cell Trait had an approximately 50-50 mixture of each. Later work showed that there was an actual chemical difference between the covalent bond structure of the two haemoglobins, and so attention was focussed on the chemical structure of haemoglobin itself. This was, in fact, the first time that any human disease had been related to a specific molecular defect.

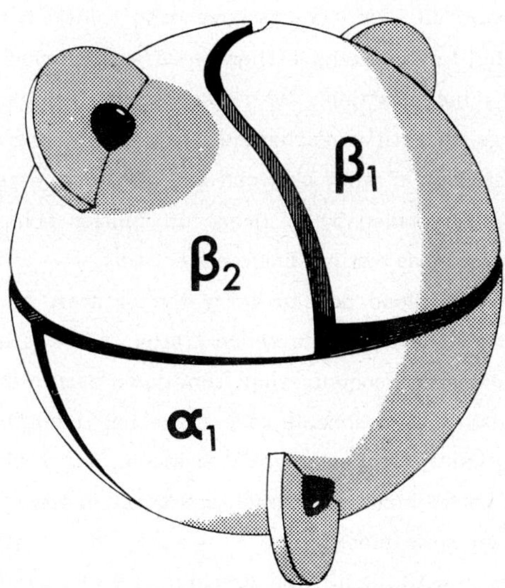


Fig 2. A diagrammatic representation of the haemoglobin tetramer. See text.

*References p. 249*

Sickle Haemoglobin

Normal Adult human haemoglobin is known as Haemoglobin A (Hb A), and consists of four distinct protein chains each of which is folded into a well-defined conformation. The four chains aggregate together to form a tetramer as shown diagrammatically in Fig 2, and each chain is folded round a haem group which contains an iron atom. Each iron atom can react reversibly with molecular oxygen, and the whole complex forms the red oxygen-carrying pigment in the blood. As shown in Fig 2, there are two distinct types of protein chain. The two alpha chains in the complex are identical, each consisting of 141 amino acid residues. The two beta chains are also identical to each other and consist of 146 residues. However these beta chains are different in the haemoglobin (Hb S) from a patient with Sickle Cell Anaemia. Whereas the sixth amino acid residue of the beta chains from a normal person is glutamate (β-6-GLU), the same position is occupied by a valine residue in someone with Sickle Cell Anaemia (β-6-VAL). This apparently trivial alteration in the haemoglobin macromolecule is quite sufficient to account for the biochemical differences between Hb A and Hb S, and also for the symptoms of Sickle Cell Disease.

Blood takes up oxygen in the lungs, and as it is pumped round the body the oxygen is delivered to the tissues. When the blood leaves the lungs it contains oxyhaemoglobin, in which each of the four iron atoms in the tetramer has accepted an oxygen molecule from the air. In deoxyhaemoglobin all four oxygens have been released, and the oxyhaemoglobin and deoxyhaemoglobin tetramers have slightly different molecular conformations. Deoxyhaemoglobin also has a higher affinity for carbon dioxide, and carries this metabolic by-product back to the lungs where it is discharged into the atmosphere. Moreover, there is a slight difference of isoelectric point between oxy- and deoxyhaemoglobin, and the deoxygenation process is accompanied by a change of solution pH. In short one must regard the oxy- and deoxy- forms as distinct chemical entities.

In order to allow each red blood cell to carry the greatest amount of oxygen, it contains haemoglobin at the highest possible concentration. This is approximately 30%, and the factor which prevents the concentration from going even higher is the solubility of haemoglobin. Indeed it is not unreasonable to suppose that solubility was an important constraint during the evolution of the haemoglobin molecule, and a reliable 30% solubility for a protein under all the varied conditions which can occur in the red blood cell during health and disease is no mean achievement.

Unfortunately for patients with Sickle Cell Anaemia, the replacement of β-6-GLU in Hb A by β-6-VAL in Hb S, alters the haemoglobin molecule in a way which reduces its solubility. Whilst Hb S is still sufficiently soluble under normal physiological conditions, a fall of pH combined with a sufficiently low oxygen partial pressure can cause tetramers of Hb S to polymerise into larger oligomers which eventually precipitate as linear polymers within the red blood cell. These polymers have the same macromolecular organization as a crystal of deoxyhaemoglobin, and one must conclude that the β-6-GLU to VAL mutation reduces the solubility of deoxyhaemoglobin S so that it can polymerise and precipitate under some physiological conditions, although oxyhaemoglobin S is still sufficiently soluble and the protein redissolves when oxygen is readmitted.

## Sickle Cells

When the linear polymers of deoxyhaemoglobin S become sufficiently long they approach the surface membrane of the red blood cell and eventually push into it. As they grow still further the shape of the cell is distorted into the characteristic sickle or holly leaf appearance which is diagnostic of Sickle Cell Anaemia. These changes can be produced in the laboratory by deoxygenation or lowered blood pH, or they can occur in the patient's body under similar conditions. For example, if blood is passing slowly through the capillary bed of a rapidly metabolising tissue, oxygen will be taken up by the tissue cells which produce lactic acid and carbon dioxide and thereby lower the pH, and provide the ideal environment for sickling to occur. Moreover, the shape of a sickled cell is much less flexible than a normal red blood cell, and it cannot slip past the obstructions which it may meet in the capillary bed. Furthermore, the solution inside a sickled cell is much more viscous when deoxyhaemoglobin S polymers are present, and this viscosity combined with the jagged outline of the sickled cells can make them obstruct the fine capillary through which they are travelling. If this causes the blood flow through the capillary to fall while the tissue continues to metabolise oxygen and produce acid, the local conditions become more and more conducive to sickling. The red blood cells will continue to sickle and build up the obstruction until a local infarct is produced with little or no effective blood flow. There is intense local pain, and if the condition spreads the patient may suffer from an acute crisis with permanent tissue scarring. Such events occur repeatedly throughout the life of the patient until the high oxygen-consuming tissues such as the heart, kidneys and the retina of the eye become permanently and irreversibly damaged and death finally ensues.

Of course any particular sickled cell may not lodge in the capillary bed, but may return through the venous circulation to the lungs where it will be reoxygenated and assume its normal biconcave shape. However, repeated sickling episodes finally produce irreversible damage to the cell membrane, giving an Irreversibly Sickled Cell which is incapable of taking up the normal biconcave form. Hence, when a blood smear from a Sickle Cell patient is studied it may contain Normal Red Blood Cells, Reversibly Sickled Cells and Irreversibly Sickled Cells.

*References p. 249*

## APPROACHES TO THERAPY

**Having described the disease, in outline, it is now necessary to consider the various possible approaches to therapy. Each must be assessed in order to decide whether it might be feasible in practice, so that the most appropriate biological experiments can be devised in order to service the chosen research strategy.** The first requirement is to draw up a fully comprehensive list of all possible therapeutic measures, and although the following list is by no means complete it serves to illustrate the wide range of different types of therapeutic approach which have been proposed.

### Gene Therapy

A fundamental way of curing Sickle Cell Disease would be to alter the relevant gene, and change the abnormal nucleic acid sequence coding for valine into the normal sequence coding for glutamate. At present, however, it is not easy to propose any strategy for carrying out this superficially simple process.

### Early Diagnosis and Abortion

If two Sickle Cell patients are expecting a baby, it is now technically feasible to examine the foetus **in utero** and establish whether it has Sickle Cell Anaemia. An abortion can be carried out if it suffers from this severe form of the disease, although the appropriateness of this approach will depend upon parental and cultural acceptability.

### Persistence of Foetal Haemoglobin

Almost all the haemoglobin in a red blood cell must be in the **deoxy**haemoglobin S form, before significant polymerisation and sickling occur. The presence of only a small amount of some other haemoglobin is quite sufficient to inhibit the polymerisation process, and oxyhaemoglobin S normally fills this inhibitory role. However other haemoglobins can be equally effective, and some patients are protected from sickling because they continue to produce significant quantities of foetal haemoglobin throughout their adult life. Foetal haemoglobin is present in the blood of all babies at birth, and is replaced by Adult Haemoglobin during the first weeks of life. The Adult Haemoglobin will be Hb S if the baby is going to suffer from Sickle Cell Anaemia, and symptoms of the disease will first appear when the production of Foetal Haemoglobin has almost ceased. If some method could be found of maintaining sufficient production of Foetal Haemoglobin throughout adult life, then the symptoms of the disease could be largely ameliorated. However it is not easy to define any strategy for doing this at present.

### Precipitating Factors

It has been claimed that various factors in the environment tend to promote sickling in patients with Sickle Cell Anaemia. These factors include a drop in ambient temperature, the onset of heavy rain and so on. Every effort should be made to educate patients to avoid such precipitating factors whenever possible.

## Antibiotic Therapy

The debilitating effects of Sickle Cell Anaemia tend to weaken the patient, and make him more liable to infection, so there is a role for antibiotics in the therapy of Sickle Cell Anaemia. However, these are already generally available.

## Nutrition, Vitamins, etc.

It may often be beneficial to improve the patient's general health by providing better nutrition or vitamin supplements. Bearing in mind that his red cells are constantly being destroyed and reformed in the bone marrow, the possibility of iron and folate supplements to the diet has been given some consideration. In broad terms anything which may benefit the patient's general health, could be of value.

## Blood Transfusion

When appropriate the patient's blood can be exchanged, and he can be transfused with fresh blood from normal donors who do not suffer from Sickle Cell Anaemia. This is already common practice, for example, prior to major surgery on a patient with Sickle Cell Anaemia. In general, however, sufficient blood is not available to treat all patients several times a year, and regular transfusions would carry additional risks such as the transmission of disease from donor to Sickle Cell patient.

## Extracorporeal Treatment of Blood

It has been shown that cyanate can react with haemoglobin S, and reduce its propensity for sickling. However, it appears that cyanate may be too toxic to be administered directly to patients, and machines have therefore been devised which should allow each patient to treat his own blood extracorporeally. This seems to be a technically feasible approach, but the cost of providing machines and the difficulties of maintaining sterile conditions may limit its usefulness on a world-wide scale.

## Anticoagulants

A critical stage is reached in any Sickle Cell patient when his cells start to block capillaries. Such blockages may clear spontaneously, but the blood clotting process will come into play if they do not clear, and clotting can transform a momentary obstruction into a permanent infarct. Anticoagulant therapy might therefore be of value and has been tried, although worthwhile effects have not yet been demonstrated in well-controlled studies.

## Vasodilators

The dilatation of peripheral capillaries is an attractive concept as a means of helping red cells to pass freely from the arterial to the venous systems, and it has been claimed that nicotinic acid may help some cases. However, so far as I am aware consistent benefit has not been obtained in well-controlled trials of vasodilators.

*References p. 249*

## Alkalosis

Since a fall of blood pH can exacerbate Sickle Cell Anaemia and initiate sickling, the possibility of raising the blood pH has been considered. However, pH control is such a crucial physiological requirement for the normal functioning of the body, that exceedingly powerful buffer systems are available in the blood and the tissues. Whilst it might be possible to raise the blood pH transiently by perhaps 0.1 pH units, no such effect can be maintained in the longer term. The effects of a single dose of alkali are quickly annulled by the body buffers, and if alkali is infused over a longer period in order to maintain a raised blood pH, the physiological buffers continue to oppose this process until they are all used up when unacceptable pathological sequelae occur to the detriment of the patient.

## Carbonic Anhydrase Inhibitors

The enzyme carbonic anhydrase in the red blood cell catalyses the equilibrium reaction between water and carbon dioxide, and it is not easy to argue on theoretical grounds whether the inhibition of this enzyme might confer benefit in Sickle Cell Anaemia, or not. On the one hand changing the equilibrium might tend to oppose the formation of deoxyhaemoglobin S. On the other hand, effects on the local pH might promote sickling. In practice a number of patients have been treated with carbonic anhydrase inhibitors, but no consistent therapeutic benefit has been observed.

## Fluid Replacement Therapy

The volume of the red blood cell is controlled by osmotic factors, and if a patient does not have a sufficiently high intake of fluids, the concentration of salts in his blood plasma may rise causing the volume of his red blood cells to shrink. Since there is no change in the weight of haemoglobin contained in the cells, the haemoglobin concentration rises and can thereby promote the polymerisation of deoxyhaemoglobin S in patients with Sickle Cell Anaemia. Patients should therefore be encouraged to drink sufficient quantities of water, and fluid replacement therapy may be of benefit during the management of Sickle Cell crises.

## Antipolymerisation Therapy

Since it is deoxyhaemoglobin S which polymerises, much basic research has been devoted to investigating the formation of the polymer and its structure. Decreasing the rate of polymer formation, or increasing its rate of breakdown, or destabilising the structure of the polymer are all processes which should tend to prevent the onset of crises.

Hyperbaric Oxygen

Patients have been submitted to high oxygen pressures, in an attempt to oppose the formation of deoxyhaemoglobin S and thereby prevent the onset of polymerisation. However, almost all the oxygen enters the blood via the lungs, and under ordinary conditions when they are inflated by air at atmospheric pressure they can adequately oxygenate all the haemoglobin which reaches them. There is some scope for extra oxygen to be carried in solution by the blood away from the lungs to the tissues, but by the time the blood has reached the relatively deoxygenated recesses of the capillary bed any benefit conferred by hyperbaric oxygen may be trivial.

Control of Diphosphoglycerate

The equilibrium between oxy- and deoxyhaemoglobin is subject to another form of physiological control which has not yet been mentioned. Glycolytic metabolism within the red blood cell produces a small molecule, 2,3-diphosphoglycerate, which reacts with haemoglobin and thereby shifts the equilibrium from the oxy- towards the deoxy- form. The concentration of 2,3-diphosphoglycerate is subject to physiological control and tends to rise during any anaemia. It therefore occurs at high concentrations in the red blood cells of patients with Sickle Cell Anaemia, and tends to promote the formation of deoxyhaemoglobin S which thereby promotes polymerisation. This is, in fact, an interesting example of a physiological feedback mechanism which works to the detriment of the patient, since he would be better off with a lower 2,3-diphosphoglycerate concentration in his red blood cells, and less deoxyhaemoglobin S. Any method of reducing the concentration of 2,3-diphosphoglycerate might therefore be of benefit.

Direct effect in oxygen affinity

An alternative approach might be to increase the oxygen affinity of the haemoglobin directly, by discovering compounds which react with the protein in the red blood cells and thereby tilt the oxygenation equilibrium in favour of oxyhaemoglobin irrespective of changes in 2,3-diphosphoglycerate levels. It has been shown that sodium cyanate has this effect, but unfortunately the compound was unacceptable on clinical trial. However, the search for compounds with similar properties still continues.

## SELECTING A THERAPEUTIC APPROACH

A number of approaches to therapy have now been considered, and it might be thought that the above list is unnecessarily long. However, it is essential to take a broad view at this stage, in order to plan biological tests which are truly relevant to the final therapeutic objectives. Some of the therapeutic approaches such as early diagnosis followed by abortion, are already practical possibilities although subject to cultural acceptability. Others, such as improved general nutrition, or the avoidance of precipitating factors like a low ambient temperature, are not amenable to drug therapy. A number of processes such as the maintained production of Foetal Haemoglobin throughout adult life offer great promise, but further fundamental research is needed before a therapeutic approach can be devised to work in this way. Some methods like the use of anticoagulants are primarily directed at the sequelae which follow after the precipitating lesion, sickling, has occurred. However, this leaves one or two approaches which could still be applied, at least in principle, when searching for new drugs to act against the precipitating lesion. The experimental requirements and limitations for each of these approaches must now be considered in more detail.

## ANTIPOLYMERISATION THERAPY

### Observations on Haemoglobin Solutions

The primary lesion in Sickle Cell Anaemia is the polymerisation of **deoxy**haemoglobin S, and by definition any therapeutic agent which works by an antipolymerisation method must act on the deoxy protein. This immediately raises an experimental difficulty because it is not always easy to remove oxygen completely from blood or from a haemoglobin solution. Yet the complete removal of oxygen may be essential. If oxygen remains it may not be possible to differentiate between a compound which prevents the polymerisation of deoxyhaemoglobin S on the one hand, and a compound which alters the equilibrium between oxy- and deoxyhaemoglobin S on the other. For example, it has already been pointed out that 2,3-diphosphoglycerate affects this equilibrium and thereby influences the ease of sickling. However any such action on the oxy-deoxy equilibrium must be clearly distinguished from the antipolymerisation approach which is now being considered.

The most fundamental method for assessing possible new antipolymerisation agents would be to observe haemoglobin solutions directly, in order to avoid complicating factors such as distribution and metabolism in blood or in the body. A reliable supply of haemoglobin S would be needed from patients with Sickle Cell Anaemia, which means in practice that close collaboration must be established with clinical haematologists who are in regular contact with a sufficient number of appropriate patients. Each patient must be sufficiently intelligent and well-informed to understand why he is being asked to donate blood for research purposes. His general health must be sufficiently good for him to donate that blood safely, and his willing agreement will be needed. The diagnosis of straightforward Sickle Cell Anaemia must also be clearly established, since misleading results would be obtained if the patient was actually suffering from another, perhaps related condition. It is also important to know whether the patient has been receiving any therapy before donating blood; he might for instance be receiving anticoagulants or be taking aspirin which could influence the final experimental results. Moreover, the possibility that he has recently received a transfusion of normal blood must be borne in mind, since a mixture of normal cells with his own sickling cells could again be misleading.

In order to check out these various factors on each blood sample as it is received, it is necessary to establish a method for **methaemoglobin determination;** a procedure for the **electrophoretic identification of haemoglobins,** and methods for the determination of **standard haematological parameters.** Methods must also be implemented for the **preparation of haemoglobin S solutions** at known concentration, pH and ionic strength. An assay must be established for **2,3-diphosphoglycerate determinations** in order to ensure that all diphosphoglycerate has been dialysed out of the haemoglobin sample, and a **total phosphate determination** on the solution should also be carried out.

Assuming that an acceptable solution of haemoglobin S has now been obtained, attention must next be turned to **control of physiological variables** during the experiment. It will either be necessary to prepare each working solution so that it is studied at an appropriate physiological pH, relying only on the buffering capacity of the haemoglobin itself, or it will be necessary to add sufficient buffer to the solutions in order to control their pH. If buffer is added, however, control experiments must be carried out to ensure that components of the buffer mixture do not directly influence the haemoglobin. Indeed this check must be made on each constituent of the solution. For example, it has been common practice for many years to add dithionite to haemoglobin solutions in order to remove the last traces of oxygen and ensure that all the protein is in the deoxy form. The assumption was that dithionite only removed oxygen, but this is not correct and it has recently been shown (ref 4) that there is a specific interaction between deoxyhaemoglobin and the dithionite molecule.

It is necessary to work at a normal physiological ionic strength, and to maintain this ionic strength with the physiological ions which are normally present in the red blood cell. These are primarily potassium, bicarbonate and chloride, with smaller quantities of sodium and magnesium. The presence of bicarbonate has a direct influence on pH control, and in order to ensure that the bicarbonate buffer system functions physiologically it is necessary to provide an appropriate partial pressure of carbon dioxide. It is also necessary to demonstrate the complete removal of oxygen from the liquid phase by measuring its solution partial pressure with a sufficiently sensitive oxygen electrode. All in all, many months of preliminary work will probably be required before these important physiological factors are brought under control.

*References p. 249*

When everything is ready attempts might be made to measure three or four relevant variables on deoxyhaemoglobin S solutions in the presence of the various compounds to be tested, with adequate controls. The most straightforward parameter would be the **determination of deoxyhaemoglobin S solubility** under the chosen experimental conditions. Alternatively one might observe the **viscosity of deoxyhaemoglobin S solutions,** or their **minimum gelling concentration,** or changes in the **rate of gelling.** An attempt could be made to determine the **affinity of each compound for deoxyhaemoglobin S** because, other things being equal, a higher affinity might contribute towards higher potency and better selectivity **in vivo.** The **stoicheiometry of binding to deoxyhaemoglobin S** should be measured. Any influence on the **isoelectric point** of the protein should be studied, and consideration should perhaps be given to the application of more sophisticated methods. For example nuclear magnetic resonance (ref 7) has been used to study the **aggregation of deoxyhaemoglobin S tetramers** when they interact to form the first small oligomeric associations which, if their growth continues unchecked, eventually grow into the long and damaging sickle haemoglobin polymers. Or again, attempts might be made to **co-crystallize deoxyhaemoglobin S** with potential anti-sickling agents, in order to find out how they interact with the deoxyhaemoglobin structure by X-ray crystallography.

Observations on Red Blood Cells

The observations on red blood cells may be divided into three general categories. First, does the compound inhibit sickling? Second, how well does it get into the cells, and third, is it metabolised inside them? These last two aspects may be dealt with fairly straightforwardly. It would be necessary to **separate red blood cells** by centrifuging them down several times, washing and resuspending them in a suitable physiological solution in order to avoid the additional complications caused by the plasma proteins of whole blood. One would need to establish procedures to **measure the concentration of compound** in the physiological saline, and set up methods to study the **distribution of compound into cells.** Necessary controls would be required, not forgetting the effects of deoxygenation. Perhaps some of the observations could be made on normal red blood cells, and in that case one might **prepare red cell ghosts** which are the reconstituted red cell membrane surrounding an appropriate experimental solution instead of the normal cell sap. This solution could contain different amounts of haemoglobin, or different proportions of Hb A and Hb S in order to study the effects of such variables upon the distribution of compound. The experiments might also be extended to cover the **rate of entry** and the **rate of efflux** of the compound into and out of the cells, and if necessary one might **prepare radioactive compound** in order to help establish whether any of the material leaving the cells was chemically changed.

Observations on Sickle Cell Patients

The step from healthy volunteers to patients with Sickle Cell Disease should not be such a jump in the dark as the earlier step from animals to man. Nevertheless, this is the time when a thorough re-evaluation of all the preceding work must be carried out, reviewing first the probable safety, and then the probable efficacy of the compound under examination. The healthy volunteers stand to gain nothing personally when they submit to experimentation, whereas the patients hope for some relief and are clearly in a risk-benefit situation. Both must be sufficiently intelligent and well-informed to understand their positions unequivocally. Moreover, the problem of deciding whether the compound confers real clinical benefit to patients has already been identified as one of the most difficult stages of the whole work. The final approach to this problem must be agreed at the animal experimentation stage or sooner, in order to ensure that appropriate doses, routes and durations of administration are studied both in animals and in human volunteers. However, it is fruitless to speculate on the details of clinical evaluation in Sickle Cell patients at this time, because no antipolymerisation compound has even reached the stage of animal evaluation in our hands.

## 2,3-DIPHOSPHOGLYCERATE THERAPY

The glycolytic pathway is of great importance in the red blood cell. It produces millimolar concentrations of 2,3-diphosphoglycerate in the cell water, and this reacts stoicheiometrically with haemoglobin thereby promoting the transition from the oxy- to the deoxy- form. This tends to promote sickling, and is an important effect because the red blood cells of patients contain unusually high concentrations of 2,3-diphosphoglycerate. If this concentration could be lowered, the symptoms of the disease would be significantly alleviated.

Enzyme Observations

The glycolytic pathway is subject to complex feedback controls, but in principle it might be possible to lower the concentration of 2,3-diphosphoglycerate by influencing one or more of the enzymes in the pathway. Graded inhibition would doubtless be necessary, because complete glycolytic blockade would be deleterious to the cell. Moreover, a specific effect on red blood cells would be required, without seriously influencing glycolysis in the rest of the body. These are difficult requirements to meet, and the attempt would probably be quite impractical were it not that an enormous body of information about glycolysis is already available in the literature. The basic jobs are to **identify a target enzyme, isolate and characterize it from human red blood cells, set up appropriate bioassays with adequate controls, confirm the mechanism of action and relevant allosteric control mechanisms, and set up biochemical screens** for evaluating the compounds to be tested.

*References p. 249*

### Observations on Red Blood Cells

Once again it would be necessary to establish whether each compound inhibited sickling, whether it got into the red blood cells and whether it was metabolised inside them. In this case, however, it would also be appropriate to determine whether the **intracellular 2,3-diphosphoglycerate concentration** was actually lowered. Any such reduction should be reflected as a change in the oxyhaemoglobin-deoxyhaemoglobin equilibrium which could be studied by observing the **oxygen dissociation curve of red cell suspensions.** A left-shift of the curve corresponding to a bias in favour of oxyhaemoglobin would be expected from compounds which significantly lowered 2,3-diphosphoglycerate levels, and these observations could probably be made on normal rather than sickle cells. In interpreting the results, however, it should be borne in mind that enzyme inhibition would not produce an instantaneous alteration in 2,3-diphosphoglycerate levels, so that some time might elapse before the desired left-shift actually took place.

### Further Observations

As before, observations would be needed on whole blood, in animals, healthy volunteers and patients. Many of the same problems would have to be dealt with, but there would be one significant difference. At every stage it should be possible to check whether the compound was depressing the 2,3-diphosphoglycerate concentration as expected, by simply observing the oxygen-dissociation curve. This is a standard physiological measurement and the dissociation curve is a **graded** response. When studying antipolymerisation therapy there were difficulties because of the need to produce complete deoxygenation in order to show that any compound was working as intended. However, such difficulties would not arise with compounds that altered the 2,3-diphosphoglycerate level, because it should be possible to use the oxygen-dissociation curve as a **graded** property at every stage of the work.

## THERAPY BY A DIRECT EFFECT ON OXYGEN AFFINITY

2,3-diphosphoglycerate reacts directly with haemoglobin, altering the oxy-deoxy equilibrium and thereby promoting the tendency of haemoglobin S to polymerise. It might be possible to discover other compounds which reacted directly with haemoglobin but produced the opposite effect. In order to evaluate such compounds some of the preceding tests would no longer be needed, but new test procedures would have to be introduced. The primary test might now be to observe the **oxygen-dissociation curve of normal haemoglobin solutions,** and pick out those compounds which produced a left-shift. This should correspond to a bias in favour of oxyhaemoglobin and should therefore oppose sickling, but the experimental detection of a left-shift might not be easy in pure haemoglobin solutions because the dissociation curve is already very left-shifted to start with. A more convenient procedure might be to right-shift the curve with 2,3-diphosphoglycerate, and then try to bring it back to its original position with the test compounds. This procedure (Fig 3) might also be more relevant to the therapeutic target, since the dissociation curve of blood from Sickle Cell patients is right-shifted by high intracellular levels of 2,3-diphosphoglycerate.

In contrast to antipolymerisation compounds, the present type can also be evaluated by studying their effects on the oxygen-dissociation curve of red cell suspensions or whole blood. Moreover, this action should appear as soon as the compounds enter the cells, unlike enzyme inhibitors which do not act until 2,3-diphosphoglycerate levels have fallen. Furthermore, the **effect upon red cell sickling** (Fig 4) could be investigated at any convenient partial pressure of oxygen, and a graded response could be observed since it would not be necessary to work under completely deoxygenated conditions. It needs to be borne in mind, however, that any compound giving a positive result in this test might be acting by an antipolymerisation mechanism, and this possibility should be ruled out if need be. The final procedures for compound evaluation are similar to those described previously, bearing in mind that the oxygen-dissociation curve can be used to monitor the blood level of the compound at every stage of the work right up to human volunteers and patients.

## THE ASSESSMENT OF TESTING PROCEDURES

Quite a large number of biological test systems have by now been considered, and it would not be reasonable to implement them all. Perhaps some would be crossed off the list because they needed too many resources to implement, but this is not a very satisfactory selection criterion. On the contrary it is more appropriate to **identify those relevant biological tests which provide the most information most reliably in the most useful form.** This approach to the selection of biological tests may be briefly exemplified by reference to Fig 3.

### Information Content

When presenting biological results, it is always desirable to **show the actual experimental observations.** In Fig 3 these are the plotted symbols, each of which represents a measurement. The findings are presented in this way so that everybody can see what was measured, and can re-interpret the observations if he wants to. Moreover, the results should if possible be shown before any mathematical transformations are carried out, since transformations can introduce bias. When the observations are shown in graphical form, which is often most convenient, the scales of the X and Y axes should be chosen so that the individual points are well displayed.

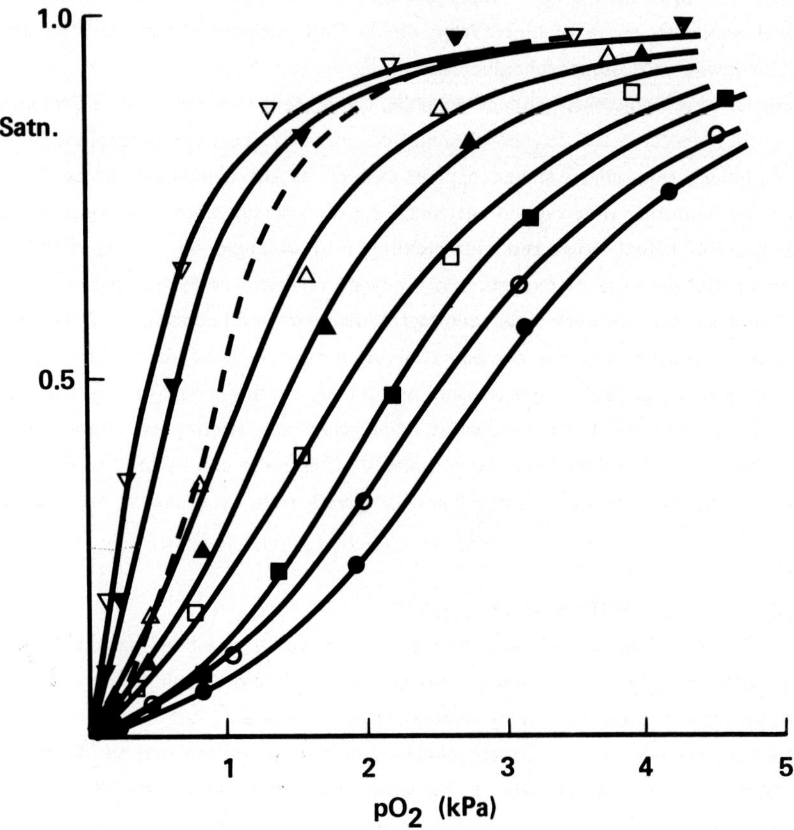


Fig 3. Oxygen saturation curves for solutions of normal human haemoglobin. The solutions were 0.12 mM in haem, 0.1 M in KCl, and 0.1 M in HEPES buffer. They were brought to pH 7.4 and the measurements were made at 37°C. All the observation points were made in the presence of 5 mM 2,3-diphosphoglycerate and various concentrations (mM) of salicylaldehyde:- ● 0; ○ 0.1; ■ 0.2; □ 0.5; ▲ 1.0; △ 2.0; ▼ 5.0; □ 10.0; the continuous curves were calculated from the best-fitting theoretical equation for the biochemical and biophysical mechanisms involved. The dashed line is the corresponding best-fit curve for haemoglobin solution in the complete absence of both 2,3-diphosphoglycerate and salicylaldehyde. It may be seen that the 2,3-diphosphoglycerate reduces the oxygen affinity of the haemoglobin and shifts the curve to the right. Salicylaldehyde opposes this effect and at the highest doses shifts the curve even further to the left than its original starting position. This effect produced by salicylaldehyde is a graded property, suitable for quantitative measurement and statistical assessment (results by Dr. R. Wootton).

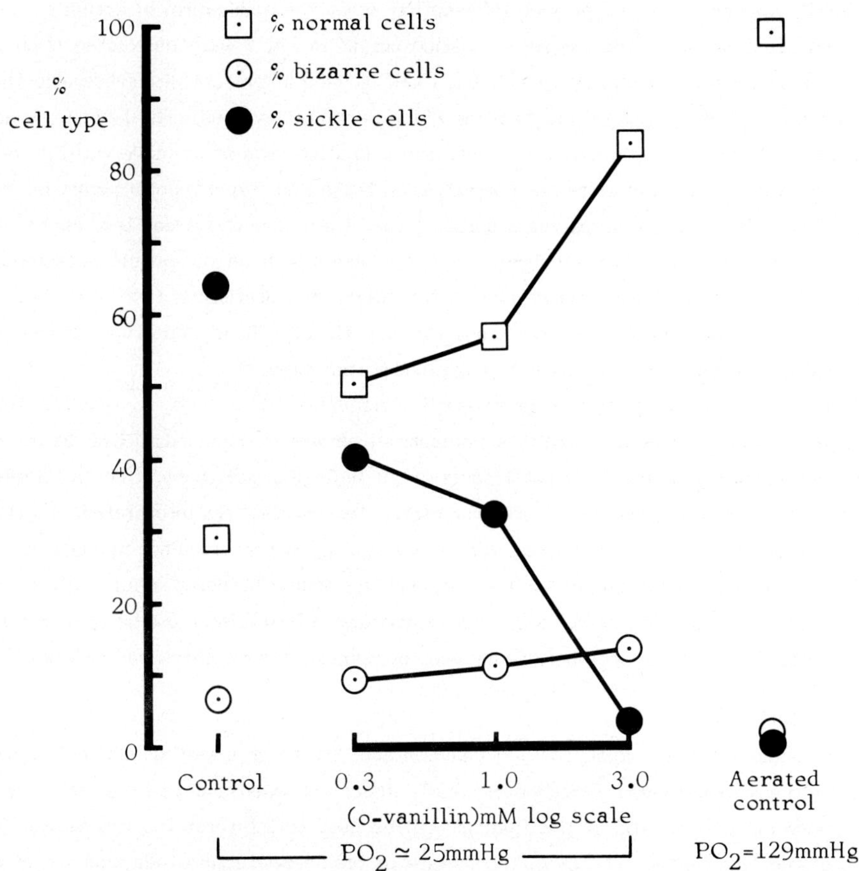


Fig 4. Observations on ortho-vanillin, a close structural analogue of salicylaldehyde which produces an anti-sickling effect by a direct action on the oxygen saturation curve of haemoglobin. Homozygous sickle blood was incubated **in vitro** for one hour at 37$^{0}$C in the presence or absence of ortho-vanillin, and the oxygen pressure was then reduced to approximately 25 mmHg. Samples were then taken and prepared for photomicrography as in Fig 1. At least 600 cells were observed under each experimental condition, and the numbers of normal discoid erythrocytes and of characteristic sickled cells were counted. Cells which fell into neither of these categories were called "bizarre", and the proportions of normal, bizarre and sickle cells were calculated.

When control observations were made in air, without reducing the oxygen pressure, almost all the cells appeared normal. However, when control observations were made at reduced oxygen pressure, without adding ortho-vanillin, more than 60% of the cells sickled and the proportion of normal cells fell to less than 30%. As the concentration of ortho-vanillin was increased, there was a fall in the fall of proportion of sickled cells, and a corresponding rise in the proportion of normal cells (results by Dr. R. D. White and Dr. G. Kneen).

A good experiment should **provide information about the mechanism of action** of the compound being studied. The oxygen saturation curves in Fig 3 were calculated from a theoretical mathematical function which was itself derived after careful consideration of the biochemical and biophysical mechanisms which might be involved. The function is an **algebraic model of the mechanisms,** and certain assumptions had to be made when it was derived. If the assumptions were not correct, then the actual experimental points might deviate from the theoretical curves suggesting that the compound under test might be acting by a different or novel mechanism. There appears to be reasonable agreement between the curves and the observations in the figure, but statistical tests are readily available to assess whether the deviations are significant. It is important to design biological tests so that the **results can be examined statistically.**

When many compounds are being assessed biologically, it is usual to tabulate the biological results in order to facilitate comparison between compounds. One or more parameters representing the different aspects of the biological activity will be calculated from the observations. The choice of parameters, the way they are interpreted, and the method by which they are calculated will all depend upon the assumed mechanism of action and the chosen mathematical function, and this should be borne in mind when the tables of results are being used. Moreover, **statistical information must be provided** so that the significance of any comparison between compounds can be statistically assessed.

## Experimental Errors

It is necessary to establish that no unacceptable errors or biases or artifacts have occurred in any experiment. This is particularly important when quantitative results are being recorded, and is vital if the findings will be used to interpret the mechanism of action of the compounds. However, the quality of biological testing today can be of a very high technical standard, and the most common mistakes are therefore small ones. Nevertheless, they can still be important and may even invalidate the final conclusions drawn from the work. For instance, it is vital to **establish that the compound is fully dissolved** throughout the experiment. The highest concentration studied must be appreciably below the saturation level, and it must be borne in mind when studying blood that the solutions can be intensely coloured, and that changes of pH occur during oxygenation and deoxygenation. There might also be chemical reactions between the compound and the constituents of the solution, and the latter might precipitate as well. Moreover, a compound could appear to be biologically inactive simply because it was all removed from the biophase by reaction with some inert constituent such as plasma albumin.

Control experiments must be carried out in order to **establish the main sources of experimental variance and error.** These controls must be devised to cover all reasonably-likely sources of variance. Does one get different results depending on the person who donates the blood? Do the results depend on the person who isolates and purifies the haemoglobin? Do they depend on whoever prepares the solution, or the person who carries out the experiment, or the spectrophotometer used to make the observations? How critical is temperature and pH control? How critical is ionic strength? Is it important to stir the solution? Does it matter if the first observations are made at the top of the dissociation curve working downwards to the bottom, or **vice versa**? Does it matter if the right-shifted curves are observed before or after the left-shifted? And what proportion of total variance is contributed by each individual factor, because **the relative importance of each source of variation will determine the final experimental design.**

**The size of the observed biological effect must be appreciable.** If the effect is "small" it might not be a real biological response at all, but just a fluctuation within the noise level of the experiment. On the other hand **compounds must not be compared when they are both producing a maximal effect. A graded property must be studied,** such as the position of the oxygen saturation curves shown in Fig 3.

**Ultimately it is the biological system which determines whether a new compound will become a worthwhile drug,** and the biological results speak for the biological system. If the Chemist has any doubts about the biological findings he should submit known compounds for testing in order to be sure that they give the expected results, and the Biologist should inspire confidence by testing them double-blind. That is to say nobody would know which compound was which until the tests had been completed and the results finally tabulated.

## Statistical Evaluation

The importance of statistical methods for evaluating biological results has already been emphasized. The necessary mathematical formulae and tables and computer programs are readily available. However, **it is often necessary to choose between different statistical approaches,** and the final conclusions can depend critically on the specific approach which is selected. It is this element of choice which lies behind the old saying that there are "lies, damned lies and statistics".

When selecting a statistical method one is very often trying to find the best overall compromise between several different factors. A particular method may be relatively powerful in the sense that very few experiments will be needed to give a clear answer. On the other hand one may have to make several assumptions in order to justify the chosen method, and the question then arises whether those assumptions can be rigorously justified. A weaker method might be more appropriate, if fewer assumptions were needed.

The assumptions influence the choice of method and they also influence the conclusions. Suppose one wishes to find out if a penny is biased. The first time that one tosses the coin it shows tails, and this could naturally happen by chance. On the most straightforward assumptions there would be a 50:50 chance that tails would show on the first toss. However, if the coin was tossed and showed tails every time, one would probably conclude that it was biased after six or seven trials. On the other hand different conclusions might have been reached if one had started with different assumptions. Suppose someone had produced the penny and said "I know this penny is biased. I have tossed it dozens of times and it always shows **heads.**" If one then did the experiment and got tails, it would not be necessary to toss six or seven times in order to reach a satisfactory conclusion. It would only be necessary to observe tails once or twice in order to throw serious doubt on the claim that the coin always showed heads. Clearly, **the choice of statistical methods and their power and the final conclusions depend upon the assumptions which are made, and it is necessary to decide on those assumptions in advance.**

## THE CHOICE OF BIOLOGICAL TESTS

It is now possible to decide which biological tests should be set up. This will depend on the relative merits of the different possible testing procedures, and the agreed therapeutic objectives. It is not necessary to make a final choice for all time. On the contrary the first experiments will be set up in order to obtain a broad range of generally relevant information about the compounds. Then, as the work progresses more detailed procedures will be needed in order to elucidate specific problems as they arise. It would be inappropriate to consider those detailed experiments here, but the first few tests will be briefly considered (Table I).

The initial observations might well be made on homozygous sickle red cells suspended in an appropriate saline at a controlled low oxygen tension. The findings would be something like those shown in Fig 4, and would give a simple straightforward graded response allowing compounds to be ranked for overall anti-sickling potency. No assumptions would be made about the mechanism of any anti-sickling effect. There should be no complications due to metabolism or protein binding, but a compound might be inactive because it did not enter the cells. The cell entry of an inactive compound would therefore be tested directly, and if it did enter the cells further testing would be inappropriate. One would conclude that it had had every opportunity to produce an anti-sickling effect by an action inside or outside the red blood cell, but had not done so. On the other hand, if the compound did **not** enter the cells it might still be able to exert a powerful effect on haemoglobin, but had been prevented from doing so. Further direct tests on haemoglobin solutions or on intracellular enzymes would therefore be called for.

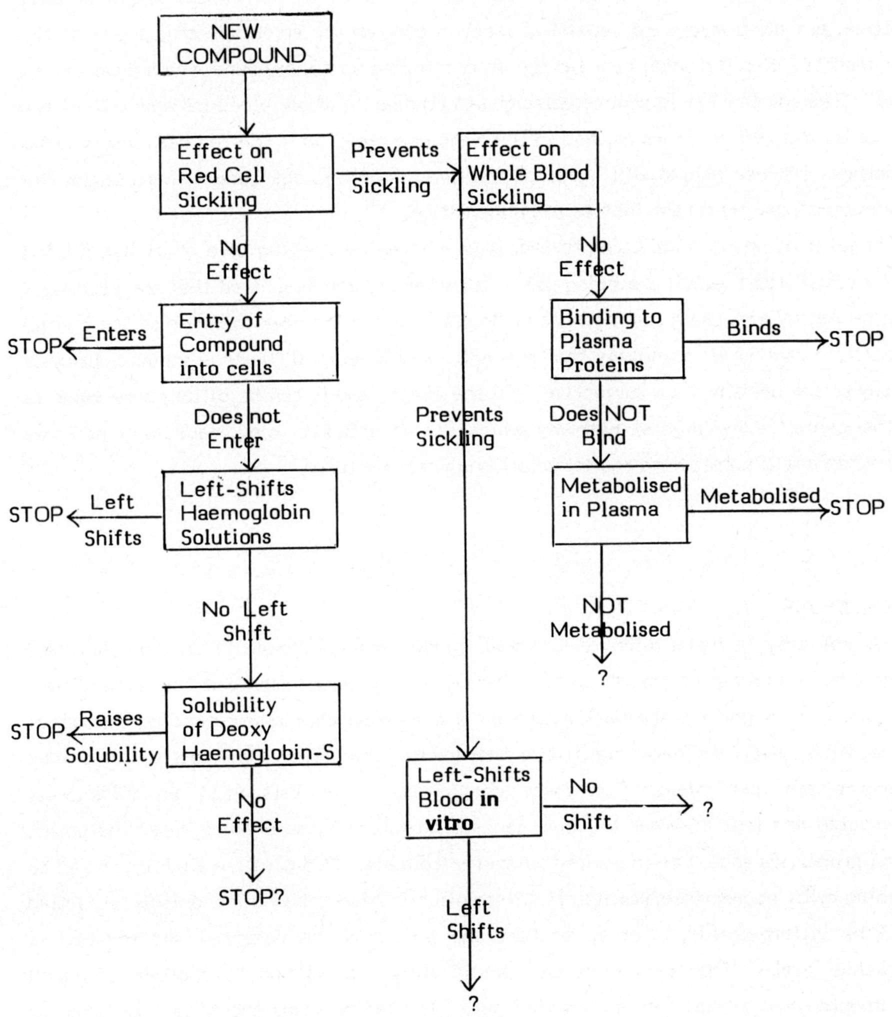


**TABLE I** A scheme for testing anti-sickling compounds. The STOP points at the side of the diagram represent reasonably informative results, which could be used when designing further novel compounds. The STOP at the bottom of the left-hand column would be reached when testing a completely inactive compound. Further testing might be appropriate if the question-marks were reached. The reader is invited to design a better scheme, using the information provided in the text. It is particularly important to include every critical decision point in such a diagram.

Table I merits careful study. It will be observed that some of the decisions are strictly objective, but other decisions depend at least in part on the scientific philosophy of the experimenter. For instance, how far should one follow up a compound which produces no effect? Perhaps one should proceed straight to studies on whole blood irrespective of the findings on red cell suspensions, and in this case one could omit the red cell observations altogether. No two people will agree on the overall policy, but general discussions will allow more of the important factors to be identified.

Whenever compounds are being tested, it is worthwhile drawing up a chart like Table I for the actual tests which are being used. It has even been suggested that the procedure might be formalised, using the methods of Boolian algebra in order to optimise the overall approach. However it is unlikely that this will yield an agreed "best" procedure, because so many of the decisions are subjective. On the other hand it can be of immense value to see the overall experimental pathway which one is actually using, especially at those times when one is considering the introduction of further tests.

## CONCLUSIONS

It is not easy to make a list of universal conclusions applicable to all biological test systems, but a number of significant requirements have been discussed and exemplified. There must be a unified approach based on a comprehensive assessment of the target disease, with clearly defined scientific or therapeutic objectives. The test systems must be appropriate and relevant to these objectives. The tests must be sufficiently reproducible and free of error to allow genuine responses to be unambiguously detected. Graded properties should be measured whenever possible. Quantitative findings should be presented with appropriate statistical information. Alternative mechanisms of action should be differentiated. Error, artifact and bias must be detected and reduced to acceptable levels. The tests must be appropriately related one to another. Control experiments must be devised and carried out. Any major snags should be identified as early as possible. If the biologist makes a reasonably successful attempt to bear such factors in mind, he may be lucky enough to find what he is seeking.

ACKNOWLEDGEMENTS

I am greatly indebted to my colleagues at the Wellcome Foundation for their help and advice, and particularly to Joan Hambidge, Geoff Kneen, Frank Norrington, Keshavlal Patel, Ralph White and Ray Wootton for their help in preparing this typescript, and providing the figures.

References

1. O. Castro, J. Cochran and S. Shukla. Clin. Res. 23(1975) 580A.
2. J.E.Cook and J.Meyer. The Archives of Internal Medicine, 16 (1915) 644-651.
3. V.E.Emmel. The Archives of Internal Medicine, 20 (1917) 586-598.
4. A. G. Ferrige, J. C. Lindon and R. A. Paterson. J. Chem. Soc. Faraday Trans. I, 75(1979) 2851-2864.
5. J.V.Neel. Science, 110 (1949) 64-66.
6. L.Pauling, H.A.Itano, S.J.Singer and I.C.Wells. Science, 110 (1949) 543-548.
7. A.N.Schechter. Hemoglobin, 4 (1980) 335-345.
8. W.H.Taliaffero and J.G.Huck. Genetics, 8 (1923) 594-598.

J.A. Keverling Buisman (Editor), *Strategy in Drug Research*



# QUANTITATIVE COMPARISONS IN CARDIOVASCULAR PHARMACOLOGY: CHARACTERIZATION OF α-ADRENOCEPTOR POPULATIONS

P.B.M.W.M. TIMMERMANS , A. DE JONGE and P.A. VAN ZWIETEN
Department of Pharmacy, Division of Pharmacotherapy,
University of Amsterdam, Plantage Muidergracht 24,
1018 TV Amsterdam, The Netherlands.

## INTRODUCTION

α-Adrenoceptors increasingly become more important as targets for agents of potential therapeutic interest. This interest is stimulated by the growing knowledge on the function of the various α-adrenoceptor populations in mammalian species. In our studies on quantitative structure-activity relationships in α-adrenergic drugs, we have attempted to characterize some α-adrenoceptor populations involved in cardiovascular processes in more detail. The ultimate goal of these efforts is a better understanding of the α-adrenergic biological response as well as of the interrelationships and classification of α-adrenoceptors in order to make them more accessible to drug design. Accordingly, quantitative relationships between the α-adrenergic effects initiated at these various α-adrenoceptors were searched for. Since all the pharmacological data have been obtained in intact animal experiments, great emphasis is put on the pharmacological aspects and the quality of the biological parameter in the interpretation of the results.

Four particular populations of α-adrenoceptors play a major role in the acute circulatory effects of most α-adrenergic agonists. Their participation in cardiovascular control is illustrated by the action of the antihypertensive drug clonidine (Catapresan®) on arterial pressure and heart rate following intravenous administration (Fig. 1). Due to its α-adrenoceptor stimulating properties, clonidine initially stimulates vascular α-adrenoceptors in the periphery, resulting in a hypertensive response. Thereafter, a long-lasting hypotensive phase develops, which is caused by the triggering of central α-adrenoceptors. Central α-adrenoceptors also mediate the bradycardic action of this drug. For detailed information on the

*References p. 266*

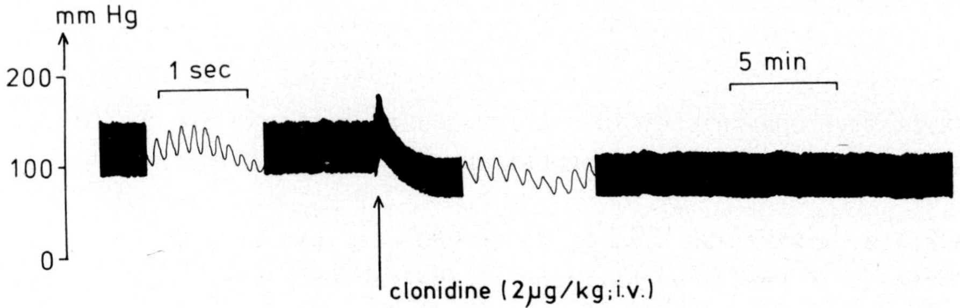


Fig. 1. Typical effect on arterial blood pressure and heart rate of the antihypertensive drug clonidine (2 μg/kg) injected intravenously into a pentobarbitone-anaesthetized normotensive rat. After a short-lasting increase, a prolonged decrease in mean arterial pressure accompanied by bradycardia is observed.

basic pharmacology the reader is referred to refs. 1-5. For reasons to be discussed a population of cardiac presynaptic α-adrenoceptors plays a significant role in the bradycardic effect of clonidine and related α-adrenoceptor stimulants.

The present paper reports on quantitative comparisons between these central and peripheral cardiovascular activities of α-adrenoceptor agonists.

## QUANTITATIVE RELATIONSHIPS BETWEEN HYPERTENSIVE AND HYPOTENSIVE ACTIVITIES.

### Procedure

Fig. 2 schematically outlines the localization of the particular α-adrenoceptors involved, the effects on arterial pressure induced by them upon activation by agonists as well as the procedure followed in obtaining the biological variables. The hypotensive action was measured following intravenous administration to anaesthetized, normotensive rats.The maximal decrease in mean arterial pressure was determined and log dose-depressor curves were constructed. Hypotensive activity was quantified by means of a $pC_{20}$, calculated from the log dose-depressor characteristics ($C_{20}$ = dose, μmol/kg, required to induce a 20% decrease in mean arterial pressure). Similarly, the hypertensive effect was measured in pithed, normotensive rats. Hypertensive potency was characterized as $pC_{60}$ ($C_{60}$ = dose, μmol/kg, associated with an increase in pressure by 60 mm Hg). The difference in accessibility to both α-adrenoceptor populations was accounted for by consideration of the apparent octanol/aqueous buffer (pH = 7.4;

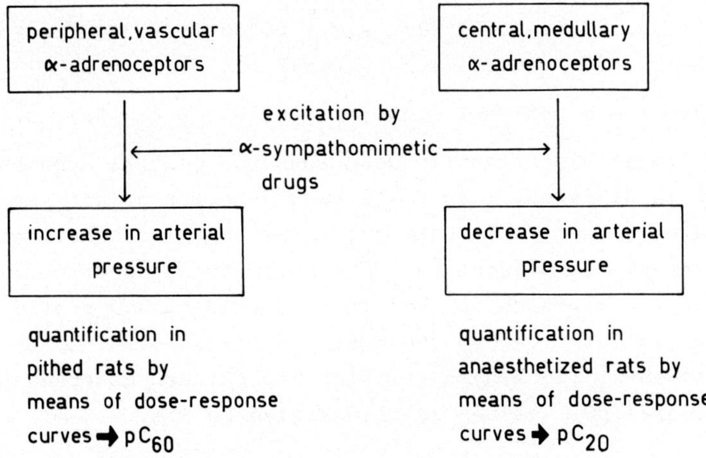


Fig. 2. Representation of the peripheral and central α-adrenoceptor populations investigated, the effects mediated by them upon activation by agonists, and the procedure followed to calculate a relationship between both α-adrenergic activities.

37°C) partition coefficient (log P'). Full details with respect to the quantification of hypo- and hypertensive activities as well as the determination of the partition coefficient have been published elsewhere [6-8].

Relationship between central hypotensive and peripheral hypertensive activities within a series of structurally dissimilar α-adrenoceptor agonists.

In case centrally induced depressor activity correlates linearly with the peripherally provoked pressor activity and the difference in accessibility to the two α-adrenoceptor populations is adequately described by log P', the following general equation 1 will be statistically relevant:

$$pC_{20} = a \log P' + b\, pC_{60} + C \qquad (1)$$

For 21 structurally dissimilar α-adrenoceptor agonists such a relationship was generated between central hypotensive activity and peripheral hypertensive potency provided that log P' was included

*References p. 266*

into the regression in a parabolic form due to the wide spread in lipophilicity of the compounds [9]:

$$pC_{20} = -0.387\ (\pm\ 0.16)\ (\log P')^2 + 0.895\ (\pm\ 0.33)\ \log P' + 0.887\ (\pm\ 0.21)\ pC_{60} - 0.098 \tag{2}$$

$n = 21;\ r = 0.945;\ s = 0.376;\ F = 47.03\ (p < 0.05)$

Equation 2 most significantly describes the central hypotensive activity of 21 different α-agonists as a function of the peripheral hypertensive potency and their overall lipophilic behaviour. The latter variable is present in a parabolic form. Equation 2 accounts for 89% of the variance in the hypotensive data and provides calculated $pC_{20}$ values close to the observed values obtained by pharmacological means. The linear relationship between observed and calculated (eq 2) $pC_{20}$ values is illustrated by Fig. 3.

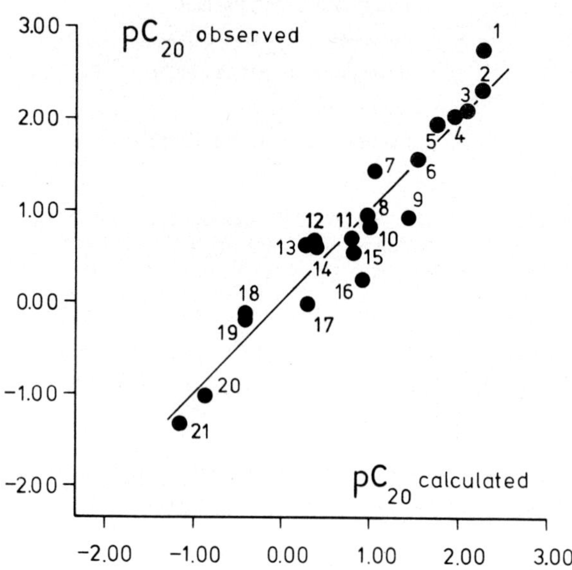


Fig. 3.Relationship between the central hypotensive activities of 21 structurally dissimilar α-adrenoceptor agonists observed after intravenous application to anaesthetized, normotensive rats and the values calculated by using eq 2.

It can be concluded from regression equation 2 that the structural requirements of the α-adrenoceptors located centrally and those of the α-adrenoceptor sites situated in the periphery at the vascular wall are apparently similar. Lipophilicity accounts for the relative difference between peripherally mediated pressor activity and centrally induced depressor potency of the α-adrenoceptor agonists. This conclusion is in agreement with our previous findings for a series of selected clonidine-like imidazolidines [10] and a limited number of α-adrenoceptor stimulants [11]. On the other hand differential agonistic and antagonistic activities have been reported for some α-adrenoceptor stimulating and blocking agents [12-15]. However, different routes of administration had been employed and the importance of lipophilicity had not been analyzed quantitatively.

Discrimination between central hypotensive and peripheral hypertensive activities among meta-substituted imidazolidines.

As a consequence of the outcome of the calculations described above, any vasopressor α-sympathomimetic agent possessing sufficient lipophilicity to penetrate into the central nervous system should also be able to decrease arterial pressure on account of the proposed similarity between central and peripheral α-adrenergic receptor sites. However, a discrepancy was encountered within a pair of 2,3- and 2,5-dichloro-substituted imidazolidines. As visualized in Fig. 4, in spite of comparable hypertensive activity and log P' values for both substitution isomers, their hypotensive potencies differ about 1.5 logarithmic units.

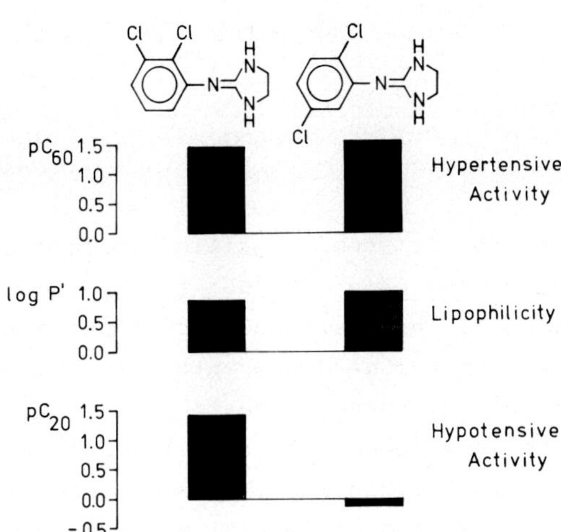


Fig. 4. Hypertensive ($pC_{60}$) and hypotensive ($pC_{20}$) activities and log P' values of 2,3- and 2,5-dichloro-substituted imidazolidines. Note that in spite of very similar hypertensive potencies as well as log P' values, their hypotensive activities differ considerably.

This result is not in accordance with the general applicability of similar α-adrenoceptor populations at peripheral and central sites

*References p. 266*

as suggested by eq 2. When the hypotensive activities of both 2,3- and 2,5-dichloro-substituted analogues are calculated according to this eq 2 and compared with the values actually measured, it is observed that the hypotensive potency of the 2,3-substituted derivative is adequately accounted for, but that the hypotensive activity of the 2,5-substituted isomer considerably deviates (Fig. 5).

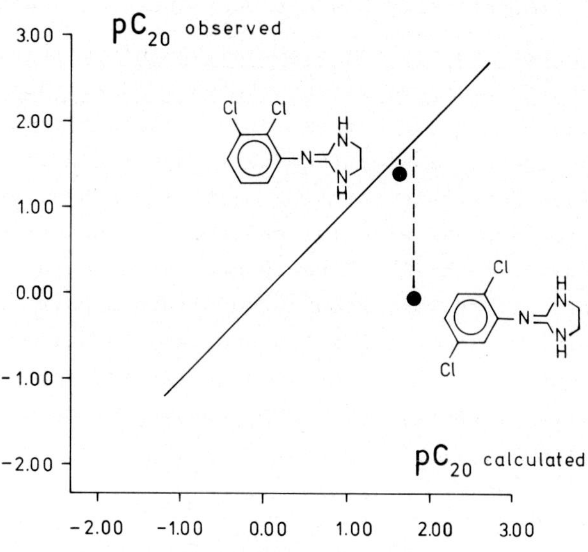


Fig. 5. Comparison between calculated (eq 2) and observed hypotensive activities within a pair of 2,3- and 2,5-dichloro-substituted imidazolidines. The straight line represents the relationship between calculated and observed values visualized in Fig. 3.

As a consequence thereof it seems justified to conclude that the 2,5-substituted derivative only does not fit in the general relationship formulated by eq 2. This particular compound discriminates between peripheral and central α-adrenoceptors in the sense that it is much less potent with respect to central (hypotensive) than to peripheral (hypertensive) receptor sites. In order to evaluate this hypothesis in more detail, quantitative comparisons were made between central hypotensive and peripheral hypertensive activities within a series of four isomeric pairs of 2,3- and 2,5-substituted imidazolidines with the 2-position occupied by chlorine [8]. The general structures have been depicted in Fig. 6.

The apparent partition coefficients (log P') of the meta-substituted derivatives as determined in the octanol/buffer (pH = 7.4) reference system at 37°C are given in Fig. 7. The data show that

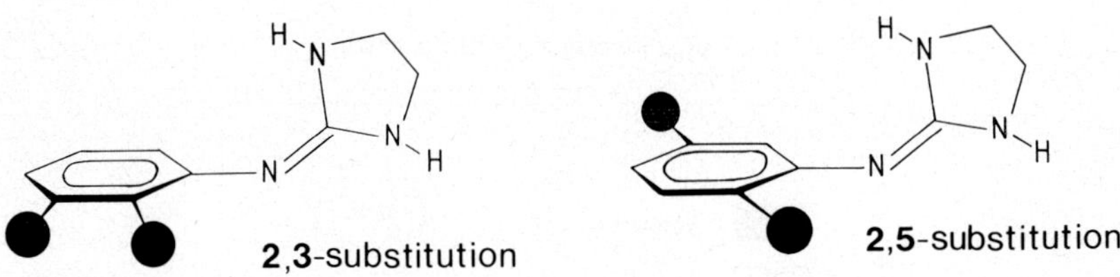


Fig. 6. General structures of 2,3- and 2,5-substituted phenyl(imino)imidazolidines. In this study the isomeric 2,3- and 2,5-substituted analogues were used in which the 2-position was occupied by chlorine. The 3- and 5-positions were substituted by either fluorine, chlorine, bromine or methyl.

lipophilicity varied by about 2.5 log P' units within this set of isomeric substitution pairs. Among the single pairs log P' of the individual members had comparable values, indicating minor differences in physicochemical properties (such as brain penetration) within each pair of isomers.

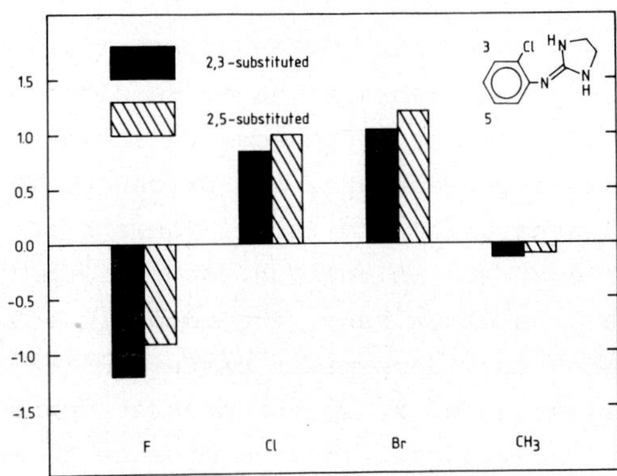


Fig. 7. Apparent partition coefficients (log P') measured between aqueous buffer (pH = 7.4) and octanol at 37°C of four isomeric pairs of 2,3- and 2,5-substituted phenyl(imino)imidazolidines.

After intravenous application to pithed normotensive rats, the compounds elicited an increase in diastolic pressure in a dose-dependent manner. From the log dose-depressor curves the peripheral hypertensive activity ($pC_{60}$) was calculated for each derivative. Fig. 8 shows that within the whole series of compounds, hypertensive activity differed less than 1 logarithmic unit. Moreover, for all isomeric pairs comparable pressor activities were obtained for the individual representatives. The 2,3-substituted analogues were generally somewhat less active than the corresponding 2,5-substituted

*References p. 266*

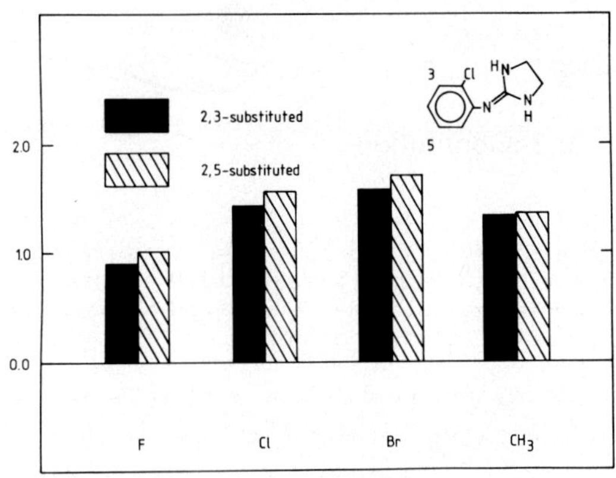


Fig. 8. Hypertensive activities of 2,3- and 2,5-substituted phenyl(imino)-imidazolidines quantified as $pC_{60}$ values following intravenous injections into pithed normotensive rats.

congeners.

After intravenous injections into anaesthetized normotensive rats, the compounds provoked a biphasic change in blood pressure (Fig. 9). In Fig. 9 the blood pressure responses are shown for the doses inducing a 20% decrease in mean arterial pressure. The 2,3-substituted imidazolidines behaved quite similarly. Their hypertensive phases preceding the 20% decrease in tension were of approximately the same magnitude. On the other hand, the isomeric 2,5-substituted molecules provoked a very dissimilar pattern of changes in blood pressure. For this group of drugs the pressor/depressor ratio increased from fluorine via chlorine and bromine to methyl. Therefore, a much more pronounced hypertensive phase preceded the development of the hypotension of the 2,5-substituted analogues, compared to the corresponding 2,3-substituted agents.

From the log dose-depressor response curves, the hypotensive activities ($pC_{20}$) of the meta-substituted imidazolidines were calculated. A comparison between these $pC_{20}$-values is made in Fig. 10. As already illustrated by Fig. 9, the hypotensive activities varied considerably (> 2 log units). Also within separate pairs of isomers, appreciable differences in depressor potency existed. The most pronounced difference was observed between the 3-bromo- and the 5-bromo-substituted analogues.

The following relationships were calculated between central hypotensive activity ($pC_{20}$) and peripheral hypertensive potency

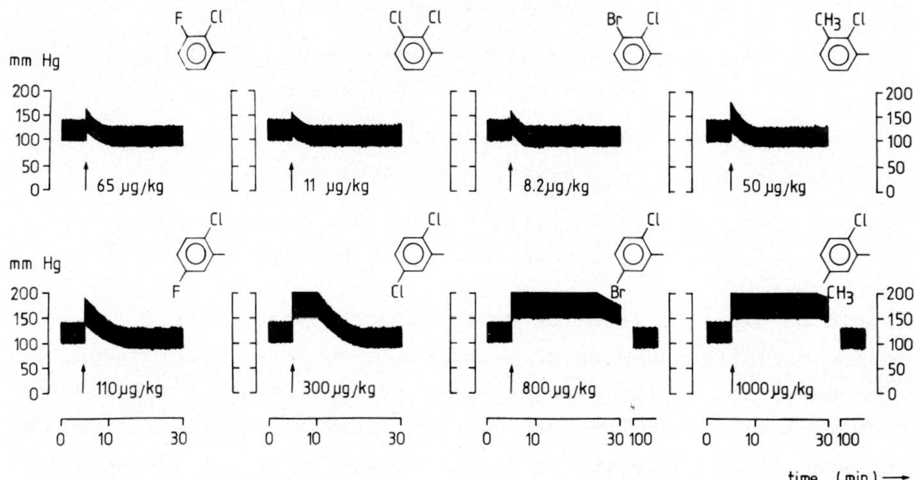


Fig. 9. Typical effects of four isomeric pairs of 2,3- and 2,5 substituted phenyl-(imino)imidazolidines on arterial pressure of anaesthetized, normotensive rats after intravenous administration. The biphasic actions are shown for the particular doses provoking a 20% decrease in mean arterial pressure.
Note the increasing pressor/depressor ratio for the 2,5-substituted analogues in the order F, Cl, Br, $CH_3$.

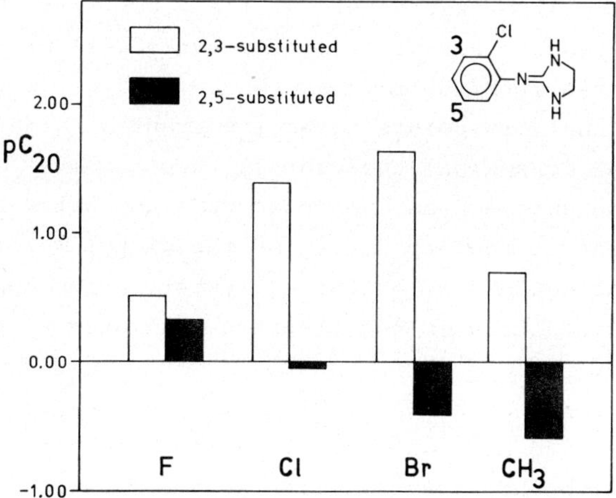


Fig. 10. Hypotensive activities of 2,3- and 2,5-substituted phenyl(imino)imidazolidines expressed as $pC_{20}$ values following intravenous administration to anaesthetized, normotensive rats.

($pC_{60}$) and log P'. Taft's steric parameter [16] of the substituent at the 5-position ($E_s$-5) was also used.

*References p. 266*

$$pC_{20} = 7.30 - 0.12\ (\pm\ 2.81) pC_{60} \qquad (3)$$
$$n = 8;\ r = -0.04;\ s = 0.86;\ F = 0.01$$

$$pC_{20} = 63.61 + 2.40\ (\pm\ 3.18)\ \log P' - 7.84\ (\pm\ 10.52) pC_{60} \qquad (4)$$
$$n = 8;\ r = 0.66;\ s = 0.71;\ F = 1.89$$

$$pC_{20} = 5.48 + 1.27\ (\pm\ 0.64)\ E_S\text{-}5 \qquad (5)$$
$$n = 8;\ r = 0.89;\ s = 0.39;\ F = 23.55$$

$$pC_{20} = 5.30 + 1.41(\pm\ 0.45)E_S\text{-}5 + 0.32(\pm\ 0.27)\log P' \qquad (6)$$
$$n = 8;\ r = 0.96;\ s = 0.25;\ F = 32.17$$

As could be expected from the data discussed above, the linear correlation between $pC_{20}$ and $pC_{60}$ (eq 3) is meaningless, due to the deviation of the 5-substituted imidazolidines. Inclusion of log P' into eq 3 also afforded a relationship (eq 4) with insignificant statistics. However, eq 5 shows that 79% of the variance in the hypotensive activity of the compounds can already be accounted for by Taft's steric constant of the substituent attached to the 5-position. This relationship was significantly ($F_{1,5}$=9.083) improved to a very acceptable level upon incorporation of log P' (eq 6). The positive signs of the coefficients in eq 6 indicate that central hypotensive activity is favored by increasing lipophilicity, but impaired by increasing steric bulk at the 5-position. Eq 6 provides calculated hypotensive activities which agree well with those measured experimentally (Fig. 11).

The present analysis points to an important structural difference among peripheral (vascular) and central (hypotensive) α-adrenoceptors. The central hypotensive α-adrenoceptor does not allow a relatively bulky substituent at the 5-position of the phenyl moiety of the imidazolidine molecule. In contrast, 5-substitution apparently does not hamper the induction of hypertension initiated at peripheral α-adrenoceptors.

What may be the reason that 2,5-substituted imidazolidines are able to discriminate between central and peripheral α-adrenoceptors? Is it an indication against a similarity among peripheral and central α-adrenoceptors as advocated in eq 2 ? The recent progress in the classification of α-adrenoceptors may offer a solution for these questions. Firm evidence exists at present that the central hypotensive α-adrenoceptors are a homogeneous population of the so-called $\alpha_2$-adrenoceptors [17-19]. However, apart from the more classical vascular $\alpha_1$-adrenoceptors an additional class of $\alpha_2$-adrenoceptors has also been identified to participate in drug-induced

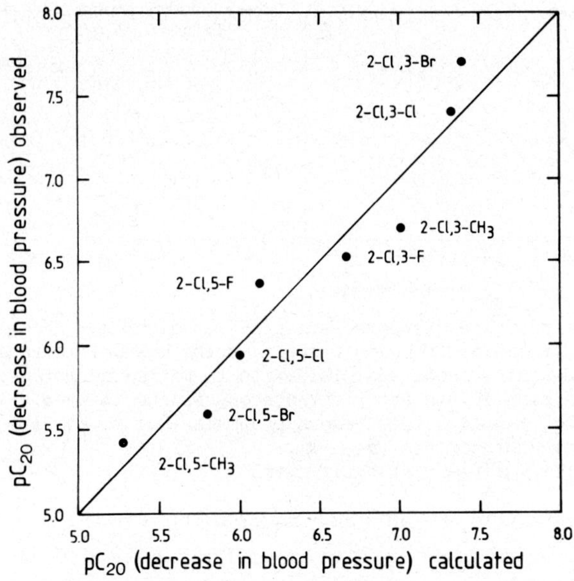


Fig. 11. Relationship between hypotensive activities obtained after intravenous application to anaesthetized normotensive rats and those calculated according to eq 6 for some meta-substituted 2-chlorophenyl(imino)imidazolidines

vasoconstriction [20-27]. Since hypotension can only be brought about by $\alpha_2$-adrenoceptor stimulation, but hypertension by both $\alpha_1$- and $\alpha_2$-adrenoceptor activation, it is likely then that phenyl-(imino)imidazolidines possessing a relatively bulky 5-substituent behave as selective stimulants of $\alpha_1$-adrenoceptors. The correctness of this supposition is illustrated by the experimental results visualized in Fig. 12 A and B. The pressor effects of the 2,3-dichloro-substituted molecule are susceptible to blockade by the selective $\alpha_2$-adrenoceptor blocking drug yohimbine [26, 28-31] as well as by the preferential antagonist of $\alpha_1$-adrenoceptors prazosin [26, 32, 33]. As a consequence thereof, the combination of both $\alpha$-adrenoceptor antagonists is found much more effective than the individual blocking drugs. On the other hand, the log dose-pressor response curve of the isomeric 2,5-dichloro-substituted imidazolidine is hardly affected by previous administration of yohimbine, but appreciably shifted to the right by prazosin. The combination of both blockers is now slightly more effective than prazosin alone. These results not only confirm the simultaneous involvement of $\alpha_1$- as well as $\alpha_2$-adrenoceptors in peripherally induced vasoconstriction, but also clearly show the $\alpha_1$-adrenoceptor selectivity of the 2,5-analogue compared to its 2,3-congener which is non-selective.

*References p. 266*

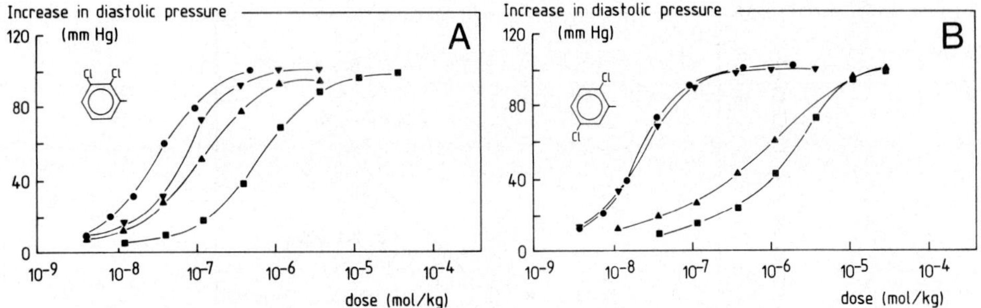


Fig. 12. Log dose-response characteristics of 2,3-dichloro- (A) and 2,5-dichlorophenyl(imino)imidazolidine (B) with respect to the maximal increase in diastolic pressure following intravenous administration to pithed normotensive rats. Measurements were made 15 min after intravenous saline (●——●), intravenous yohimbine (1 mg/kg, ▼——▼), intravenous prazosin (0.1 mg/kg, ▲——▲) and the combination of both antagonists (■——■).
Means of 5 to 8 separate experiments.

Based on the observation that increasing steric dimensions favor $\alpha_1$-adrenoceptor agonistic activity we have extended the series with the 2-chloro, 5-trifluoromethyl-substituted analogue (St 587). As shown in Fig. 13, the increase in diastolic pressure observed in pithed rats following intravenous administration of St 587 is solely mediated by vascular $\alpha_1$-adrenoceptors. The absence of $\alpha_2$-adrenoceptor agonistic activity is further illustrated by the observation that St 587 is devoid of central hypotensive (bradycardic) activity [34]. This particular imidazolidine derivative completely lacks agonistic activity at $\alpha_2$-adrenoceptors due to its bulky 5-$CF_3$-substituent. The combination of $\alpha_1$-adrenoceptor selectivity and lipophilic character is new at present and makes St 587 a valuable pharmacological tool for identifying and characterizing central $\alpha_1$-adrenoceptor populations.

The presence of a heterogenous $\alpha$-adrenoceptor population in the vasculature consisting of $\alpha_1$- as well as $\alpha_2$-adrenoceptors also explains the significant relationship between peripheral and central $\alpha$-adrenergic activities derived for structurally dissimilar $\alpha$-adrenoceptor agonists and other imidazolidine derivatives [9, 10], since the majority of these compounds are non-selective agonists of $\alpha_1$- and $\alpha_2$-adrenoceptors or selective stimulants of $\alpha_2$-adrenoceptors [15, 23, 24, 27, 35-52]. Non-selective $\alpha_1/\alpha_2$-adrenoceptor agonists as well as selective agonists of $\alpha_2$-adrenoceptors fit such a relationship, because $\alpha_2$-adrenoceptors are present at central as well as peripheral sites. However, it cannot be accomplished for pure agonists of $\alpha_1$-adrenoceptors. These particular drugs can induce

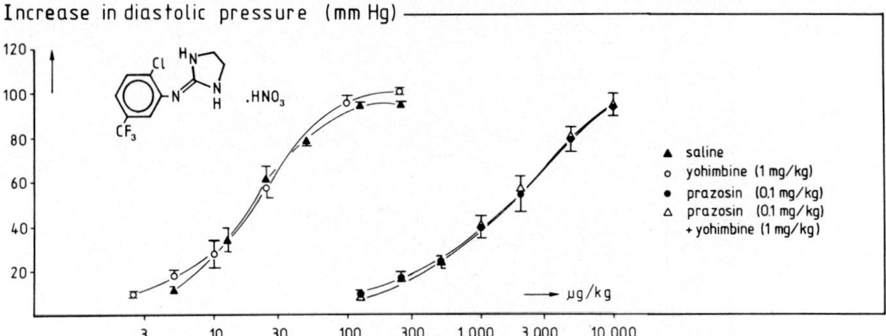


Fig. 13. Log dose-response curves of the maximal hypertensive effect of St 587 following intravenous injection into pithed normotensive rats.
Means ± standard estimation of the means (n = 5-8).

vasoconstriction via excitation of vascular $\alpha_1$-adrenoceptors, but fail to decrease blood pressure, since they are devoid of stimulating properties of (central) $\alpha_2$-adrenoceptors.

CENTRAL AND PERIPHERAL BRADYCARDIA.

The action of α-sympathomimetic drugs, e.g. clonidine, on arterial pressure is accompanied by a decrease in heart rate (bradycardia) as demonstrated by the typical example of Fig. 1. It is generally accepted that, like the induction of hypotension, the bradycardia also results from a central nervous origin, and is caused by the stimulation of central $\alpha_2$-adrenoceptors. The argument in favour of this presumption is the observation that the potency of α-sympathomimetic drugs to provoke hypotension parallels their bradycardic activity [6] Fig. 14 confirms such a relationship, in which the depressor potency, $pC_{20}$(BP), of 8 imidazolidines correlates with their bradycardic activity, $pC_{20}$(HR) [8]:

$$pC_{20}(BP) = -1.05 + 1.16\ (\pm\ 0.35)\ pC_{20}(HR) \qquad (7)$$
$$n = 8;\ r = 0.98;\ s = 0.18;\ F = 124$$

In generating eq 7, bradycardia was quantified as the dose (mol/kg) required to elicit a 20% decrease in heart rate after intravenous administration to anaesthetized normotensive rats. In case eq 7 is generally applicable, this would mean that bradycardia and hypotension will be found simultaneously for any α-sympathomimetic drug, since apparently they are inherent mechanisms. However, it was noticed for the derivative 3,4-dihydroxyphenyl(imino)imidazolidine (DPI), that this drug was able to decrease heart rate (maximal reduction

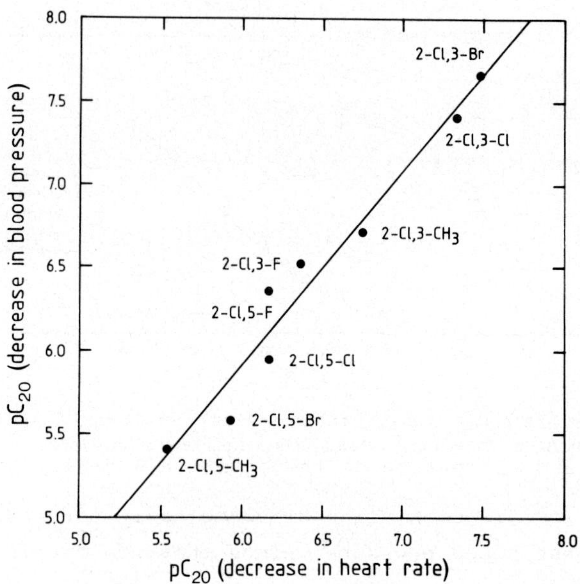


Fig. 14. Relationship between bradycardic and hypotensive activities of 8 phenyl-(imino)imidazolidines. The biological variables were quantified as $pC_{20}$ values obtained from log dose-response curves following intravenous administration to anaesthetized, normotensive rats.

about 15% at already low doses, but that it lacked hypotensive activity over a large dose range following intravenous administration to anaesthetized normotensive rats [53]. It was recognized that the limited lipid solubility of DPI could have unmasked a peripheral mechanism of bradycardia.

In order to obtain more information, bradycardia was quantified for a series of imidazolidines covering a wide range of lipophilicity. In anaesthetized, normotensive rats, the bradycardic effects of the lipophilic 2,6-dichloro(= clonidine)- and the 2,3-dibromo-substituted compounds were characterized by monophasic log dose-bradycardic response curves (Fig. 15). In contrast, the log dose-response curves of the less lipophilic drugs displayed a bisigmoidal shape (Fig. 15).

The dual nature of the bradycardic effect of the compounds was evaluated by two variables. The potency of the drugs to induce a decrease in heart rate was quantified by calculating the molar doses required to provoke a 10 as well as a 20% decrease in cardiac frequency; $pC_{10}$ (HR) and $pC_{20}$ (HR), respectively. Correlation studies showed that $pC_{20}$ (HR) could be described as a linear combination of $pC_{10}$ (HR) and log P'. Furthermore, $pC_{20}$ (HR) almost perfectly correlated with $pC_{20}$ (BP), whereas log P' had to be incorporated to

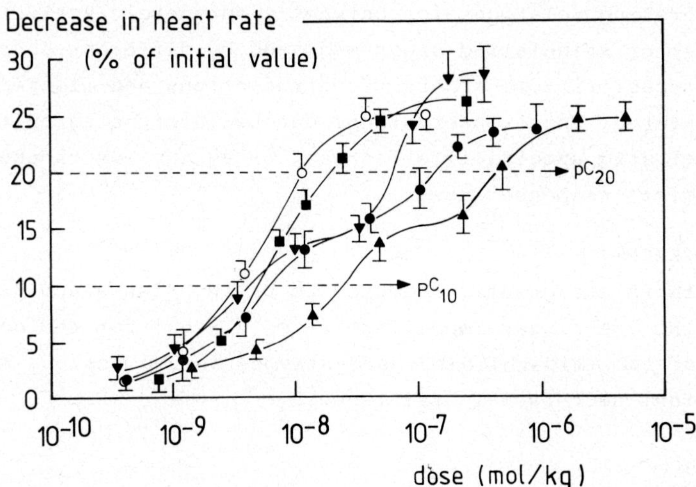


Fig. 15. Log dose-bradycardic effect curves of some imidazolidine derivatives determined in anaesthetized normotensive rats after intravenous administration. ○——○: 2-Cl,6-Cl (= clonidine); ■——■: 2-Br,3-Br; ▼——▼: 2-Me,3-Br; ●——●: 2-Cl,3-Me; ▲——▲: 2-Cl,3-F. Data are presented as mean values ± S.E.M. (n = 5-6).

verify such a relationship for $pC_{10}$ (HR). The appearance of log P' to make the correlation between $pC_{20}$ (HR) or $pC_{20}$ (BP) with $pC_{10}$ (HR) statistically relevant, strongly suggests that $pC_{10}$ (HR) identifies a peripherally induced bradycardic effect and that $pC_{20}$ (HR) stands for central bradycardia.

The question as to whether there exists a peripheral mechanism by which bradycardia can be accomplished can be answered positively. Presynaptically located $\alpha_2$-adrenoceptors in the heart itself are involved in a negative feedback mechanism in the regulation of transmitter release [54-58]. The activation of these prejunctional $\alpha_2$-adrenoceptors reduces the amount of neurotransmitter (noradrenaline) released from the sympathetic nerve endings. Final proof for the proposition that $pC_{10}$ (HR) is a measure of this peripheral sympatho-inhibition, was provided by the linear relationship observed between $pC_{10}$ (HR) and the potency at cardiac presynaptic $\alpha_2$-adrenoceptors established in a separate experimental animal model [59].

It is concluded that bradycardia elicited by α-sympathomimetic drugs may consist of a peripheral and a central component. Central bradycardia can only be elicited by agonists possessing sufficient lipid solubility to penetrate into the central nervous system.

## CONCLUSIONS

In generating relationships between α-adrenergic activities of α-adrenoceptor stimulating drugs mediated by different populations of α-adrenoceptors some apparent contradictions and discrepancies are encountered. These observations can be interpreted on the basis of distinct drug specificities as well as by the events underlying the biological response itself.

## ACKNOWLEDGEMENT

The authors are greatly indebted to Dr. H. Stähle and Dr. W. Hoefke (C.H. Boehringer Sohn, Ingelheim, F.R.G.) for the generous donation of the imidazolidine derivatives, and to Mrs. E. Zeeman for competent secretarial assistance.

## REFERENCES

1 P.A. van Zwieten, Prog. Pharmacol., 1(1975)1-63.
2 H. Schmitt, in F. Gross (Ed.), Antihypertensive Agents, Springer, Berlin, 1977, pp. 299-396.
3 W. Kobinger, Rev. Physiol. Biochem. Pharmacol., 81(1978)39-100.
4 P.A. van Zwieten and P.B.M.W.M. Timmermans, Trends Pharmacol. Sci., 1(1979)39-41.
5 P.B.M.W.M. Timmermans, W. Hoefke, H. Stähle and P.A. van Zwieten, Prog. Pharmacol., 3(1) (1980)1-104.
6 P.B.M.W.M. Timmermans and P.A. van Zwieten, Arch. int. Pharmacodyn., 228(1977)237-250.
7 P.B.M.W.M. Timmermans, A. Brands and P.A. van Zwieten, Naunyn--Schmiedeberg's Arch. Pharmacol., 300 (1977)217-226.
8 A. de Jonge, F.P. Slothorst-Grisdijk, P.B.M.W.M. Timmermans and P.A. van Zwieten, Europ. J. Pharmacol., 71(1981)411-420.
9 P.B.M.W.M. Timmermans, A. de Jonge, J.C.A. van Meel, F.P. Slothorst-Grisdijk, E. Lam and P.A. van Zwieten, J.Med.Chem., 24(1981) 502-507.
10 P.B.M.W.M. Timmermans and P.A. van Zwieten, Europ. J. Pharmacol., 45(1977)229-236.
11 P.B.M.W.M. Timmermans and P.A. van Zwieten, Life Sci., 28(1981) 653-660.
12 H. Schmitt and S. Fénard, Arch. int. Pharmacodyn., 190(1971) 229-240.
13 D. Bogaievsky, Y. Bogaievski, D. Tsoucaris-Kupfer and H. Schmitt, Clin. Exp. Pharmacol. Physiol., 1(1974)527-539.
14 H.A.J. Struyker Boudier, G. Smeets, G. Brouwer and J. van Rossum, Life Sci., 15(1974)887-899.
15 H.A.J. Struyker Boudier, J. de Boer, G. Smeets, E.J. Lien and J. van Rossum, Life Sci., 17(1975)377-386.
16 C. Hansch, in J. Cavallito (Ed.), Structure-Activity Relationships, Pergamon Press, London, 1973, Vol. 1, p. 75.
17 S. Berthelsen and W.A. Pettinger, Life Sci., 21(1977)595-606.
18 A.S. Hersom, L.Finch and G. Metcalf, Proc. 7th Intern. Congr. Pharmacol., (1978) abstr. 2713.
19 P.B.M.W.M. Timmermans, A.M.C. Schoop, H.Y. Kwa and P.A. van Zwieten, Europ. J. Pharmacol., 70(1981)7-15.
20 J.R. Docherty, A. MacDonald and J.C. McGrath, Brit. J. Pharmacol., 67(1979)421P-422P.

21 G.M. Drew and S.B. Whiting, Brit. J. Pharmacol., 67(1979)207-215.
22 P.B.M.W.M. Timmermans, H.Y. Kwa and P.A. van Zwieten, Naunyn--Schmiedeberg's Arch. Pharmacol., 310(1979)189-193.
23 P.B.M.W.M. Timmermans and P.A. van Zwieten, Europ. J. Pharmacol., 63(1980)199-202.
24 P.B.M.W.M. Timmermans and P.A. van Zwieten, Naunyn-Schmiedeberg's Arch. Pharmacol., 313(1980)17-20.
25 P.B.M.W.M. Timmermans and P.A. van Zwieten, J.Auton. Pharmacol., 1(1981)171-183.
26 P.B.M.W.M. Timmermans, J.C.A. van Meel and P.A. van Zwieten, J. Auton. Pharmacol., 1(1980)53-60.
27 W. Kobinger and L. Pichler, Europ. J. Pharmacol., 65(1980)393-402.
28 K. Starke, E. Borowski and T. Endo, Europ. J. Pharmacol., 34(1975) 385-388.
29 E. Borowski, K. Starke, H. Ehrl and T. Endo, Neuroscience, 2(1977) 285-296.
30 R. Weitzell, T. Tanaka and K. Starke, Naunyn-Schmiedeberg's Arch. Pharmacol., 308(1979)127-136.
31 A. de Jonge, P.N. Santing, P.B.M.W.M. Timmermans and P.A. van Zwieten, J. Auton. Pharmacol., (1981) in press.
32 D. Cambridge, M. Davey and M.J. Massingham, Brit. J. Pharmacol., 59(1977)514P-515P.
33 J.C. Doxey, C.F.C. Smith and J.M. Walker, Brit. J. Pharmacol., 60(1977)91-96.
34 A. de Jonge, J.C.A. van Meel, P.B.M.W.M. Timmermans and P.A. van Zwieten, Life Sci., 28(1981)2009-2016.
35 P.A. van Zwieten, Pharmacology, 13(1975)352-355.
36 H.J. Schümann and U. Werner, Naunyn-Schmiedeberg's Arch. Pharmacol., 268(1971)71-82.
37 F. Jacobs, U. Werner and H.J. Schümann, Arzneim. Forsch., 22(1972) 1124-1137.
38 R. Giudicelli and H.J. Schmitt, J. Pharmacol., 1(1970)339-358.
39 R. Hammer, W. Kobinger and L. Pichler, Europ. J. Pharmacol., 62(1980)277-283.
40 W. Kobinger and L. Pichler, Naunyn-Schmiedeberg's Arch. Pharmacol., 291(1975)175-191.
41 W. Kobinger and L. Pichler, Europ. J. Pharmacol., 40(1976)311-320.
42 P.B.M.W.M.Timmermans, J.C.J. Mackaay, P.H.M. Fluitman and P.A. van Zwieten, Pharmacology, 19(1979)294-300.
43 E. Lindner and J. Kaiser, Arch. Int. Pharmacodyn., 211(1974) 305-325.
44 P. Simon, R. Chernat and J.R. Boissier, Thérapie, 30(1975)855-861
45 H. Schmitt, G. Fournadjiev and H. Schmitt, Europ. J. Pharmacol., 10(1970)230-238.
46 A. Heise and G. Kroneberg, Arch. Pharmacol., 266(1970)350-354.
47 M.J. Antonaccio, R.D. Robson and L. Kerwin, Europ. J. Pharmacol., 23(1973)311-315.
48 L. Finch, Brit. J. Pharmacol., 52(1974)333-338.
49 W. Kobinger and L. Pichler, Naunyn-Schmiedeberg's Arch. Pharmacol., 300 (1977) 39-46.
50 D.E. Hutcheon, A. Scriabine and V.N. Niesler, J. Pharmacol. Exp. Ther., 122(1958)101-109.
51 P.B.M.W.M. Timmermans and P.A. van Zwieten, Pharmacology, 16 (1978)106-114.
52 J.C.A. van Meel, A. de Jonge, P.B.M.W.M. Timmermans and P.A. van Zwieten, J. Pharmacol. Exp. Ther., (1981) in press.
53 A. de Jonge, P.N. Santing, J.C.A. van Meel, P.B.M.W.M. Timmermans and P.A. van Zwieten, Europ. J. Pharmacol., (1981) in press.
54 S.Z. Langer, Brit. J. Pharmacol., 60(1977)481-497.
55 K. Starke, Rev. Physiol. Biochem. Pharmacol., 77(1977)1-124.
56 T.C. Westfall, Physiol. Rev., 57(1977)659-728.

57 S.Z. Langer, K. Starke and M.L. Dubocovich (Eds.), Presynaptic Receptors, Pergamon Press, Oxford, 1979.
58 D.M. Paton (Ed.), The Release of Catecholamines From Adrenergic Neurons, Pergamon Press, Oxford, 1979.
59 A. de Jonge, P.B.M.W.M. Timmermans and P.A. van Zwieten, Naunyn--Schmiedeberg's Arch. Pharmacol., 317(1981)8-12.

J.A. Keverling Buisman (Editor), *Strategy in Drug Research* 


# EXAMPLES OF THE ROLE OF COMPUTERS IN NEW COMPOUND DESIGN IN A PHARMACEUTICAL COMPANY

Y. C. MARTIN
Abbott Laboratories, No. Chicago, Ill. (U.S.A.)

## ABSTRACT

The analysis in our laboratory of the quantitative relationship between physical properties and biological potency of cannabinoids, 5'-adenosine analogues, and trimethoprim analogues has resulted in correct predictions of potency in all three types of molecules. Both regression and discriminant analysis led to correct predictions. In our experience, not every type of data led to a quantitative structure-activity equation, and not every equation was predictive. This report provides examples that illustrate that the principal reasons for such failures of prediction are improper series design and lack of consideration of conformational changes within the set of compounds.

## INTRODUCTION

In this paper attention will be focused on specific examples, as yet unpublished, of uses and extensions of linear free energy relationships (ref. 1) in medicinal chemistry programs at Abbott. Linear free energy relationship analysis involves the statistical analysis of the relationship between the biological potency of compounds and their physical properties such as hydrophobicity, electronic nature, and the size of the variable substituents. We will show how linear free energy analysis has been useful to us in new drug discovery. Finally, the extensions of this approach into considerations of conformation and shape will be discussed.

## CANNABINOID ANALOGUES

### Regression Analysis

For a number of years in the early 1970's Abbott maintained a program of synthesis and testing of cannabinoid analogues (refs. 2-5). In 1971 we performed a Hansch QSAR analysis on literature dog ataxia potency of compounds of Structure Ia (ref. 6). The side chain had been modified extensively with various alkyl substituents, so there was a satisfactory variation in lipophilicity (pi) and steric bulk ($E_s$), but no variation in electronic properties ($\sigma$*).

*References p. 284*

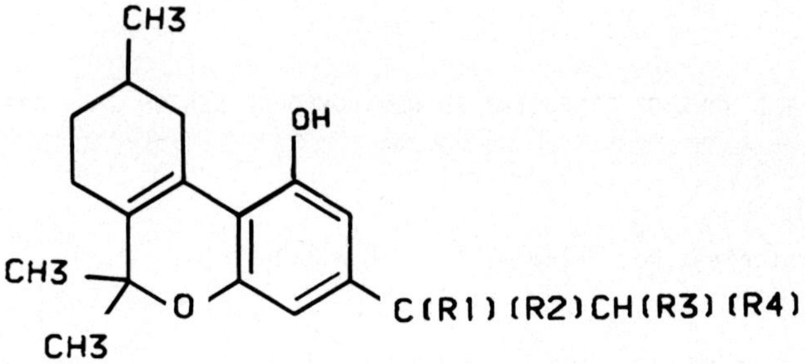

CH3

OH

CH3 O C(R1)(R2)CH(R3)(R4)

CH3

I

Ia, vary R1, R2, R3, and R4
Ib, R1 = $CH_3$, R2 = R3 = H, R4 = $(CH_2)_3C_6H_4F$
Ic, R1 = $CH_3$, R2 = R3 = H, R4 = $(CH_2)_3C_6H_5$
Id, R1 = $CH_3$, R2 = R3 = H, R4 = $(CHCH_3)(CH_2)_2C_6H_4F$
Ie, R1 = $CH_3$, R2 = R3 = H, R4 = $(CHCH_3)(CH_2)_3C_6H_4F$

The following equation was derived for all analogues of the indicated structure, i.e. the analogue with a methyl side chain was omitted.

$$\log(1/C) = -1.53 + 0.32\,(\underline{pi}_1 + \underline{pi}_2) + 0.36\,\underline{pi}_3 + 1.39\,\underline{pi}_4 - 0.27\,(\underline{pi}_4)^2 \tag{1}$$

$n = 25$, $R^2 = 0.77$, $s = 0.38$, optimum $\underline{pi}_4 = 2.6$.

In Eq. 1, C refers to the molar dose that produces ataxia in the dog, the various pi values to the hydrophobicity of the indicated substituent, n to the number of analogues, R to the multiple correlation coefficient, and s to the standard deviation of observed vs calculated activities. The corresponding equations with pi summed over all positions or with $E_s$ values substituted for some of the pi values were not statistically significant.

Eq. 2 was derived from the data on those compounds for which $R_1 = R_2 = R_3 = H$:

$$\log(1/C) = -1.29 + 0.60\,\underline{pi}_4 - 0.14\,(\underline{pi}_4)^2 \tag{2}$$

$n = 10$, $R^2 = 0.79$, $s = 0.17$, optimum $\underline{pi}_4 = 2.1$

It was concluded from Eqs. 1 and 2 that there is a specific hydrophobic effect of each of the R groups of Ia, and that there is an optimum hydrophobicity of the chain.

Aralkyl analogues were then designed to bracket the optimum calculated hydrophobicity. The equations correctly predicted the potency of the new analogues: analogues Ib, Ic, and Id have approximately the same hydrophobicity (0.0 to 0.8 log units higher) as the most potent Ia analogue and their potencies in the dog ataxia test are equal to it; on the other hand Ie is 1.4 log units more lipophilic than Ia and it is also 10X less potent in the dog ataxia test (ref. 2).

This relationship was verified by a regression analysis of a set of data generated at Abbott. The set consisted of 12 analogues of Ia in which the side-chain had been modified. The biological activity S is the score on the rat hyperirritability test.

$$\log(S) = -2.98 + 2.13\,\underline{pi} - 0.25\,(\underline{pi})^2 \qquad (3)$$

$$n = 12,\ R^2 = 0.84,\ s = 0.11,\ \text{optimum}\ \underline{pi} = 4.28.$$

The optimum pi calculated for the whole side chain agrees favorably with that calculated for it in Eqs. 1 and 2. The equation in which $E_s$ was substituted for pi had an $R^2$ of 0.69, and so it was concluded that the effect is truly a hydrophobic and not a steric one.

Table 1

Discriminant Analysis of Cannabinoid Analogues

| Property | Coefficient Analgetic Activity | Coefficient Irritability Activity |
|---|---|---|
| Physicochemical Properties | | |
| pi of side chain | 1.8 | 2.4 |
| pi of phenolic substituent | | |
| pi of C-ring | | 2.5 |
| $E_s$ of side chain | | |
| Indicator Variables | | |
| Free phenol | | |
| Additional aromatic ring substitution | | |
| Phenol is converted to an ester | 3.0 | 4.5 |
| Phenol is converted to a carbamate | -4.3 | |
| Phenol is converted to an ether | | |
| X is =O | -2.9 | -5.1 |
| C-ring contains S | | |
| C-ring contains O | | |
| C-ring contains N | -2.3 | |
| C-ring contains C only | | |
| C-ring is aromatic | 13.0 | -6.3 |
| Double bond in C-ring is moved or absent | | |
| C-ring is substituted to hinder the -OH | | |
| C-ring is five-membered | -2.9 | |
| C-ring is substituted | 2.2 | |
| Intercept | -7.6 | -15. |

Table 2

Predictive Ability of the Discriminant Functions

Classification of Data Used to Derive the Discriminant Functions

| | Analgetic Data: Calculated Active | Analgetic Data: Calculated Inactive | Irritability Data: Calculated Active | Irritability Data: Calculated Inactive |
|---|---|---|---|---|
| Observed | | | | |
| Active | 34 | 10 | 51 | 7 |
| Inactive | 14 | 78 | 15 | 36 |
| Percent Correct | 82 | | 79 | |

Classification of Data Used to Test the Discriminant Functions

| | Analgetic Data: Calculated Active | Analgetic Data: Calculated Inactive | Irritability Data: Calculated Active | Irritability Data: Calculated Inactive |
|---|---|---|---|---|
| Observed | | | | |
| Active | 18 | 0 | 24 | 2 |
| Inactive | 5 | 12 | 22 | 41 |
| Percent Correct | 86 | | 73 | |

## Discriminant Analysis

The synthetic program in this project involved preparing not only side-chain analogues, but also modifications in the left (or C) ring of I and pro-drugs of the phenol (refs. 2-5). The final products and some of the pyrone precursors were tested as possible analgesic agents, hypnotics, antidepressants, antipsychotics, tranquilizers, antiulcer agents, antidiarrheal agents, antihypertensives, and anticonvulsants as well as for the typical hyper-irritability side effect.

Because the structural variation between compounds was so dramatic and the animal testing was generally dichotomous, these data were analyzed with discriminant analysis (ref. 7). Table 1 lists the variables considered and the coefficients of these variables in the discriminant function for analgetic activity and hyper-irritability in rats. The observation that the two activities generally have opposite coefficients means that the same structural variations influence both activities. However, substitution in the C-ring, especially if it "protects" the phenolic-OH group, increases analgetic activity without increasing the side effect.

Table 2 demonstrates that the discriminant functions were truly predictive, that is, the percentage of compounds correctly classified does not significantly decrease i the set of compounds tested after the discriminant functions were described. The increase in efficiency if the discriminant functions had been used to guide synthesis can be calculated by comparing the percentage of active analgetics without the side effect in the total set of new compounds as opposed to the percentage of such compounds within the set predicted to have this profile:

Total set: 18/35 X 43/89 = 20%

Predicted set: 18/23 X 41/43 = 75%

This calculation suggests that the use of the QSAR method of discriminant analysis more than doubled the chance of finding the desired compound.

### Lack of Equations for Antidepressant, Tranquilizer and Anticonvulsive Activity

The QSAR efforts in this program were not without limitations and disappointments, however. We were never able to develop a QSAR description of the requirements for antidepressant, tranquilizer, or anticonvulsive activity in spite of the fact that more than 200 analogues had been tested in each of these screens. (We did show that there was no significant correlation among these activities nor between them and analgetic and hyper-irritability responses.) The only information that this negative result supplied was that the structural properties that seem to determine analgetic activity and the hyper-irritability response are not important determinants of the other activities: that is, that the goal of separating activities should be possible to attain. The lack of QSAR equations may be due to noise in the biological data or because the series was designed on the basis of structural rather than statistical and physicochemical considerations (ref. 8). However, it must be also admitted that the problem may lie in the fact that the QSAR analyses did not explicitly consider the role of the three-dimensional shape of the molecules in the analysis. Earlier conformational calculations showed that the modifications in the ring to the left in I could lead to different molecular profiles (ref. 9). If the program were active today it is possible that the predictive design of antidepressants, tranquilizers, and anticonvulsants would be improved because of more ready availability of the computer software and hardware necessary to study molecular shape.

## ADENOSINE ANALOGUES

Also in the early 1970's Abbott was involved in a program the goal of which was to prepare an antianginal agent that increased the partial pressure of oxygen in the coronary sinus blood. The synthetic program involved modifications of the 5'-group of adenosine carboxylate, II (refs. 10-12).

### Discriminant Analysis

In terms of therapeutic usefulness it was considered desirable to prepare a compound that not only increased coronary sinus $P_{O_2}$ but that also decreased blood pressure, without being too toxic. To study the relationship between structure and the biological properties we used discriminant analysis. The results of the two-group discriminant functions are reported here; however, in some

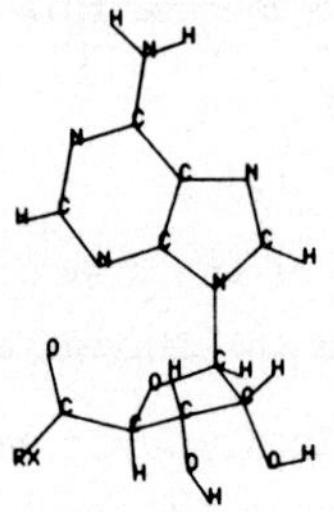

II

cases three categories of activity were also considered.

The results are summarized in Table 3.

The discriminant function for lowering of dog blood pressure shows that only amides lowered blood pressure and that amides with branched or cyclic side chains did not have this property. The function has good predictive ability.

Two discriminant functions were derived for increase in coronary sinus $P_{O_2}$ (measured simultaneously with the blood pressure responses above). The one with four variables indicates that amides and esters are both likely to be active, but only if their side chain has a small pi value: this equation is of no predictive value. The simpler equation includes only the pi value of the substituent: it has acceptable predictive ability.

Two discriminant functions were derived for mouse toxicity. Only the simpler one, which included no indicator variables, had predictive utility.

Table 3

Discriminant Analysis of the Antihypertensive, Antianginal, and Toxic Properties of 5'-Adenosine Analogues

| Property | Lower Dog Blood Pressure | Increase Dog $P_{O_2}$ a | b | Mouse Toxicity a | b |
|---|---|---|---|---|---|
| Structural | | | | | |
| Amide | 4.9 | | 3.2 | | 6.9 |
| Branched side-chain | -6.5 | | | | |
| Cyclic side-chain | -7.6 | | | | -4.0 |
| Ester | | | 4.0 | | |
| pi-value | | -1.3 | -1.2 | -0.6 | -0.6 |
| pi-squared | | -1.0 | -0.9 | | |
| Intercept | -1.0 | 2.4 | 0.0 | -0.3 | -3.6 |
| Percent correct | | | | | |
| Original | 89 | 76 | 78 | 70 | 82 |
| Predicted | 86 | 70 | 50 | 71 | 50 |

The predictive success in one case and failure in two cases of discriminant functions that contain indicator variables should lead to caution in the use of such descriptors. They may fool us into thinking that we understand the physical basis for the activity or inactivity of a certain type of compound.

For each biological activity studied a discriminant function with predictive value was obtained. The result underscores the utility of such work, even though, as will be seen in the next section, we are a long way from understanding the molecular basis for the structure-activity relationships in this series.

Regression Analysis

When a number of analogues had been prepared we derived the following equation

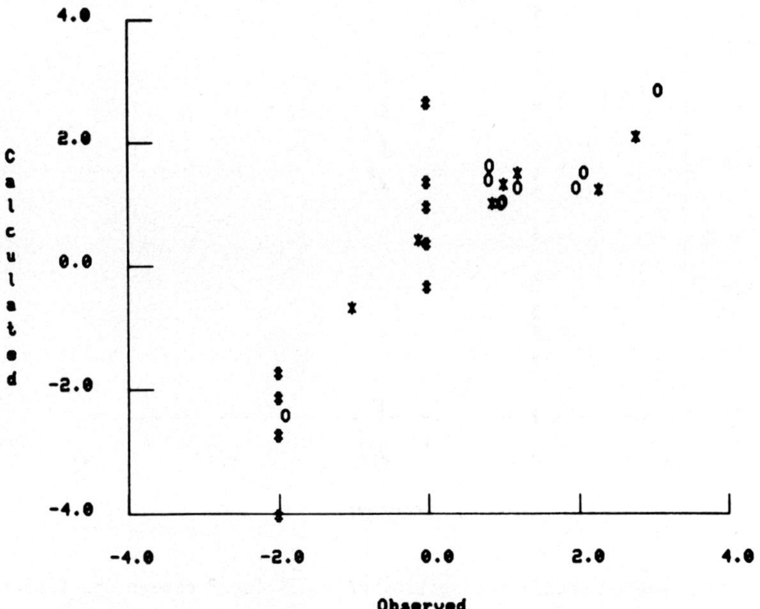


Figure 1. The ability of Eq. 4 to predict the potency of newer 5'-carboxamides of adenosine. O represents the compounds used to derive Eq. 4, * the predicted compounds for which an accurate dose-response curve was measured, and # the predicted compounds for which only a rough estimate of potency is available.

References p. 284

for the series for which X = NH, that is for secondary amides:

$$\log(1/C) = 0.77 - 2.22\ \underline{pi} - 1.32\ (\underline{pi})^2 + 1.47\ I \quad (4)$$

$$n = 9,\ R^2 = 0.86,\ s = 0.43.$$

In Eq. 4, C refers to the intravenous micromolar dose that produces an area under the time-response curve of 250 and the I indicator variable is assigned a value of 1.0 for cyclic analogues and 0.0 for non-cyclic analogues. This equation correctly predicted the potency of an additional seven analogues and also classified the potency of eight analogues that had not been tested in a full dose-response test. Fig. 1 illustrates these predictions.

Although the equation had good predictive ability for secondary amides, it was less successful for esters, and it incorrectly predicted that tertiary amides should also be active. Fig. 2 illustrates these points.

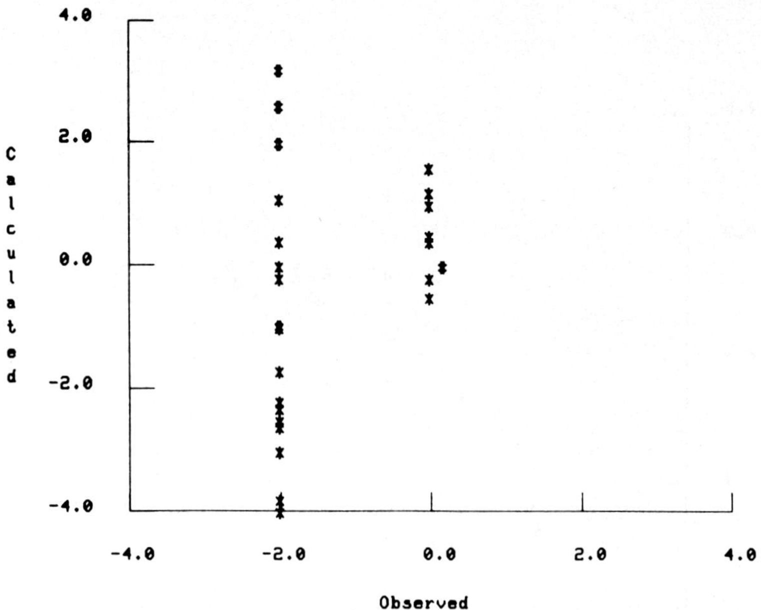


Figure 2. The lack of predictive ability of Eq. 4 for * esters and # tertiary amides.

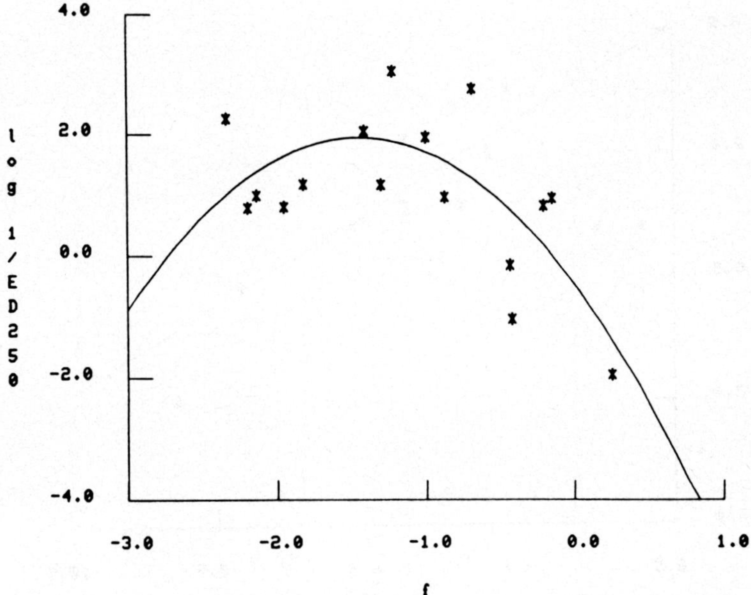


Figure 3. The fit of the potency of the secondary amides to Eq. 5.

When we reexamined these data early this year we could use the lessons that had been learned in the past eight years to try to understand why Eq. 4 was restricted in applicability to only one sub-set of the compounds. Five potential reasons why a regression equation may not be predictive have been identified: (a) the biological activity may have been improperly transformed (ref. 15), (b) the influence of ionization may have been ignored or improperly handled (ref. 15), (c) the relationship between physical properties and biological potency may have been fit by an incorrect function (ref. 15), (d) the data set may have been improperly designed for such analysis (ref. 8), or (e) incorrect molecular descriptors may have been chosen (ref. 1). Since the biological activity was calculated from a dose-response test, point _a_ was ruled out. The degree of ionization does not vary in the series so point _b_ was ruled out. The chemists had prepared a wide series of analogues that passed the proposed statistical criteria for a well-designed series, (ref. 8) so point _d_ was not the cause of the lack of predictability. Points _c_ and _e_ were considered in concert.

The regression analysis was repeated on the potency of the 16 secondary amides. For physical properties Leo f-values (ref. 16) and STERIMOL steric parameters (ref. 17) were used. Both linear and nonlinear equations (ref. 15) were considered. Fig. 3 illustrates the relationship between potency and the Leo hydrophobicity

*References p. 284*

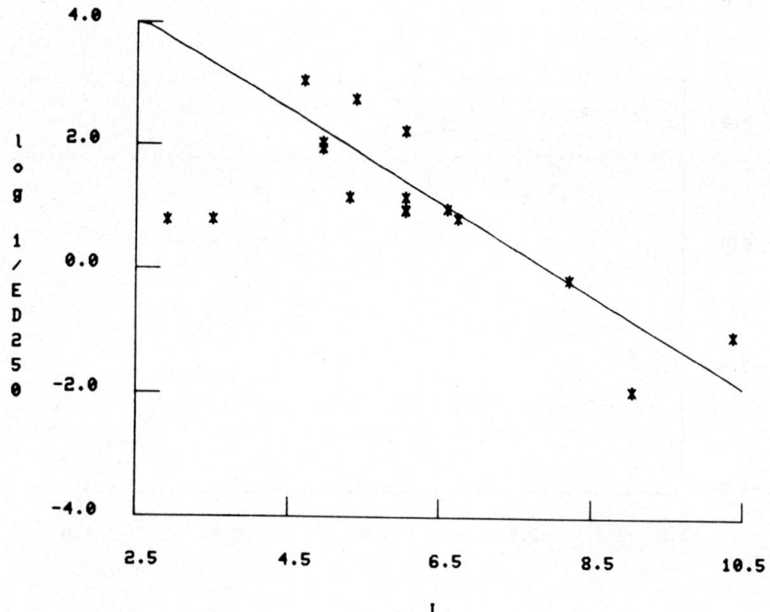


Figure 4. The fit of the potency of the secondary amides to Eq. 6, except the two points at low L values were not adjusted with the indicator variable.

parameter. The equation that describes the relationship is the following:

$$\log(1/C) = -0.44 - 3.31\ f - 1.16\ f^2 \tag{5}$$

$$n = 16,\ R^2 = 0.48,\ s = 1.00.$$

Clearly this relationship is not very precise, nor is the data obviously fit by another function. The indicator variable for cyclic compounds does not improve the correlation. Eq. 6 (Fig. 4) is a substantially better fit of the data:

$$\log(1/C) = 1.68 - 1.30\ L - 2.70\ I \tag{6}$$

$$n = 16,\ R^2 = 0.80,\ s = 0.62.$$

The L refers to the length of the substituent in the direction of the bond to the parent structure, and the I to an indicator variable that was set to 1.0 for the compounds for which $R_2$ is H or $CH_3$, that is for the two smallest substituents.

## Conformational Analyses

Five different types of evidence led us to propose that the difference in potency of the different analogues relates to conformational or shape differences between the compounds. The first concerns the original regression equation: the need for

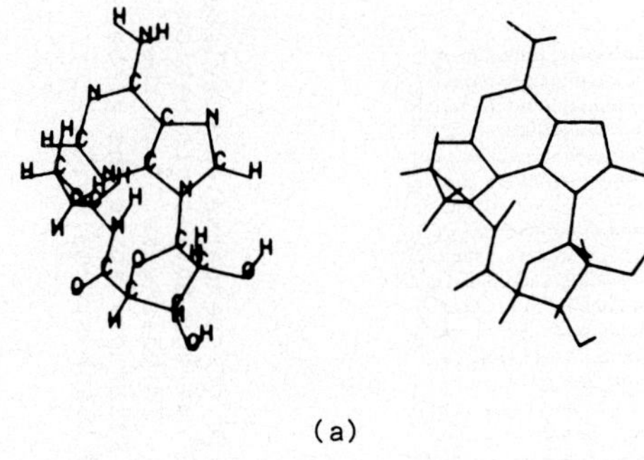

(a)

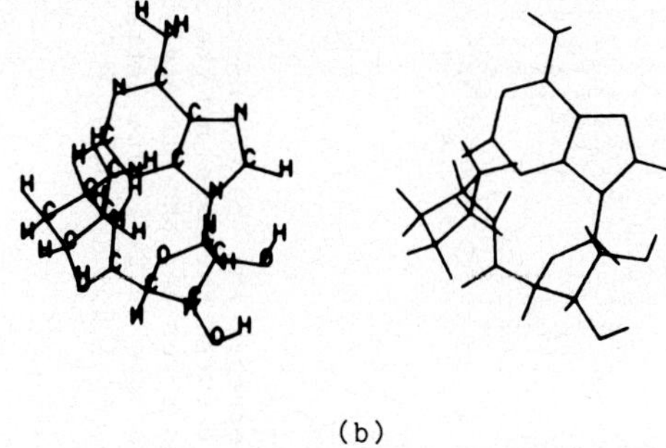

(b)

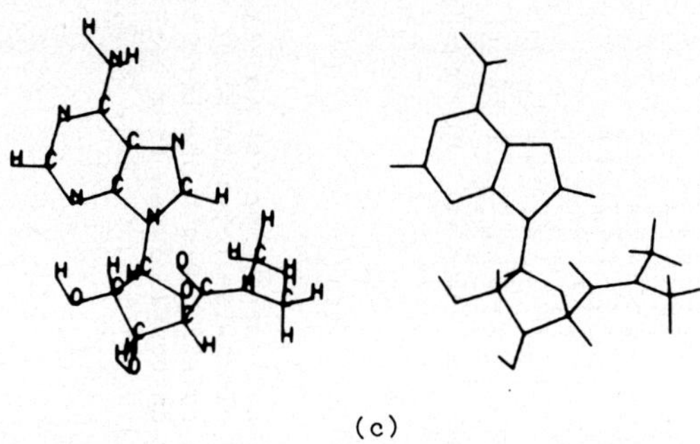

(c)

Figure 5. Computer-generated stereo-pairs of the low-energy conformations of some adenosine 5'-carboxamides: (a) the cyclopropyl amide, (b) the cyclopentyl amide, and (c) the dimethyl amide.

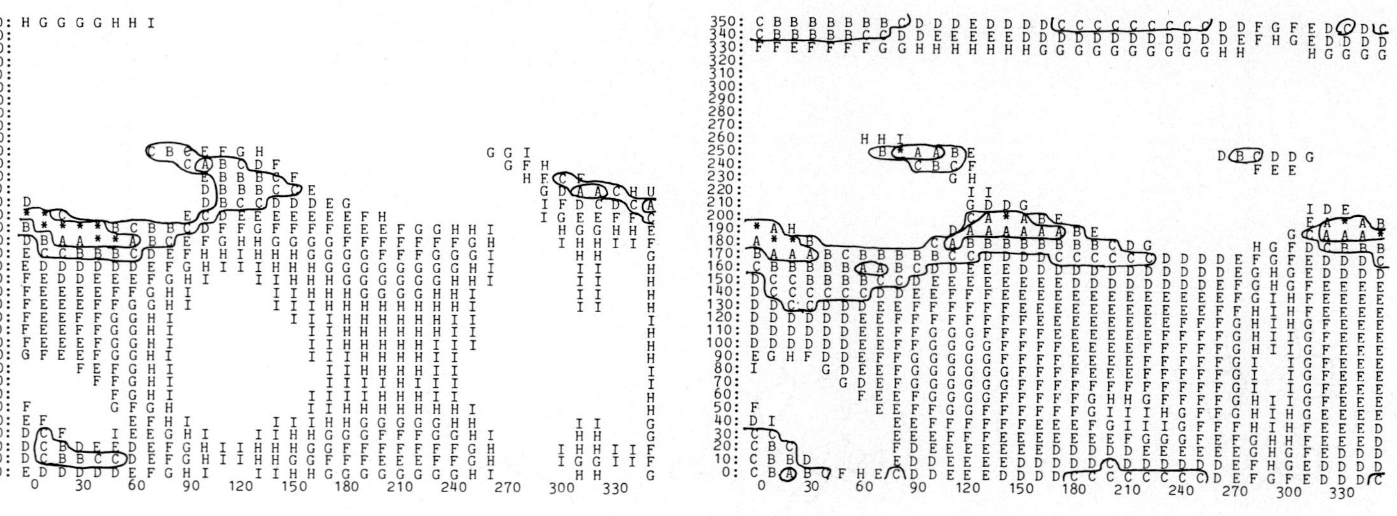

Figure 6. Conformational energy maps of (a) the 5'-cyclopropyl and (b) the unsubstituted amide of adenosine carboxylate. The Y-axis represents clockwise rotation about the bond between the base and the sugar with $0^{o}$ as the anti-conformation. The X-axis represents rotation about the bond between the sugar and the carbonyl carbon atom. In this case $0^{o}$ is the conformation with the carbonyl oxygen atom cis to the hydrogen at C4'. The letters refer to Kcal/mole above the global minimum: *< 0.5, A< 1.0, B< 1.5, C< 2.0, D< 2.5, E< 3.0, F< 3.5, G< 4.0, H< 4.5, I< 5.0, and blank spaces >5.0.

the indicator variable for cyclic substituents, and the lack of predictive ability for tertiary amides and esters. The second piece of evidence is that the parameter L seems to describe the relative potency of the secondary amides, but it alone is not enough to predict the lack of activity of the tertiary amides and most esters. The third evidence is that the slope of the equation with L is negative (larger groups lead to less activity) and the equation doesn't include the unsubstituted and methyl analogues. The fourth evidence comes from published NMR studies that suggest a totally different conformation for the dimethyl and the methyl analogues (ref. 12). Both the conformation of the sugar with respect to the base and the carbonyl with respect to the sugar are different in the two compounds. At the time of those studies we had no facilities to examine this relationship in other compounds theoretically. Since we now have such programs operational, we decided to investigate theoretically the conformational properties of some of the key analogues. We wanted to see if we could establish the spatial requirements of the receptor for these compounds.

While this work is only in its early stages, some preliminary results are obvious. These were obtained by the use of the potential energy program CAMSEQ (ref. 18) operating on geometry optimized by MM2 (ref. 19) and charges generated by CNDO/2 (ref. 20). Fig. 5a shows the preferred conformation of the most potent analogue of the set, the cyclopropyl amide (it produces a 136% increase in coronary sinus $P_{O_2}$ that lasts for over 150 min. at a dose of 0.01 mg/kg intravenously). The potency of the cyclopentyl amide is decreased by two orders of magnitude. Its preferred conformation is shown in Fig. 5b. Note the shift in the angle of the sugar with respect to the base and the dramatic change in the rotation angle of the side chain with respect to the carbonyl oxygen. The slight differences in distances between the hydroxyl sugars and the $NH_2$ group, which is required for activity, between the two analogues is enough to account for the differences in potency. The inactivity of the tertiary amides is explained by the fact that they exist almost exclusively as the anti-conformer, Fig 5c.

The lower activity of the $NH_2$ analogue compared to the NH-cyclopropyl analogue is best understood by a comparison of their energy maps, Figs. 6a and b. Clearly, the cyclopropyl analogue is more conformationally restricted, apparently to the optimum conformation. The $NH_2$ analogue is more flexible and the smaller proportion of the molecules in the active conformation decreases the binding constant to the receptor. Currently in progress is a more detailed analysis of an extensive set of 5' analogues.

## SERIES DESIGN

Over the course of several years we had occasion to attempt to find quantitative

*References p. 284*

structure-activity relationships for many series of compounds. Although we were successful approximately 75% of the time, nagging problems were both series for which we could not find equations and those for which several equations fit the data equally well. These experiences led to our considerations of the properties of a well-designed series (ref. 8). Besides being synthetically accessible, three statistical criteria may be used to evaluate a proposed series: (a) the relevant physical properties should be varied widely enough that their influence on potency would be detectable in the biological test (b) the physical properties should be varied in a manner that each is independent of the others and (c) each analogue should be unique in physical properties. Point c may be relaxed in evaluating literature series.

Trimethoprim analogues

As part of our antibacterial program we performed a QSAR analysis on a published series of trimethoprim analogues (ref. 21). In 1974 we found two equations, the first for activity against *P. vulgaris*:

$$\log(1/C) = 1.32 - 0.62\,\underline{pi} \qquad (7)$$
$$n = 31,\ R^2 = 0.48,\ s = 0.52$$

and the second for activity against *S. aureus*:

$$\log(1/C) = 4.57 + 0.30\,\underline{pi} - 3.58\ \mathrm{EHOMO} \qquad (8)$$
$$n = 31,\ R^2 = 0.42,\ s = 0.58$$

In Eq. 8 the variable EHOMO is the energy of the highest occupied molecular orbital as calculated by the Hückel method.

In 1975 we re-examined the data and found again two equations, the first for activity against *P. vulgaris*:

$$\log(1/C) = 0.93 - 0.76\,\underline{pi} + 1.06\ \mathrm{FM} \qquad (9)$$
$$n = 31,\ R^2 = 0.79,\ s = 0.35$$

and the second for activity against *S. aureus*:

$$\log(1/C) = 0.67 + 0.11\ \mathrm{MRO} + 0.15\ \mathrm{MRM} + 0.026\ \mathrm{MRP} \qquad (10)$$
$$n = 31,\ R^2 = 0.80,\ s = 0.34$$

The variable FM describes the field effect of the meta substituents. The MR variables are molar refractivity, which is thought to parameterize dispersion binding. The last letter of the variable name indicates the position of substitution. Eqs. 7 and 9 are compatible; Eq. 9 simply indicates that an electronic effect is operating in addition to a hydrophobic one. The correspondence between Eqs. 8 and 10 is more troublesome because the two could suggest different analogues to be synthesized. The reason for the problem can be understood from Table 4. In this table the variable R describes the resonance effect of the substituent and F its field effect. The first thing to note is that four of the

Table 4

Evaluation of Trimethoprim Series

| Variable | Mean ± Standard Deviation | $R^2$ |
|---|---|---|
| pi (sum) | 0.95 ± 0.78* | 0.90 |
| MRO | 3.60 ± 3.07* | 0.63 |
| MRM | 7.18 ± 3.24* | 0.60 |
| MRP | 11.77 ± 7.08 | 0.90 |
| FM | 0.33 ± 0.22 | 0.90 |
| FP | 0.21 ± 0.12* | 0.44 |
| RM | -0.49 ± 0.31 | 0.90 |
| RP | -0.40 ± 0.23 | 0.72 |

* The variable has a standard deviation much lower than that which can be achieved by careful selection of substituents.

variables (pi, MRP, FM, and RM) have a multiple correlation coefficient with the other physical properties of 0.90. This says that the properties could substitute for one another in a regression equation. The second point of interest in Table 4 is that four of the eight properties were not varied enough to investigate their possible effect on potency.

The point of this analysis is not to criticize the original publication, after all it was published almost twenty years ago and other analogues have been reported on since. Rather, it is to suggest that a statistical investigation of the physical properties themselves may lead to insights as to why a quantitative structure-activity analysis is not successful and more importantly to see the deficiencies in the design of the original set of compounds. One could perhaps find an improved analogue of one's own or a competitor's compound if (s)he knew the deficiencies in the design of the original series.

In the meantime, our chemists prepared a series of trimethoprim analogues based on our predictions. They wisely made analogues of constant electronic character and with a perfect correlation between pi and MR. The predictions of Eqs. 9 and 10 were verified, that is that larger substituents decreased potency against *P. vulgaris* and increased it against *S. aureus*.

*References p. 284*

## OVERVIEW

The role of quantitative structure-activity relationship analysis in a medicinal chemistry program has been described previously (ref. 1). Briefly, such considerations can be used in series design and in the analysis of the relationship between physical and biological properties. Outliers from such an analysis may mean that one is in a new series, that (s)he has a new "lead". Both the cannabinoid and adenosine examples suggest that outliers and lack of predictability may lead one to consider computer-based conformational analysis of the structure-activity analysis. Such approaches are today much more time-consuming than the simpler quantitative structure-activity analyses, but they hold much promise.

## REFERENCES


1 Y. C. Martin; J. Med. Chem., 24 229-237, 1981.

2 M. Winn; D. Arendsen; P. Dodge; A. Dren; D. Dunnigan; R. Hallas; K. Hwang; J. Kyncl; Y. Lee; N. Plotnikoff; P. Young; H. Zaugg; J. Med. Chem., 19 461-471, 1976.

3 H. G. Pars; F. E. Granchelli; R. K. Razdan; J. K. Keller; D. G. Teiger; F. J. Rosenberg; L. S. Harris; J. Med. Chem., 19 445-454, 1976.

4 R. K. Razdan; B. Z. Terris; H. G. Pars; N. P. Plotnikoff; P. W. Dodge; A. T. Dren; J. Kyncl; P. Somani; J. Med. Chem., 19 454-461, 1976.

5 R. K. Razdan; G. R. Handrick; H. C. Dalzell; J. F. Howes; M. Winn; N. P. Plotnikoff; P. W. Dodge; A. T. Dren; J. Med. Chem., 19 552-554, 1976.

6 R. Adams et al.; J. Am. Chem. Soc., 70 662-664, 664-668, 1948.

7 Y. C. Martin; J. B. Holland; C. H. Jarboe; N. Plotnikoff; J. Med. Chem., 17 409-413, 1974.

8 Y. C. Martin; H. N. Panas; J. Med. Chem., 22 784-791, 1979.

9 R. A. Archer; D. B. Boyd; P. V. Demarco; I. J. Tyminski; N. L. Allinger; J. Am. Chem. Soc., 92 5200-5206, 1970.

10 H. H. Stein; J. Med. Chem., 16 1306-1308, 1973.

11 R. N. Prasad; A. Fung; K. Tietje; H. H. Stein; H. D. Brondyk; J. Med. Chem., 19 1180-1186, 1976.

12 R. N. Prasad; D. S. Bariana; A. Fung; M. Savic; K. Tietje; H. H. Stein; H. Brondyk; R. S. Egan; J. Med. Chem., 23 313-319, 1980.

13 M. C. Bindal; P. Singh; R. P. Bhatnagar; S. P. Gupta; Arzneimittel-Forsch., 30 924-928, 1980.

14 R. Marumoto; Y. Yoshioka; O. Miyashita; S. Shima; K. Imai; K. Kawazoe; M. Honjo; Chem. Pharm. Bull., 23 759-774, 1975.

15 Y. C. Martin; in "Physical Chemical Properties of Drugs" S. H. Yalkowsky, A. A. Sinkula, S. C. Valvani, eds. Dekker, New York, 49-110, 1980.

16 C. Hansch; A. J. Leo; "Substituent Constants for Correlation Analysis in Chemistry and Biology", Wiley, New York, 1979.

17 A. Verloop; W. Hoogenstraaten; J. Tipker; in "Drug Design" E. J. Ariens, ed., Academic, N. Y., 7 165-207, 1976.

18 R. Potenzone; H. R. Weintraub; A. J. Hopfinger; Comput. Chem., 13 187-194, 1977.

19 N. L. Allinger; Y. H. Yuh; QCPE 395 1-87, 1980.

20 CNDO/2 was incorporated into the CAMSEQ program, ref. 18.

21 B. Roth; E. Flaco; G. Hitchings; S. R. M. Bushby; J. Pharm. Med. Chem., 5 1103-1123, 1962.

J.A. Keverling Buisman (Editor), *Strategy in Drug Research*



# COMPUTER-ASSISTED DRUG DESIGN. STRATEGY AND ALGORITHMS

A.B.ROZENBLIT
Institute of Organic Synthesis, Latvian Academy of Sciences, Riga, USSR

## ABSTRACT

Computer-assisted methods are applicable during all stages of drug design, however, nowadays they are becoming increasingly important for the establishment of empirical relationships, both quantitative and qualitative.

Logico-structural approach (LSA) permits the determination of logical relationships between structure and type of biological activity and the selection of features, possible pharmacophores, on the basis of which new compounds can be designed. LSA can be used for different chemical notation languages e.g., fragmentary codes and graphs representing both topology and topography of the molecule. Systems using LSA programs are described and the scheme of an integrated system for computer-assisted drug design is discussed.

## INTRODUCTION

Perspectives of computer-assisted drug design are closely connected with the more general problem of application of artificial intelligence methods to scientific investigations. This implies the creation of computer programs capable of performing certain functions that are traditionally considered to be manifestations of a scientist's intellectual capacity. A fairly wide circle of investigators has been engaged in the development of such programs over the last years. For example, the "Heuristic Dendral" and "Methadendral" programs elaborated by the Feigenbaum group at Stanford University[1] are well known. Other examples which should be mentioned are the programs for planning the synthetic routes leading to new chemical compounds.

These problems have been always regarded by chemists as creative and are characterized by certain particularities, naturally posing

*References p. 307*

the question of their computerization. Firstly, these are mass and, to a certain extent, routine investigations and secondly, they involve the processing of a great amount of information for their optimal execution.

The elaboration of new drugs also belongs to this kind of investigation. Let us examine the general scheme of the drug design process (Fig.1). Note that any scientific investigation, especially of applied character fits this scheme.

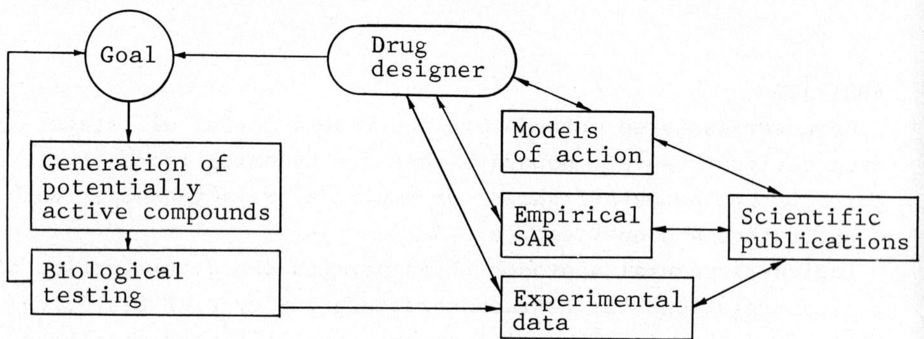


Fig.1. General scheme of the drug design process.

In accordance with his goal the drug designer "generates" chemical structures which are expected to possess the target activity. In the course of his work the investigator is guided by the prior information he has on hand. Based on experimental data the empirical structure-activity relationships (SAR) are established; more frequently these relationships are not formalized but are presented as logical rules and even as intuitive reasoning. In only a few cases does the investigator have at his disposal a model for certain types of pharmacological activity which more or less adequately describes the real process.

According to the above design a new compound may be synthesized and subjected to biological testing. If the results are accordant with the goal, the investigation can be suspended temporarily or continued to obtain a more effective drug.

In the event of negative results, new structures may be generated. The results of experiments can be stored in experimental data files and may serve to improve theory, both empirical relationships and models.

The analysis of such simplified schemes helps to clarify the role played by computerized methods and allows one to assess their capabilities. It is apparent that computers can be used for storage, systematization and retrieval of experimental structure and biological activity data available for chemical compounds. Convenient hardware facilities for the input of structural data in graphic form are commercially available now. Data base management systems permit the organization of fast retrieval processes using various structural components and their combinations, biological activity, etc., as keys.

Indeed, no technological or program problems exist. The problem is what data should be fed into the computer. Biological activity data are heterogeneous and results obtained by different investigators are hardly comparable. That is what makes the creation of a large biological data bank oriented to the establishment of structure-activity relationships so complicated.

The simulation of pharmacological action of drugs using computers involves conformational analysis with semi-empirical potentials or quantum chemistry methods. Only in some cases, when a hypothesis concerning the receptor structure can be put forward, can the above methods permit the construction of a model which illustrates the process of "recognition" and binding of the molecule by the receptor [2].

Computerized methods for the determination of empirical structure-activity relationships have become widespread. However, the majority of examples are concerned with retrospective analysis of SAR in "closed" chemical series, i.e. they involve well-known series of compounds, with a very low probability of finding a really interesting new drug.

The abbreviation QSAR widely used in the literature, is usually understood as "quantitative structure-activity relationship". It must be pointed out, however, that it can be also understood as "qualitative structure-activity relationship". These are no less important and, as found in practice, they can also be solved by computer-assisted methods. A logico-structural approach has been developed which may serve as a methodological basis for the establishment of qualitative relationships.

## THE LOGICO-STRUCTURAL APPROACH

The logico-structural approach (LSA) is based on the rules of Mill's inductive logic [3,4]. In fact, every investigator uses similar logic when trying to establish SAR and select features responsible for certain types of biological activity. This logic is clearly demonstrated by Austel and Kutter [5].

*References p. 307*

We shall discuss below the essence of LSA.

Suppose there exists a given set of compounds $C_1$, $C_2$, ... $C_n$, the structures of which are described (in terms of a certain language L) as $S_1$, $S_2$, ... $S_n$. Let all of these compounds manifest a certain biological activity, A. Then, this type of action may be attributed to a structural fragment, $\varphi^r$, present in the structures of all given compounds. The structure description of this fragment is then the intersection of the structure descriptions of all given compounds:

$$\varphi^r = \bigcap_{i=1}^{n} S_i$$

One can suppose that this structural fragment is the potential feature of activity, $A_k$, i.e. the potential pharmacophore. In practice, the intersection of all compounds manifesting a particular type of activity can turn out to be nil, i.e. there exists, within the framework of the chosen description language, no fragment which is common to all compounds under question. In other cases, although the intersection of structure description may not be nil, this activity feature may be insignificant if it frequently occurs in inactive compounds.

The above situations can be explained by the existence of several different pharmacophores responsible for a given type of activity or by an inability to establish a similarity between the compounds given. In such cases an intersection may be found for som compounds only. The intersection formed must be assessed statistically.

The quality of features, their essential values, depend crucially on the structure description language used. Nevertheless, the structure of feature selection algorithms remains basically unchanged and can be described by the following scheme.

1. Potential features of each class of activity are selected by pair-by-pair intersection of compound structure descriptions:

$$\varphi^r = S_m \cap S_n$$

where $S_m$ and $S_n$ are structure representations of the m-th and n-th compounds, respectively;

2. Occurrence numbers, $l_k$, are calculated for potential features of compounds in every class of biological activity, $A_k$;

3. Statistical estimation of selected intersections on the basis of $l_k$ values is performed and statistically significant features for each activity class are selected.

One of the principal criteria of feature estimation is the probability that the new compound with the feature $A_k$ activity will really belong to this class. The mean value of this probability in the case of two activity classes, can be computed from the expression:

$$P(A_k/\varphi^r)=\frac{l_k + 1}{l_r + 2}$$

where $l_k$ is the occurrence number for feature $\varphi^r$ on compounds of class $A_k$;

$l_r$ - the occurrence number for feature $\varphi^r$ on all compounds under examination.

When considerable variation in prior probability is observed among the classes, it is advisible to use in the place of probability $P(A_k/\varphi^r)$ a relative value, i.e. prognostic utility of the feature:

$$U_k^r = P(A_k/\varphi^r)/P(A_k)$$

where $P(A_k)$ is prior probability of the class, i.e. the probability of finding a compound with activity of $A_k$ among randomly selected compounds.

The definition of intersection depends on the structure representation used. The languages employed for structure description of chemical compounds must be considered in detail because of their importance.

LANGUAGES FOR STRUCTURE DESCRIPTION

The present approach to chemical structure notation was devised at the Scientific Research Institute for Biological Testing of Chemicals (Moscow Region) and the Institute of Organic Synthesis (Riga). It is based on our current understanding of the processes under way during the pharmacodynamic stage which is mainly responsible for the specificity and type of therapeutic action of compounds.

1. The type of pharmacological activity is determined by the capacity of a compound to bind complementarily and interact with the functional chemical structure in the living organism, i.e. the "receptor".

2. Interaction of chemical compounds with a receptor involves only part of the molecule, i.e. the "pharmacophore". This process is determined by the formation of weak chemical bonds - hydrogen, electrostatic, van-der-Waals', hydrophobic.

3. Compounds carrying identical or similar pharmacophores are

capable of exerting identical specific effects.

Based on these assumptions one can state that the chemical notation language oriented to drug design problems should provide:
(1) adequate representation of the pharmacophore;
(2) efficient procedures for the identification of pharmacophores and for the generation of new structures based on the found pharmacophores.

## Descriptor centers

As judged by the principles of language design outlined above, it appears advisable to select among chemical structures potentially active centers, i.e. atoms or groups of atoms functioning as centers of "weak" interaction or reaction centers. These centers, further referred to as "descriptor centers" (DC), first of all include atoms and groups of atoms containing valence p and d-electrons or an integer electrostatic charge. Distances between DC are essential for compound-receptor interaction, so they must be included as elements of the language.

All heteroatoms (N, O, S, P, etc.), cycles and also carbon atoms connected with multiple bonds are respected as DC. Clearly, the electronic pattern of heteroatoms and consequently their participation in the formation of "weak" bonds is strongly affected by their valent state and the types of atoms connected with them. For this reason, the same heteroatoms may be regarded as various DC according to their environment. For instance, quaternary nitrogen carrying an integer positive charge (DC 01) differs drastically from tertiary nitrogen (DC 03), which, in its turn, is different from secondary or primary nitrogen (DC 02) in that it is incapable of acting as proton donor during hydrogen bonding. Conversely, primary and secondary nitrogens can belong to the same DC since they both can serve as proton donors. It is apparent that an oxygen atom attached by a double bond (DC 13) differs significantly from the same atom having two simple bonds (DC 12 and 11). These differ in that an OH group (DC 11) being a proton donor can undergo ionization and participates in hydrogen bonding , but ester oxygen (DC 12) cannot do so.

On the other hand, atoms of various elements can belong to the same DC. For example, the effects exerted by Cl, Br and I (DC 31) on biological activity differ quantitatively rather than qualitatively, fluorine atom (DC 32) being unlike them, because it is capable of forming a fairly strong hydrogen bond. Terminal CH groups are also regarded as DC to characterize the lipophylic ability.

The list of atomic descriptor centers can be redefined by taking into account more delicate differences between atoms according to their environment.

Any single cycle not exceeding 9 atoms is considered to be a descriptor center. The code (label) of such a descriptor center indicates the cycle size and the number of $\pi$-electrons in the conjugated cyclic system. If any of the atoms in the cycle lacks $\pi$-electrons (conjugated cyclic system is absent), zero is indicated. For example, cyclic systems in the structures

O or S etc. are designated 5,6

but

NH or S etc. are designated 5,0

In the cases when a single cycle is part of a fused aromatic system, the code of this cycle indicates in all cases 6 $\pi$-electrons (which is in compliance with the Hückel rule). Thus it is possible to indicate that a given cycle consists of aromatic bonds only. E.g., the cycles constituting the azulene molecule are

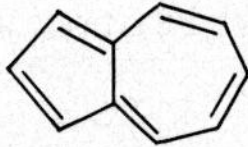

designated as DC "5,6" and "7,6".

## Systems of chemical notation based on the concept of descriptor centers

The concept of descriptor centers was applied by elaborating two systems of chemical structure representation.

The first system, Substructure Superposition Fragmental Notation (SSFN) was suggested by Avidon et al [6,7]. The definition of cyclic descriptor centers in the original version of SSFN differs from that described above.

The coding procedure involves the listing of all chains in the compound initiated and terminated by DC, but having no intersection. Linear descriptors describe all such chains, consisting of DC codes, and serve as an index for the length of the carbon chain from one DC to another, expressed in the number of carbon atoms. The descriptor also indicates the presence of conjugation along the chain. There are special descriptors indicating the geometry of the cyclic frame, the number of $\pi$-electrons in the cyclic conjugated system, and the position of heteroatoms.

The main advantage of SSFN resides in its simplicity and linear structure. Hence, it is suitable for statistical pattern recognition algorithms and for quantitative evaluation of structural similarity among biologically active compounds.

On the other hand, SSFN, as do other fragmental notation systems, "disintegrates" structure, i.e., the information stored by means of this notation concerns the structural fragments of the molecule only but fails to provide information on their interconnections. Therefore, a new method for structural representation was developed that retains the DC idea and describes the topology of a molecule as a whole, called the DCAM method.

Using this notation the structure of a compound is represented by an undirected labeled graph, its vertices corresponding to descriptor centers and its edges showing the paths between descriptor centers. Vertex labels correspond to types of descriptor centers, and edge labels to path length (number of atom-atom bonds). The label may also contain information on the nature of chemical bonds along the route (presence of multiple bonds or aromatic bonds, conjugation between DC). The adjacency matrices of such a graph will be referred to as the descriptor centers adjacency matrix (DCAM) [8].

There exist in DCAM language some DC consisting of several atoms. Besides cyclic DC they include pairs of carbon atoms connected by double or triple bonds. These DC can have one or more common atoms shared with other DC. In this case, the edge of the graph connecting two DC (and, respectively, the element of DCAM) has a label indicating the number of common atoms of these DC. E.g., in the structure of pyridine two DC are selected: nitrogen ("05") and cycle ("6,6"). These DC are considered as mutually overlapping to give the label - 1.

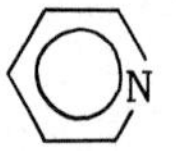

$$\begin{vmatrix} 05 & -1 \\ & 6,6 \end{vmatrix}$$

The minus sign serves to indicate mutual overlapping.

Let us consider DCAM for quinoline and iso-quinoline (see next page)

Comparison of DCAM permits us to see that the similarity and differences between these two structures are in agreement with chemical intuition. Both of them contain two aromatic 6-membered cycles including a nitrogen atom. The matrix element 1,3 indicates

N

| | 1 | 2 | 3 |
|---|---|---|---|
| 1 | 6,6 | -2 | 1 |
| 2 | | 6,6 | -1 |
| 3 | | | 05 |

N

| | 1 | 2 | 3 |
|---|---|---|---|
| 1 | 6,6 | -2 | 2 |
| 2 | | 6,6 | -1 |
| 3 | | | 05 |

the difference between them.

DCAM contains ample information on the topology of active centers but gives only qualitative reference to the electronic structure of some atomic groups.

It is possible to further develop graph representations of chemical structures, described by DCAM by taking into account more precisely the spatial and electronic structure of the molecule, which is ultimately crucial for the manifestation of their biological activity and other properties.

Instead of by code, descriptor centers can be represented by means of numerical parameters describing, for example, the effective atomic charge, $\pi$-electron density, van-der-Waals' radius, donor-acceptor properties, etc.

Bonds can be characterized by means of geometric length, bond order, etc.

The label of the graph edge indicates the geometric distances between DC. In many cases the distances between DC can vary due to the possibility of structure group rotation around bonds. In such cases it is useful to indicate the range of variation. Using different DC characteristics one can obtain a variety of graph representations for chemical structures. The simplest way is to retain the DC representation as used by DCAM and to introduce geometric distances between them. We call such representation a descriptor center geometry matrix (DCGM).

## PRINCIPLES OF PHARMACOPHORE SELECTION USING STRUCTURAL NOTATION LANGUAGES

As I have said before, pharmacological activity features, i.e. potential pharmacophores, can be discerned by finding the intersection of active structures. Hence, any structure representation language must include the definition of intersection.

For SSFN language, this intersection is identical with the definition of the intersection of sets, i.e. intersection of compound descriptions in the SSFN results in common descriptors for these compounds.

For DCAM and other graph representations, a more precise definition of the intersection of graphs has been introduced, viz. a maximal subgraph which is common to all intersected graphs. A maximal subgraph is a graph such that the addition to it of at least one vertex or edge makes it unable to be a subgraph for at least one of the intersected graphs. It must be pointed out that unlike a single possible intersection of sets, there can exist several nonisomorphous intersections of labeled graphs. Procedures for the identification of maximum common subgraphs are rather sophisticated, but now efficient programs are available which provide comparatively fast solutions to the problems [8].

During the execution of intersection procedures it is possible to check the coincidence of elements of the intersected graphs only up to a given limit. A such modification of the procedure is necessary especially when DCGM or other topographical notation systems are used.

To demonstrate the possibilities of different languages described in this paper we will consider the intersections of various structure notations of compounds manifesting neurotropic activity.

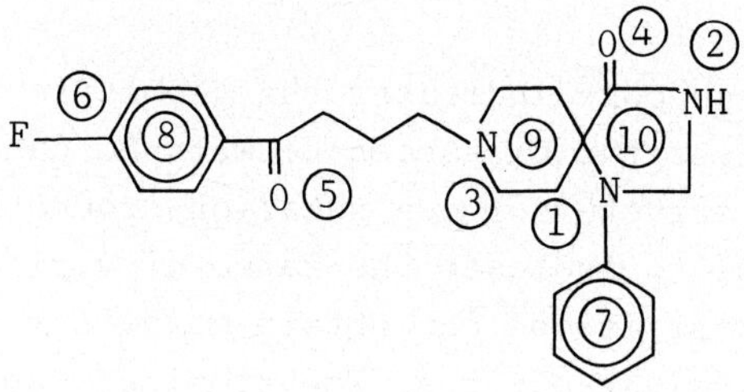

(I)

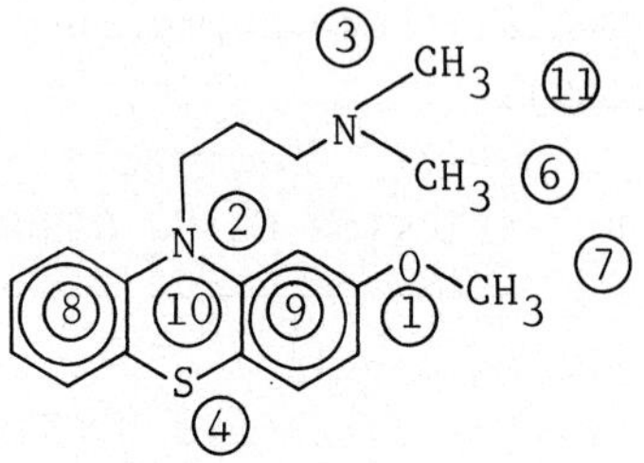

(II)

Intersection of SSFN codes results in the substructures shown in Table 1.

TABLE 1

Substructures given by the intersections of SSFN codes of the compounds I and II

| Structural fragments | 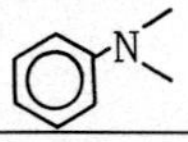 Ph–N(Me)₂ fragment | 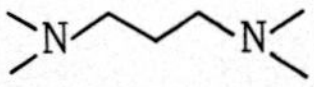 N–C–C–N fragment |
|---|---|---|
| Descriptors of the first compound | ⑦—① | ①—③ |
| Descriptors of the second compound | ⑧—② or ⑨—② | ②—③ |

These substructures in the above compounds are combined in a single fragment

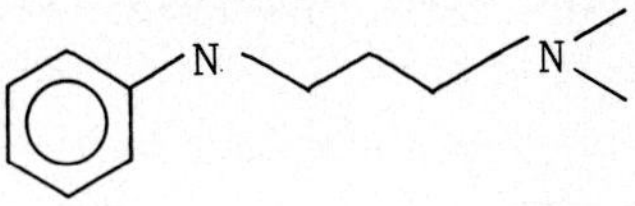

but the intersection procedure does not formally lead to this conclusion.

Intersection of DCAM for compounds I and II results in the following submatrices

$$\begin{vmatrix} 03 & 4 & 1 \\ & 03 & 5 \\ & & 6,6 \end{vmatrix} \; SM_1 \qquad \begin{vmatrix} 03 & 5 \\ & 6,6 \end{vmatrix} \; SM_2$$

The descriptor centers in the given compounds corresponding to the diagonal elements of $SM_1$ and $SM_2$ are shown in Table 2.

TABLE 2

Descriptor centers corresponding to the submatrices $SM_1$ and $SM_2$

| Diagonal element | 03 | 03 | 6,6 | 03 | 6,6 |
|---|---|---|---|---|---|
| Compound I | ① | ② | 7 | ③ | ⑦ or ⑧ |
| Compound II | ② | ③ | ⑧ or ⑨ | | |

Both the matrix $SM_1$ and $SM_2$ in compound II correspond to the fragment

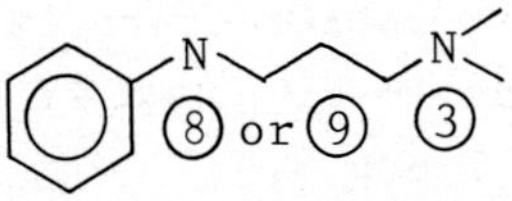

⑧ or ⑨ ③ (F1)

The same fragment corresponds to matrix $SM_1$ in compound I, while matrix $SM_2$ in this compound may correspond to the fragment F1 and to the fragment

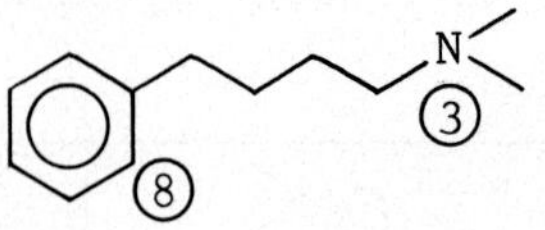

(F2)

Hence, matrix $SM_2$ corresponds to the fragment

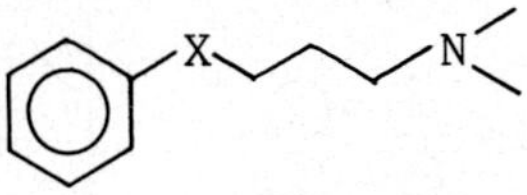

(F3)

where x stands either for nitrogen or carbon.

If we take another compound, a well-known pharmaceutical, haloperidol, belonging to the same heterocyclic butyrophenone series as compound I

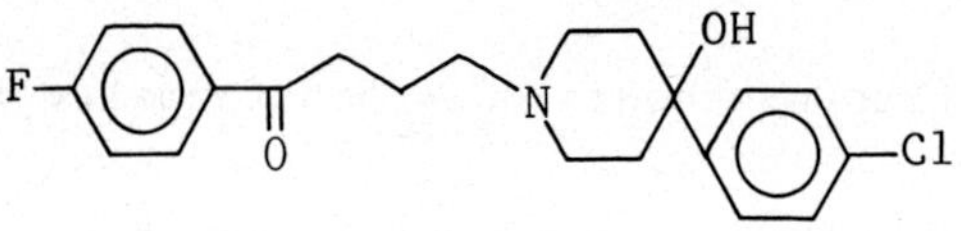

(III)

then the intersection of compounds I, II and III will yield matrix $SM_2$, i.e. fragment F3. This fragment serves as a potent feature responsible for neuroleptic activity.

Now, we will examine the intersection of DGGM of compounds I and II. We assume that variation in the distances between the corresponding descriptor centers in the graphs to be intersected must not exceed 5 %. Intersection of these DCGM will then give submatrices

$$\begin{vmatrix} 03 & 2.81 \\ & 6.6 \end{vmatrix} \text{ and } \begin{vmatrix} 03 & 6.35\text{-}6.64 \\ & 6.6 \end{vmatrix}$$

The first submatrix corresponds to the fragment

~2.8 Å

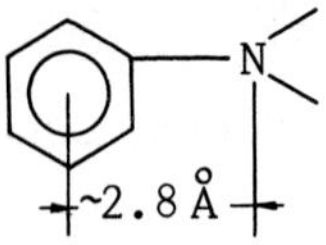

In the first compound this substructure is obtained for descriptor centers 1 and 7, whereas in compound II it is found for descriptor centers 2 and 8 or 2 and 9.

The second matrix corresponds to the fragment

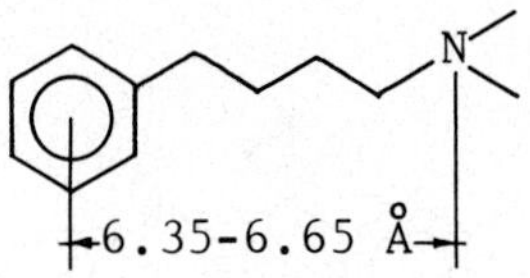

6.35-6.65 Å

In compound I this substructure corresponds to descriptor centers 3 and 8, connected by a chain of carbon atoms (the distances between DC are equal to 6.46 Å), whereas in compound II they are descriptor centers 3 and 8 or 3 and 9 connected by a chain of atoms, a nitrogen atom 2 being included therein. The distances between the centers amount to 6.35 and 6.64 respectively.

Interestingly, nitrogen 3 and benzene ring 7 in compound I are spaced 5.8 Å apart, and, consequently, this substructure is not included in the intersection, as opposed to the results obtained using DCAM notation.

EXTENSION OF THE STRUCTURE REPRESENTATION LANGUAGES

It is not infrequent that the language chosen for chemical structure description appears inadequate for the solution of a given problem and fails to select meaningful biological activity features. In this case, it is expedient to introduce generalizations for some language elements. These generalizations must be based on the meaningful analysis of data. After the investigator has provided precise definitions of such generalizations, redescription of chemical structures must occur automatically.

The generalization procedure is carried out as shown below. If we assume that some notation fragments $f_1$, $f_2$, ... $f_n$ share common properties, a new element can be introduced which is the disjunction of the above elements:

$$\varphi = f_1 V f_2 V \dots V f_n,$$

where V is the sign of disjunction (logical "or").

This new element, $\varphi$ , which will serve to replace elements $f_i$, can be described either by enumerating its elements or by applying some formal rule that enables the association of element $f_k$ with the set $\{f_i\}$.

Some examples are given here:

Example 1. Descriptor centers 02, 04, 11 (see p. 6 ) can be grouped together according to their ability to act as proton donors in the formation of hydrogen bonds.

Example 2. It is assumed that the manifestation of biological activity depends on the total size of the $R_1$ substituent in fragment

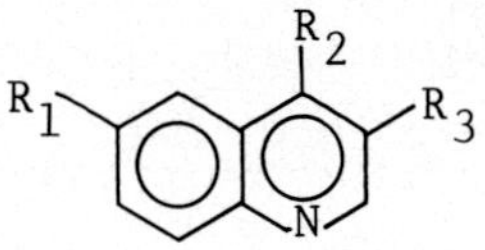

Then, a new element, $R_v$, is introduced to replace the $R_1$ substituent in the above fragment, if its van-der-Waals' volume falls within the given range $V_{min}<V<V_{max}$.

Generalization procedure conducted in the interactive mode allows the improvement of the language of chemical structure description by adapting it to the solution of a specific problem, and provides rapid verification of hypotheses concerning the mechanism of biological action of chemical compounds.

## PROGRAM SYSTEMS BASED ON LSA

Using the logico-structural approach, several software systems have been developed at the Institute of Organic Synthesis in Riga.

The STRAC program system uses the most primitive notation - vector representation (similar to Marcush formula). An interesting peculiarity of STRAC is the possibility to add new structural parameters to compound descriptions through an interactive man-computer procedure [4]. The STRAC system has been successfully applied to the analysis of SAR in several series of chemical compounds and is still used now and then.

The ORACLE program system is based on a fairly large data base for the structure and activity of chemical compounds. The data base specifically designed for SAR analysis was set up in 1976 at the Scientific Research Institute for Biological Testing of Chemicals (Moscow Region) and at the Institute of Organic Synthesis in Riga [9].

The data base (by now enumerating approximately 9000 compounds) contains information on 57 major types of pharmaceutical activity. The chemical structures are coded by means of SSFN described earlier.

A special program looks through the bank and compiles a listing of all descriptors occurring in the bank (with an occurrence number attached to every descriptor). These data are stored in the statistical file together with the coefficients of prognostic feature utility calculated by the formula

$$U_k^r = \frac{l_k + 1}{l^r + 2} \cdot \frac{L + 2}{L_k + 2}$$

where $l_k$ is the occurrence number of descriptor $\varphi^r$ on $A_k$ activity;
$l^r$ is the occurrence number of descriptor $\varphi^r$ in the whole bank;
$L_k$ is the occurrence number of the compound exhibiting activity $A_k$ in the bank;
L is the total number of compounds in the bank.

When $U_k^r > \lambda_k$, where $\lambda_k$ denotes a certain threshold value, the descriptor $\varphi^r$ is considered responsible for activity $A_k$. The threshold value $\lambda_k$ is chosen for every activity by means of a prediction procedure applied to the compounds of the bank using the leave-one-out technique. The prediction and, hence, the threshold, is considered acceptable if it satisfies two conditions.

(1) $P_{Ak} > 0.9$, where $P_{Ak}$ is the probability of correct recognition being calculated from the expression

$$P_{Ak} = \frac{M_k}{L_k}$$

where $M_k$ is the number of compounds being correctly classified as having activity $A_k$.

(2) Among the threshold values $\lambda_k$ meeting the first requirement one has to choose those with the maximum efficiency coefficient $K_{ek}$ being calculated from the formula

$$K_{ek} = \frac{L\ M_k}{L_k\ M_{pk}}$$

where $M_{pk}$ is the total number of compounds that can be classified as possessing activity $A_k$;
L, $L_k$, $M_k$ are as described earlier.

The efficiency coefficient demonstrates a reduction in costs to obtain a single prospective compound by applying the prediction system.

The ORACLE system can be used in two ways:

(1) The investigator trying to find a new drug with a certain activity can be supplied with a list of structural features of this activity, i.e. descriptors, and their statistical estimations.

References p. 307

(2) The chemist who intends to synthesize or has already synthesized a new compound can obtain a summarizing prediction: the list of most probable activities with their statistical characteristics $P_k$ and $K_{ek}$, complete with the list indicating what descriptors in the structure of the given compound are considered responsible for certain activities.

The ORACLE system was carefully investigated over a wide range of activity prediction experiments [10]. Now it is being widely used by scientists all over the USSR.

The TOPLOG program system is based on graph representations of chemical structure and the main principles and algorithms of the logico-structural approach. This system was designed only recently

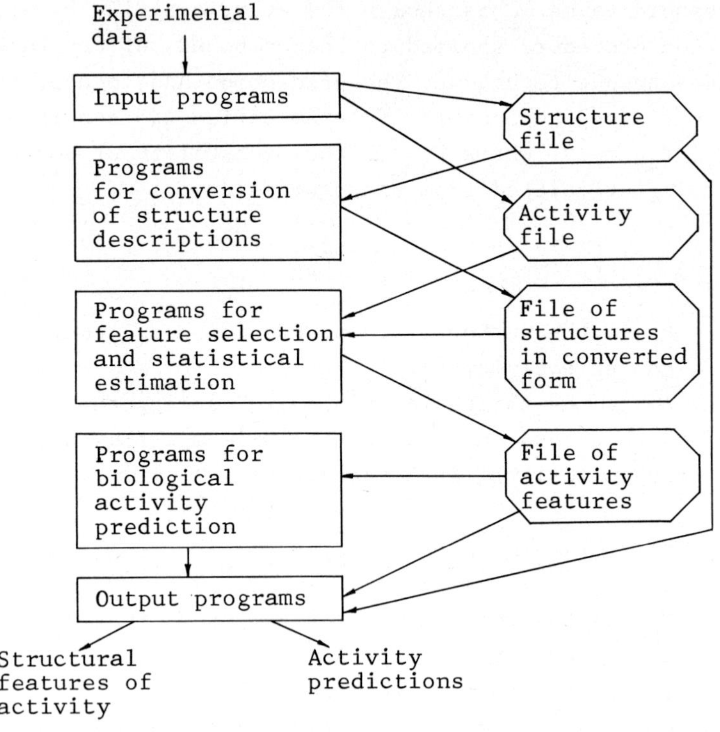


Fig. 2. The scheme of a program system realized using logico-structural approach.

and is still in the process of development. Hence, we have not accumulated a sufficient amount of experimental data for the application of this system. However, available experimental evidence indicates that graph representation is advantageous for the selection of meaningful activity features. In addition, some important practical problems have been solved using TOPLOG.

Both ORACLE and TOPLOG can be represented schematically as shown in Fig. 2.

The input programs permit feeding of structures and activities in conventional form,i.e. structural formulae can be fed into the computer via a display in the usual graphic form and the input of activities is performed by filling table entries. These data are stored in files or used for current prediction processes.

To be used in programs the structural data must be transformed into special representational forms, e.g. SSFN or DCAM.

Using structural and biological activity data the appropriate programs select structural features of certain types of activity, i.e. possible pharmacophores. These substructures are also stored in special files.

The activity features used as guidelines by drug designers can be retrieved in convenient form, i.e. as structural formulae of certain fragments of the molecule.

In other cases the file of selected features is used by prediction programs.

## LEAD GENERATION: IS IT POSSIBLE?

The question naturally arises as to the possibility of gaining anything by the mere analysis of data relating to compounds.

Indeed, sometimes the computer finds well-known, trivial features. More interesting is the case when it finds a known feature masked by the structural environment. For instance, for the structure

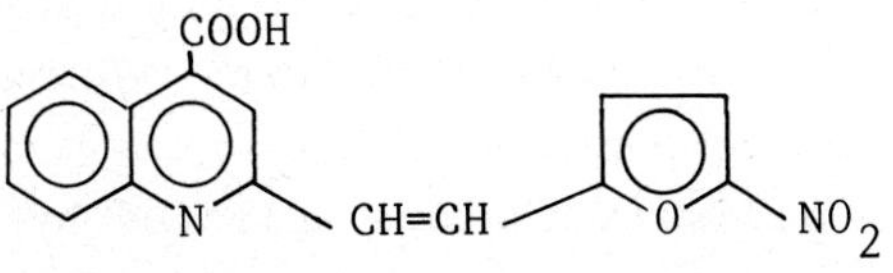

COOH
N CH=CH O $NO_2$

antituberculotic activity was predicted, among others [4,10] . This prediction was confirmed by testing. However, this structure can hardly be considered as representative of a new lead, because the feature that served as grounds for prediction was the main substructure of the well-known tubazide and its derivatives:

*References p. 307*

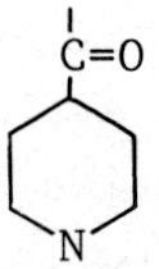

C=O

N

The most interesting results can be reached when comparing structures belonging to different chemical series but manifesting similar activity.

To illustrate the point one can examine two known anti-inflammatory nonhormonal compounds [12]

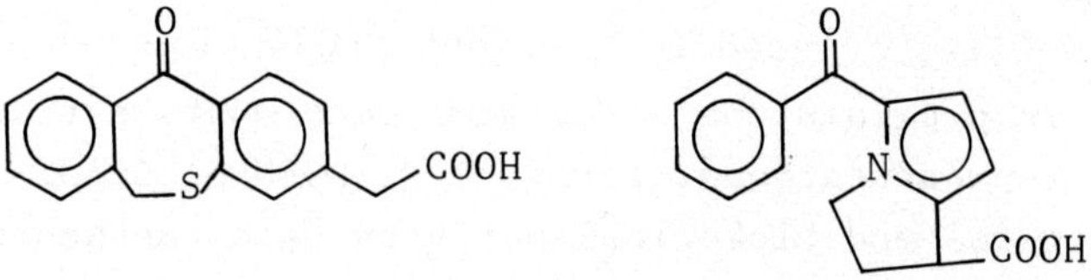

O S COOH O N COOH

You can see that these compounds belonging to different series share a common fragment

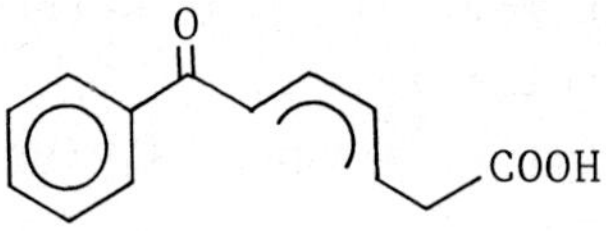

O COOH

Naturally, it can be only a freak of chance, but there exists a reasonable possibility that using such a fragment, one can find a new interesting lead.

## DESIGN OF NEW STRUCTURES

Computer programs can be also applied to the design of new structures using the interactive mode for this purpose. Combinatorial programs can generate possible structures making use of desirable activity features as components. The program must take into account not only the activity feature selected by the computer but also the experience of pharmacology expressed in the form of logical rules of "if-then" type. As a good example, we can mention the summary of practical rules given in the paper by Ariëns and Simonis [13] , which can be elaborated for computer storage and manipulation.

## INTEGRATED COMPUTER SYSTEM

To be capable of serving as an optimal "assistent" for the drug designer a computer system must consist of four main subsystems (Fig.3).

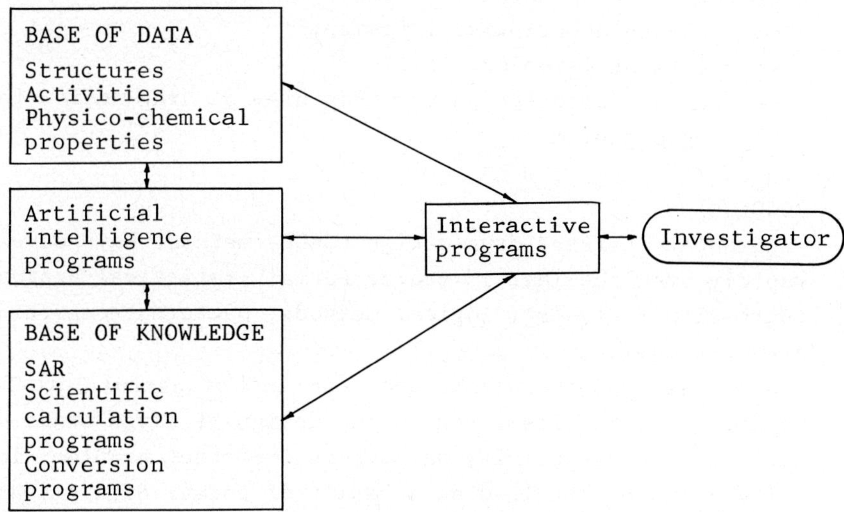


Fig. 3. The scheme of an integrated system for computer-assisted drug design

1. Data base - stores experimental facts: structures, activities, physico-chemical properties etc.

2. Base of knowledge - stores empirical SAR (both qualitative and quantitative) and programs for theoretical calculations like conformational analysis, calculations of physico-chemical parameters.

3. Artificial intelligence programs - permit purposeful manipulations with the contents of data and knowledge bases to obtain new information (to be stored then in the base of knowledge).

4. Programs providing investigator-computer interaction make use of the natural scientific language, such as structural formulae, molecular models, graphs, tables, directives and messages.

The computer system described above has not been realized yet. Nevertheless, it is quite possible to create such a system integrating the systems which solve only partial problems, but more or less approach the "ideal" complex system. One may mention PROPHET [14], SET [15], ADAPT [16], CIS [17] and also STRAC, ORACLE, TOPLOG, described on the previous pages.

Application of computer systems does not change, in general, the scheme, shown in Fig.1, but the role of the investigator changes essentially. The investigator, leaving to the computer routine operations, not only controls the program and estimates the intermediate results but performs superior creative functions as well:

- establishes the goal of investigations;
- formulates description language;
- corrects decision criteria;
- proposes hypotheses on the mechanism of drug action in the living organism.

## CONCLUSION

Computer-assisted drug design (CADD) methods have developed rapidly over the last 15 years. Formal statistical approaches like regression analysis*, logical methods, pattern recognition, etc. are most common.

All these methods permit the retrieval of useful information from voluminous data files. Hence, the design of large banks of comparable structure-activity data is an important problem. The structural features obtained as a result of formal data elaboration can then be meaningfully explained and give the drug designer clues to the discovery of new highly effective drugs.

Methods of formal analysis will evidently be developed in the future, however, having reached culmination, they will gradually be replaced by meaningful computer methods, based on the modelling of real biological processes. The current trend of modern pharmacological science is to use quantum chemistry methods and conformational analysis to simulate processes of drug-receptor binding. One can see, in perspective, a variety of models describing the different stages of drug action.

Nevertheless, formal analysis methods will, apparently, retain a certain significance as the natural stage of scientific development moves from fact storage to empirical rules and further on to the theory.

CADD has passed the process of initial formation and the investigation program managers and drug designers can expect to use CADD as their working instrument along with, e.g., physico-chemical analysis. The results of wide practical application of CADD

*In this paper we do not tackle the quantitative aspects of the problems and the methods involved. A great number of publications has appeared in this field including several reviews, among which one can recommend the book by Franke [11] and the paper by Unger [12].

will have a large impact on the improvement and further development of these methods.

REFERENCES


1 B.G.Buchanan, D.H.Smith, W.C.White, R.J.Gritter, E.A.Feigenbaum, J.Lederberg and C.Djerassi, J.Am.Chem.Soc., 98 (1976), 6168-6178.
2 H.Broch, D.Cabrol and D.Vasilescu, Int.J.Quantum Chem., 7 (1980), 283-295.
3 V.E.Golender and A.B.Rozenblit, Computer-Assisted Methods of Drug Design, Zinātne, Riga, 1978, p.232 (in Russian).
4 V.E.Golender and A.B.Rozenblit, in E.J.Ariëns (Ed.), Drug Design, vol. IX, Academic Press, N.Y., 1980, pp.299-337.
5 V.Austel and E.Kutter, in E.Kutter (Ed.), Arzneimittelentwicklung, Grundlagen, Strategien-Perspektiven, G.Thieme Verlag, Stuttgart, 1970, p.113.
6 V.V.Avidon and L.A.Leksina, Nauch.-Tekhn.Inform., Ser.2, No 3 (1974), 22-25 (in Russian).
7 V.V.Avidon, S.P.Kozlova and V.S.Arolovich, Nauch.Tekhn.Inform., Ser.2, No 12 (1974), 21-23 (in Russian).
8 L.S.Gitlina, V.E.Golender, V.V.Drboglav, A.B.Rozenblit, R.A.Eihenberga, V.V.Avidon, Methods of Representation and Elaboration of Structural Information for Structure-Activity Relationships Analysis, preprint, Institute of Organic Synthesis, Riga, 1981, p.75 (in Russian).
9 L.A.Piruzyan, V.V.Avidon, A.B.Rozenblit, V.S.Arolovich, V.E.Golender, S.P.Kozlova, E.M.Michailovsky and E.G.Gavrishchuk, Khim.-Farm. Zh., No 5, 11 (1977), 35-39 (in Russian).
10 V.V.Gavrilova, V.E.Golender, A.B.Rozenblit, N.M.Sukhova, M.J.Lidaks and E.J.Lukevics, Khim-Farm.Zh., No 2, 13 (1979), 45-53 (in Russian).
11 R.Franke, Optimierung Methoden in der Wirkstoff-Forschung. Quantitative Struktur-Wirkung Analyse, Akademie-Verlag, Berlin, 1980, p.454.
12 S.Unger, in E.J.Ariëns (Ed.), Drug Design, Vol.IX, Academic Press, N.Y., 1980, pp.47-119.
13 E.J.Ariëns and A.-M.Simonis, in Topics in Current Chemistry, Vol.52, Springer-Verlag, Berlin, 1974, pp.1-61.
14 W.F.Raub, Federation Proc., Vol.33 (1974), 2390-2392.
15 C.Hansch, A.Leo, D.Elkins, J.Chem.Doc., No 2, 14(1974), 57-69.
16 A.J.Stuper and P.C.Jurs, J.Chem.Inf.Comput.Sci., No 2, 16(1976), 99-104.
17 G.W.A.Milne and S.R.Heller, J.Chem.Inf.Comput.Sci., No 4, 20(1980), 204-211.

J.A. Keverling Buisman (Editor), *Strategy in Drug Research* 


# STRATEGY IN DRUG RESEARCH
## SUMMING UP

E.J. ARIËNS
Institute of Pharmacology and Toxicology, University of Nijmegen, the Netherlands

The Symposium was preceded by an outline given by a World Health Organization expert on tropical diseases. He outlined the great need, especially for drugs to be used in the treatment of tropical infectious diseases. This category of drugs often is indicated as "orphan drugs", suggesting that they are to a certain extent neglected. No doubt a good deal of research in the area is performed by both Industrial and Governmental Research Institutions but in proportion to the tremendous needs - hundreds of millions of sick people are involved - whatever one does in this respect, for the moment falls short. We should be aware of the fact that the people of the world, especially of the developing world, are not much interested in our scientific research efforts, but are looking forward with hope to the products thereof.

The name of this Symposium "the Second Noordwijkerhout IUPAC-IUPHAR-Symposium" emphasizes the participation of both medicinal or pharmacochemists and pharmacologists. If I would put the question: "Where are medicinal chemists and pharmacologists meeting?", the answer undoubtedly would be at Noordwijkerhout. This is true for this week but there is another more general answer, namely: they meet there where the bioactive agent, the drug, representing a complex of particular chemical properties, meets its pharmacological counterparts, the receptors or enzymes, to which the drug is chemically complementary. There the information introduced into the drug molecule by the medicinal chemist is translated into signals starting the events studied by the pharmacologist. At this level medicinal chemistry and pharmacology so to say merge and the differences between the two professions disappear. Here a common language is spoken.

The Organizing Committee has been well aware of this situation which is clearly reflected in the program. Major topics are drug receptors, enzymes as targets for drugs as well as drugs as targets for enzymes (pharmacon metabolism) and pharmacokinetics, determining the degree in which the drug molecules and their target molecules reach eachother.

With regard to the receptors, there can be mentioned the lecture on benzodiazepines, outlining recent developments in which agonists and antagonists are concerned. An interesting aspect is that, although these receptors only exist as a concept - little or nothing is known on their chemistry, neither on their possible endogenous messenger - they are a useful tool in the development of new agents on the basis of receptor binding studies.

The lectures on the adrenergic receptors on the other hand, gave a detailed analysis of receptor biochemistry and kinetics. Undoubtedly the biological receptor is much more complex than what was postulated in the simple receptor concept applied in the discussion of drug action on a molecular level. The adrenergic receptors, known in much detail,have, in fact, not been exploited as tools in drug development; on the contrary, in this case new drugs developed on basis of structure-action relationship studies, have essentially contributed to the detailed knowledge on adrenergic receptor systems as elucidated in the last contribution of the Symposium.

A highlight in the study of drug-receptor interaction was presented in a discussion of the action of diphosphoglycerate (DPG) on hemoglobine. Here the receptor is known in detail, even so that the spatial arrangement of the major, predominantly basic amino acid side-chains, involved in binding of DPG and thus constituting its receptor, is known. This opens perspectives for drug design in optima forma. An interesting aspect is that both the receptor and the effector system are part of one relatively simple macromolecular complex and that the effect, the binding of oxygen, can be measured very accurately. The discussion of this receptor-effector system served as a basis for a critical review of the various aspects that are relevant in the analysis of drug action and the development of new drugs.

The presentation on the strategy in the development of peptide drugs made clear that structure-action relationship in this field allows much more freedom than originally assumed, and, may be, even more than peptide chemists like. Often only a small sequence of amino acids of a large polypeptide molecule is essential for the action whereas substitution of the natural amino acids by unnatural ones,particularly those with isosteric side chains, is well tolerated. This even to such a degree that one gradually moves from the field of peptides into that of hemipeptides, thus bridging the gap between bioactive peptides and "nonpeptidic peptidomimetics".

The lectures on enzymes as tools and targets in drug research outlined schematically the various possibilities and limitations in this field. Emphasis was put on the class of "suicide enzyme inhibitors". Here, besides the requirements for the binding to the particular active site, also the requirements for the covalent coupling between the inhibitor and the active site are determinant. In this way high selectivity and on basis of the irreversibility in action a high potency are warranted. Clear-cut examples of the step-by-step development of the aforementioned type of inhibitors were given, reaching from the paper concept up into the clinical testing.

This session was closed by the elucidation of the B-type monoamine-oxidase inhibitors and their possible practical use; these inhibitors effectively reduce the enzyme's capacity but apparently regenerate various capacities, essential to "life" in senescence.

In the session devoted to drug metabolism in relation to drug efficacy and toxicity, the first speaker emphasized the possibilities of the "soft drug approach". This approach implies the introduction into the drug molecules of vulnerable groups, that are suitable for particular, preferably hydrolytic, enzymatic attack. This allows control of drug metabolism and thus e.g. avoidance of systemic action, or ultrashort action, in case this is wanted. Practical examples of the soft drug approach were given.

In a following presentation a survey of the many negative aspects of drug metabolism was given. Not only the risks involved in particularly oxidative conversions (via electrophilic, biologically alkylating, reactive intermediates) as a factor in drug toxicity were discussed, but emphasis also was put on the many more general undesirable aspects of drug metabolism. As such were mentioned: the need of frequent dosing, in fact implying a waste of drug, drug interactions, species dependence, patient-to-patient variance, and in relation therewith the need for highly expensive therapeutic monitoring of plasma levels of drugs, etc. It was concluded that in many cases metabolically stable drugs are advantageous over drugs cleared along metabolic pathways. Such drugs are in their pharmacokinetics predominantly dependent on the balance between lipophilicity and hydrophilicity and their elimination is predominantly dependent on excretion processes.

Pharmacokinetics too got proper attention. QSAR for absorption, distribution and elimination was shown to be possible on the basis of regression analysis. The predominant role of the lipophilicity and in relation therewith the $pK_A$ of the compounds was emphasized although for particular aspects of pharmacokinetics such as metabolism and active transport of drugs, also the electronic and steric properties of particular substituents in the molecules count. Examples were given of the prediction of plasma concentration curves in relation to the dose on basis of regression analysis. Integration of quantitative approaches for structure-activity relationships in the strict sense - based on measurement of receptor binding or dose-response relationships on isolated organs - "QSAR" in the strict sense, and quantitative "structure-pharmacokinetic" relationships, "QSPR", will allow for fargoing rationalization in drug development. What is still lacking to a fargoing extent is knowledge on the quantitative "structure-metabolism" relationship, "QSMR".

Drug biotransformation as a source for new drugs was discussed by Dr. Oelschläger. The fact that in many cases drug metabolic products appeared to be biologically active, and in some cases in fact constitute the only active molecular species, implies the possibility of the use of such metabolic products directly as drugs, or possibly after further molecular manipulation such as prodrug formation. The various mechanisms involved in the generation of active metabolites and their potential practical application were exemplified.

From the discussion on drug metabolism in relation to toxicity it was suggested that the choice of a therapeutically active metabolite in the most advanced oxidized state, is advantageous since this will reduce the risk involved in oxidative conversions and simplify pharmacokinetics.

The role of computers in QSAR, and therewith in the design of new drugs was clarified on the basis of various practical examples and elucidated by a cinematographic demonstration of matching spatial configurations of structurally related compounds with indication of the distribution of properties such as lipophilicity and polarity on the molecular surfaces.

Finally Dr. P. Timmermans, as a "last minute stand-in" for a speaker prevented from coming, presented a highly instructive overview of work dealing with structure-action relationship in the field of α-adrenergic imidazole derivatives. These compounds served as a tool in the classification and identification of various types of α-adrenergic receptors, while the insight thus gained in its turn served as a basis in the considerations that are essential for the development of new, in their action more selective α-adrenergic agents.

In conclusion, for this "IUPAC-IUPHAR Symposium", the choice of the various topics and speakers by the Organizing committee was close to optimal. This illustrates that not only in drug development, but also in properly organizing a meeting a sound concept - in this case that of the confrontation of medicinal chemists and pharmacologists with views and problems arising around the molecular interactions at the basis of drug action - can essentially contribute to the success.

# "THE VALUE OF PREDICTIONS IN STRUCTURE–ACTIVITY ANALYSIS"

## PROCEEDINGS OF THE SATELLITE SYMPOSIUM QSAR

J.A. Keverling Buisman (Editor), *Strategy in Drug Research* 


# THE PREDICTIVE MERITS OF ANTIHISTAMINE-QSAR STUDIES

R.F. REKKER

Vakgroep Farmacochemie, Vrije Universiteit, Amsterdam, The Netherlands

## ABSTRACT

Diphenhydramines are the most intensively investigated series of anti-$H_1$-active structures: ring substitutions of different type, elongation of the ethylenic part connecting O and N, as well as a number of alterations in the cationic head, have been applied to improve activity or to modify the activity pattern which besides anti-$H_1$-activity includes anti-cholinergic (atropine-like), local-anesthetic, central dopaminergic and anti-arrhythmic activities as well.

The greater amount of research on diphenhydramines and related classes of antihistaminic compounds (ethylene diamines, 1,1-diaryl-3-aminopropanes, 1,1-diaryl-3-aminopropenes and 1,2-diaryl-4-aminobutenes) dates from the period in which QSAR was far from maturity so that an evaluation of the obtained results was more often done in a retrospective rather than in a prospective way.

An attempt is made to 'rewind' a number of facts and to perform a 'play-back'.

## INTRODUCTION

The history of antihistamine drugs started in 1937, when Ungar et al. (ref. 1) described the antihistamine action of 2(1-piperidinomethyl)-1,4-benzodioxane (F933), a compound known since 1933 and tested by Fourneau and Bovet (ref. 2) for possible antagonism to adrenaline.

The weak antihistamine activity was found to be improved markedly by changing over to open-chain ethers including their analogs in which O had been replaced by N (Bovet and Staub (1937), ref. 3).

Thymoxyethyldiethylamine (F929) and N,N-diethyl-N'-phenyl-N'-ethyl-ethylenediamine (F1571) proved most effective and they may be considered the predecessors of two important antihistamines, diphenhydramine and phenbenzamine, respectively.

Phenbenzamine was first mentioned in an article written by Halpern in 1942 (ref. 4). Diphenhydramine stems from investigations performed by Rieveschl in 1944 and was patented in 1947 (ref. 5).

*References p. 335*

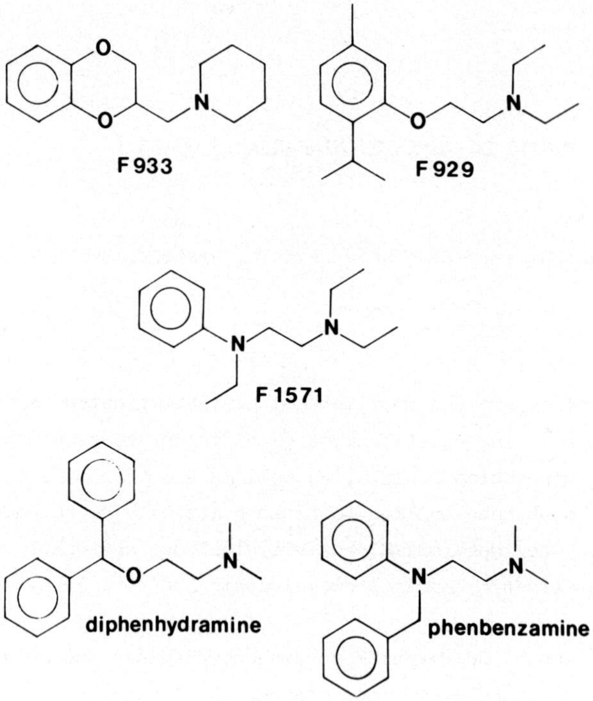

F 933 F 929

F 1571

diphenhydramine phenbenzamine

Fig. 1. Structures of interest in the history of antihistamines

An explosive development in the last few decades has afforded a plethora of structures having antihistamine activity. The following survey provides a compilation of the major categories, while stating for each of them the oldest representative.

| | | |
|---|---|---|
| $(Ar{-}CH_2)(Ar)N{-}CH_2{-}CH_2{-}N\langle$ <br> ethylenediamines | phenbenzamine | Halpern, 1942 (ref. 4) |
| $Ar_2C(R){-}O{-}CH_2{-}CH_2{-}N\langle$ <br> ($R = H$ or $CH_3$) <br> aminoalkylethers | diphenhydramine | Rieveschl, 1944 (ref. 5) |
| $Ar_2CH{-}CH_2{-}CH_2{-}N\langle$ <br> 1,1-diaryl-3-aminopropanes | fenpipran | Schaumann, 1942 (ref. 6) |
| $S(C_6H_4)_2N{-}CH_2{-}CH(CH_3){-}N\langle$ <br> phenothiazines | promethazine | Halpern, 1946 (ref. 7) |
| $Ar{-}C(CH_2{-}Ar){=}CH{-}CH_2{-}N\langle$ <br> 1,2-diaryl-4-amino-$\Delta^2$-butenes | $R = C_6H_5$ | Stoll et al., 1950 (ref. 8) |
| $Ar_2C{=}CH{-}CH_2{-}N\langle$ <br> 1,1-diaryl-3-aminopropenes | $Ar = C_6H_5$ | White et al., 1951 (ref. 9) |

Especially since 1970, attempts have been made to clarify the relations between chemical structure and antihistamine activity. There is no denying that this endeavour has been fruitful in certain structures because it has deepened our insight considerably (refs. 10,11,12,13,14,15,16,17,18). Nevertheless, many problems have remained unsolved.

In the context of this satellite symposium a 'playback' may be useful, and armed with current knowledge, a number of major issues can be marshalled.

FROM F933 TO DIPHENHYDRAMINE

Interesting information is obtained by inspection of the superpositions given in Fig. 2.

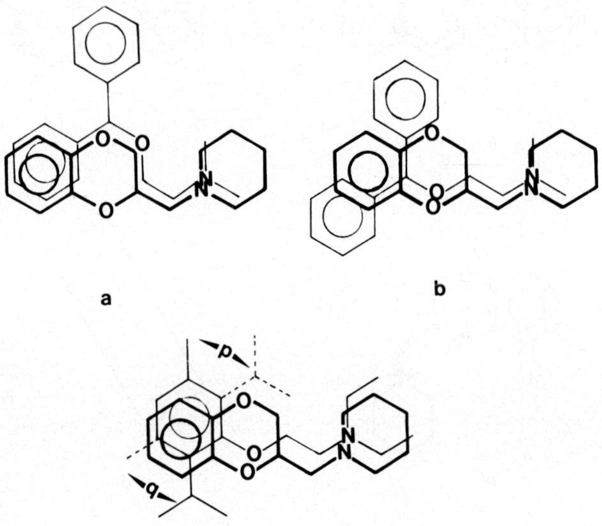

a

b

c

Fig. 2. Superpositions of some compounds from Fig. 1:
a. superposition of F933 on diphenhydramine with the N-C-C-O unit of the latter covered by the N-C-C-C-(O) unit of the former;
b. superposition of F933 on diphenhydramine with the N-C-C-O unit of the latter covered by the N-C-C-O unit of the former;
c. superposition of F933 on F929 with the N-C-C-O unit of the latter covered by the N-C-C-O unit of the former; the phenylring of F929 is given in two positions, one with fully drawn valences and the other with broken valences; p and q indicate regions of bulk or hydrophobicity.

The markedly improved activity of F929 as compared to F933 would accentuate the necessity of 2 rather than 3 C atoms to be present between O and N accompanied by a demand for bulk or hydrophobicity in flanks p and q of the benzene ring.

Superpositions other than those illustrated in Fig. 2 can also be easily achieved, however; see, for example, Fig. 3, in which two variants b' and b" are added to the superposition of F933 and diphenhydramine.

On inspection of the overall pattern of these superpositions, it would appear that the outline presented in d of Fig. 3 is essential to antihistamine activity, involving a rather extensive hydrophobic region (designated by h.r.) and a fairly large space where a (charged) nitrogen atom finds its location.

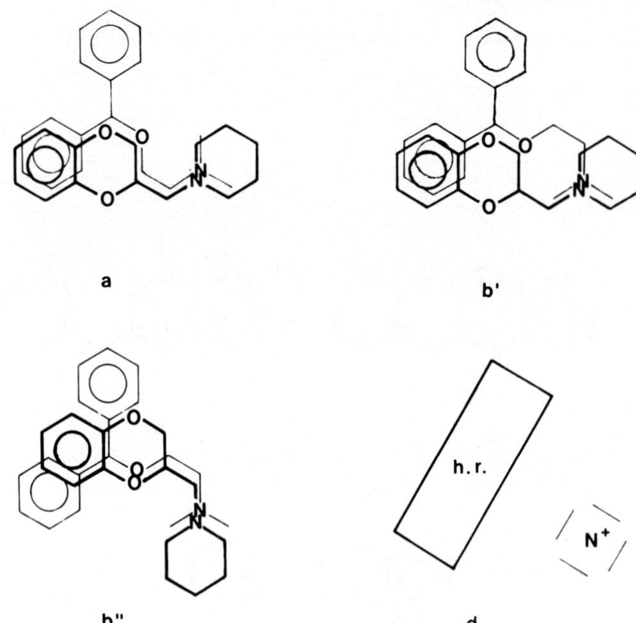


Fig. 3. Superpositions of F933 and diphenhydramine, and a tentatively derived schematic structure pattern of an antihistamine:

a. identical to a) from Fig. 2;

b'. b) from Fig. 2 with an O/N cisoid instead of a transoid conformation in which the N-C-C-O unit of diphenhydramine is no longer optimally covered by the N-C-C-C-(O) unit of F933;

b". a situation comparable to b', except that the N-C-C-O unit of diphenhydramine is covered by the N-C-C-O unit of F933;

d. schematic structure pattern of an antihistamine; h.r. = hydrophobic region; $N^+$-location designated by a broken square.

At this stage three rather important conclusions can be drawn about diphenhydramine:

a) the ether-O atom no longer has a fixed position, and it is even pertinent to ask if it does have a real binding function. If not, it could be replaced by, for example, NH or S, and might even be omitted or replaced by an additional $CH_2$ group:

TABLE 1

Antihistamine and anticholinergic activities of a few compounds derived from or connected with diphenhydramine

$CH_2$-$CH_2$-$N(CH_3)_2$

| X and Y | ring-subst. | $pA_2$(antihistamine) | $pA_2$(anticholinergic) |
|---|---|---|---|
| X = H H | unsubst. | 6.1 (8.0) | 7.1 (6.7) |
| Y = CH-S | 4-$CH_3$ | 7.1 (8.8) | 6.3 (6.1) |
| | 2-$CH_3$ | 6.3 (6.4) | 7.2 (6.8) |
| X = S<br>Y = N | unsubst. | $pA_2$-values are not available; antihistamine activity significantly higher than that of diphenhydramine (ref. 24) | |
| X = $CH_2$-$CH_2$<br>Y = CH-O | unsubst. | 8.9 | 8.0 |
| X = $CH_2$-$CH_2$-$CH_2$<br>Y = CH-O | " | 6.9 | 6.9 |
| X = CH=CH<br>Y = CH-O | unsubst. | 9.5 | 7.6 |

Note: in brackets activities of corresponding 'O-ethers' (X = O); $pA_2$: see ref. 27.

- replacement by NH provides ethylene diamines, which are also antihistamines;
- replacement by S affords aminoalkyl-thioethers, which also have a reasonable antihistamine activity and were examined by Timmerman et al. in 1971 (see Table 1 and ref. 19);
- omission of O leads to the 1,1-diaryl-3-aminopropanes, which are quite active antihistamines.

b) the gap between the two phenyl rings of diphenhydramine can in all likelihood be filled up by additional hydrophobicity from several sources. This automatically gives rise to the following classification of structures:

- phenothiazines, which were examined for the first time in 1946 by Halpern (ref. 7). The two phenyl rings are linked together by an S bond, the CH-O combination has been replaced by N and the aliphatic side-chain may possibly show branching (see Table 1 and Fig. 4e);
- tricyclic derivatives of the type denoted in Fig. 4f. A saturated bridge composed of two C atoms has been inserted between the two phenyl nuclei of diphenhydramine. These derivatives were described by Van der Stelt et al. in 1973 (see Table 1 and ref. 20);

O tricyclic derivatives of the type denoted in Fig. 4g. An unsaturated bridge made up by two C atoms has been placed between the two phenyl nuclei. The derivatives thus obtained were also described by Van der Stelt et al. (see Table 1 and ref. 20).

c) since neither the O nor the N atom no longer seem to have an entirely fixed location a certain chain lengthening between O and N must be permissable. A study by Harms et al.(ref. 14; see Fig. 4h) has revealed that an intercalation of 3 C's between N and O is certainly justified and that with increasing lengt of the intercalant an obvious decrease in antihistamine activity becomes manifest.

WHAT IS THE PRECISE FUNCTION OF THE SECOND PHENYL RING IN DIPHENHYDRAMINE AND ITS DERIVATIVES ?

It is becoming obvious that questions concerning the precise function of the phenyl ring used for the transformation of the benzodioxane derivative (F933) or of thymoxyethyldiethylamine (F929) into diphenhydramine, strongly suggest themselves.

In the above paragraphs we heavily opted for the view that it was merely a

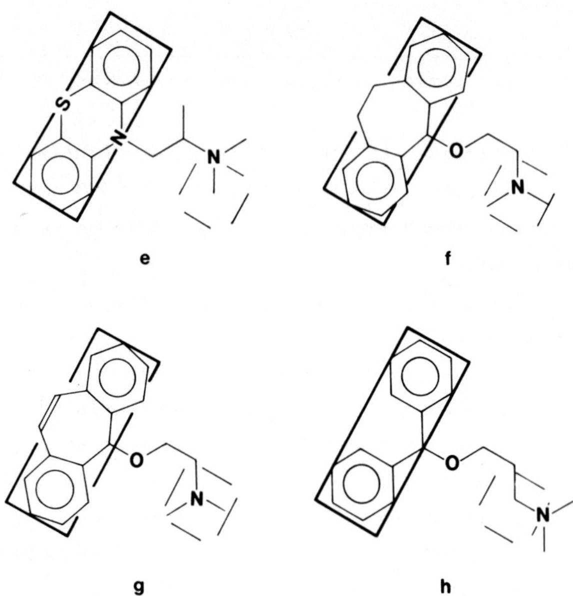


Fig. 4. Structures derived from diphenhydramine by filling up the gap between the two phenyl nuclei with extra hydrophobicity (e, f and g) or by extending the aminoethyl chain (h).

matter of an extra amount of hydrophobicity introduced at the proper location, but what other factors, it may be asked, are additionally involved?

Table 2 presents the results of a study which, performed in 1966, was not published until 1975. Its objective was to ascertain any effect of replacing a phenyl group in diphenhydramine by a group whose susceptibility to inductive factors could be likened to that of a phenyl group. Tabulated are not only the observed $pA_2$ values but also the Taft $\sigma^*$ values and it will at once be clear that there is no relation at all between $pA_2$ and $\sigma^*$.

Once that study had been extended to include the cyclohexyl derivative and some of the compounds derived from it, it did become obvious that perhaps something like the bulkiness of the substituents could be of importance but at that time there were virtually no means yet of checking this mathematically.

The $\pi$-method of Hansch introduced in 1962 (ref. 21):

$$\log P(SX) / P(SH) = \pi(X) \qquad (1)$$

where the partition coefficients of SH and SX are indicated by P(SH) and P(SX), respectively, and the hydrophobic substituent constant by $\pi(X)$, could have provided the $\pi$ values of the substituents tested by us. However, as this method did not allow for the existence of proximity effects, i.e., of rises in lipophilicity in cases where two electronegative groups are separated by 2 or 3 C atoms, for example $(\delta^-)\text{-O-}CH_2CH_2\text{-O-}(\delta^-)$, any attempt to correlate $pA_2$ with $\pi$ would have been fruitless.

The concept of the hydrophobic fragmental constant was not introduced until 1973, and does take into account the proximity effects just mentioned (ref. 22):

$$\log P = \sum_1^n \underline{a}_n f_n + \Sigma\,\text{anom.} \qquad (2)$$

where $f$ represents the hydrophobic fragmental constant, $\underline{a}$ is a numerical factor expressing the number of times that a given fragment occurs in the structure under investigation, and $\Sigma$ anom. stands for the total of all anomalies encountered during the development of the $f$ system. These include proximity effects for 2 C and 3 C separations between electronegative groups (0.57 for each 3 C separation and 0.87 for each 2 C separation).

The $f$-value of any substituent appears to be very suitable for tracing possible links between $pA_2$ and hydrophobicity. The correlation of $pA_2$ with $f$ does not look very elegant (r = 0.779) but the parameter combination $f$ and $f^2$ affords the following, quite acceptable, equation:

$$pA_2 = 1.316(\pm.532) f - 0.272(\pm.156) f^2 + 5.010(\pm.355) \qquad (3)$$

$n = 12 \quad r = 0.894^{\dagger} \quad s = 0.351^{\dagger} \quad F = 20.0$

†) All regression equations in this paper are provided with r and s values adjusted for the number of degrees of freedom (ref. 23).

*References p. 335*

TABLE 2

Antihistamine activities in a series of diphenhydramines with one phenyl group replaced by a nonaromatic group

$C_6H_5$–CH(R)–O – $CH_2$ – $CH_2$ – $N(CH_3)_2$

| R | $pA_2$ obs. | $pA_2$ est. | $f$ | $f^2$ | $\sigma^*$ | $\pi$ |
|---|---|---|---|---|---|---|
| –H | 5.6 | 5.24 | .18 | .03 | .49 | .00 |
| $-CH_2OH$ | 4.4 | 4.48 | -.37 | .14 | .55 | -.66 |
| $-CH_2-O-CH_2CH_3$ | 5.3 | 5.82 | .72 | .52 | .52 | .53 |
| $-C(=O)-O-CH_2-CH_3$ | 6.1 | 5.92 | .84 | .70 | 2.00 | .23 |
| $-CH_2-CH=CH_2$ | 6.2 | 6.31 | 1.38 | 1.89 | .23 | 1.20 |
| $-CH_2-C\equiv CH$ | 6.1 | 6.06 | 1.01 | 1.02 | .76 | .98 |
| | 7.0 | 6.53 | 2.93 | 8.60 | -.15 | 2.46 |
| $CH_3$ | 6.4 | 6.31 | 3.45 | 11.91 | a | 2.66 |
| | 6.9 | 6.60 | 2.57 | 6.60 | a | 2.16 |
| $CH_3$ | 6.2 | 6.48 | 3.09 | 9.53 | a | 2.36 |
| $CH_2$ | 6.1 | 6.48 | 3.09 | 9.53 | a | 2.56 |
| $CH_2$ | 6.5 | 6.57 | 2.72 | 7.42 | a | 2.26 |
| | 8.0 | 6.51 | 1.84 | 3.39 | .60 | 2.13 |

[a]) Not available

where $f$ is the hydrophobic fragmental constant of substituent R, taking into account any corrections that may be needed for proximity effects. The relationship established is depicted graphically in Fig. 5.

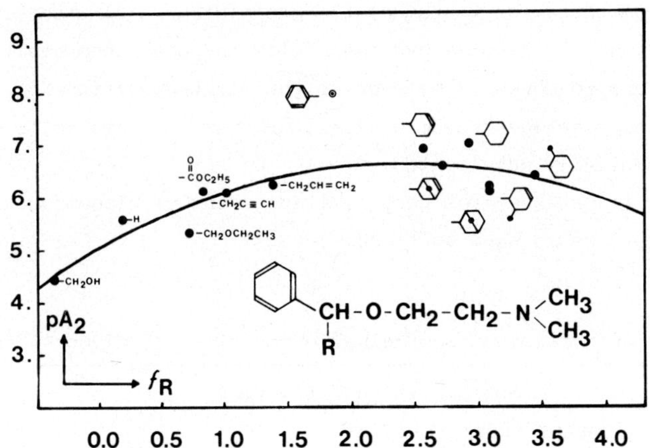


Fig. 5. $pA_2$ (antihistamine activity) plotted versus $f_R$ for compounds included in Table 2; $f_R$ denotes the hydrophobic fragmental value of R, while taking into account any required corrections for proximity effects.

The above equation will be deteriorated markedly by including the phenyl derivative (= diphenhydramine itself), the correlation coefficient dropping from 0.894 to 0.811. As suggested by eqn 3, the $pA_2$ of diphenhydramine should have been 6.5, or 6.8, if each phenyl nucleus were, for some reason, to be accounted for separately. Its $pA_2$ value is, however, 8.0*, which is far higher than the predicted $pA_2$ optimum of 6.6 attained at $f$ = 2.42.

It will be clear that any prediction of a $pA_2$ for the derivative with one more phenyl group extra (the triphenylmethylether of dimethylaminoethanol) on the basis of eqn 3 will come to nothing. A $pA_2$ value has not been published for this ether, but Leonard and Huttrer (ref. 24) report that the product falls into the category of "weakly actives"; by implication, diphenhydramine would be among the "actives", and this simply means that the activity of the triphenyl derivative is below expectations.

The reason that the monophenyl ether of dimethylaminoethanol undergoes such a singular rise in antihistamine activity following introduction of the second phenyl ring is probably to be found in a mechanism of interaction lying outside the proper sphere of hydrophobicity.

One may think of, for example, a $\pi - \pi$ interaction of this phenyl group with

*) This $pA_2$ value is decidedly of a better quality than the one published previously (see, for instance, ref. 14).

another phenyl group inhering in a receptor, for instance the phenyl group from a phenylalanine unit (ref. 10). Actually, this picture should be completed with Witiak's statement (ref. 25) that strongest competitive histamine antagonism seems to occur when at least one ring is capable of attaining a position 5-6 Å away from the amino N-atom of the antihistamine structure.

If as early as the fifties hydrophobicity had been adequately documented, the straightforward moves to be made in the right direction for understanding the relationships between structural features and antihistamine activity could have been essentially accelerated.

In the first instance, the very limited series of diphenhydramine derivatives shown in Table 3 would have sufficed.

TABLE 3

Antihistamine activities of some alkyl-derivatives of diphenhydramine

| substituents | antihistamine activities | | *f* | |
|---|---|---|---|---|
| | 'MAGNUS-test' (ref. 26) | $pA_2$ | para + para' | R |
| none | 1 * | 8.0 | 0.36 | 1.84 |
| 4-methyl | 3.7 | 8.7 | 0.88 | 2.36 |
| 4,4'-dimethyl | 0.5 | 7.2 | 1.40 | 2.36 |
| 3-methyl | 0.2 | 7.2 | 0.88 | 2.36 |
| 2-methyl | 0.2 | 6.7 | 0.88 | 2.36 |
| 4-ethyl | 2.4 | 8.2 | 1.40 | 2.88 |
| 4-isopropyl | 1.4 | 7.6 | 1.92 | 3.40 |
| 4-tert. butyl | 0.6 | 6.0 | 2.44 | 3.92 |

*) reference substance; R denotes the (heaviest) substituted phenyl ring

What the chosen substituents have in common is that they all enhance the lipophilicity of the diphenhydramine molecule. Next, a study of the antihistamine activities of the derivatives selected would have revealed the following:

a) ortho and meta substitutions with $CH_3$ groups diminish antihistamine activity considerably, in spite of their positive contributions to lipophilicity, which will approximately reach the optimal value of the R-unit.

b) a single para substitution with $CH_3$ raises antihistamine activity considerably. As the resulting increase in lipophilicity is exactly the same as that following one ortho or meta $CH_3$-substitution (see Table 3), more factors than those connected with eqn 3 must be thought of. It is tempting to suggest that while the width of the hydrophobic field* in Fig. 3d permits no scope for ad-

*) The designation "hydrophobic field" is used throughout on purpose, as the illustrations in Figs. 3d and 4 make it clear that one has to do with a real plane. It stands to reason that the actual pattern of this hydrophobic field may also be vaulted in shape.

ditional lipophilic bulk the length does, provided that this bulk is restricted in size, for single para $C_2H_5$ just like double para $CH_3$ substitution does not serve a useful purpose. The para isopropyl and tert.butyl derivatives quite fit into this picture; any positive contribution to antihistamine activity is precluded for these derivatives on account of either eqn 3 or the limited length of the hydrophobic field.

The group of structures described in Table 3, as limited as it is, would, therefore, be of ample proportions to serve as a source of valuable information next to eqn 3. Also the desirability of synthesis followed by study of compounds with ortho $-CH_2-CH_2-$ or $-CH=CH-$ bridge would have clearly brought out.

Yet it must be remembered that the data in Table 3 stem from the years 1955 - 1956, when a compilation as tabulated here could merely serve as an initial step towards any adequately thought-out research program. This explains why the first phase of the researches comprised even more than 30 compounds in which the chosen phenyl substituents, none excepted, were all alkyl groups.

A first quantitative relationship for this series was that proposed by Kutter and Hansch (ref. 25).

$$\log BR = 0.326\,E_s^{o,m} - 0.346\,(E_s^{p})^2 - 0.189\,E_s^{p} + 0.563\,E_s^{p'} - 1.878 \qquad (4)$$

$$n = 30 \quad r = 0.945 \quad s = 0.231$$

where the symbols are denoted as follows:

BR = biological response: the relative antagonistic activity of the compound in comparison with diphenhydramine, toward a standard dose of histamine, by the Magnus technique (ref. 26); $pA_2$ values as determined according to Ariëns (ref. 27) were not available at that time;

$E_s^{o,m}$ = sum of the ortho and meta substituent Taft $E_s$ values on the highest substituted ring;

$E_s^{p}$, = $E_s$ value of the para substituent in the same ring;

$E_s^{p'}$ = $E_s$ value of the para substituent in the other ring in the case of para-para' disubstitution. If the structure is not of the para-para' disubstituted type, the hydrogen $E_s$ value is used.

The equation makes an exclusive use of Taft's $E_s$ parameter. Bearing in mind that in the series under investigation there exists a clear parallel between bulk - and thus $E_s$ - of the substituent tested and its lipophilicity, the equation can in the first instance simply be regarded as a variant of eqn 3. Both a squared and a linear occurrence of one of the $E_s$ parameters is observed and in fact they can be considered as substitutes for $f^2$ and $f$, respectively.

The inequality of the two phenyl rings emerges from this equation as a new element. A distinction is made on the basis of the heaviness of substitution actually implying that the most lipophilic ring is singled out. Of this ring, the $E_s$ parameters are taken into consideration or, putting it in another way, lipophilicity is accounted for as a deteriorating factor; a bulkier substituent

– with decreasing $E_s$ – will add less and less to the right-hand part of eqn 4 or even subtract from it, leaving the remaining log BR smaller and smaller*. Actually, this will imply that in ortho and meta positions only H is allowed to occur, and that any alkyl group must be avoided.

The para substituent in the heaviest substituted – or most lipophilic – ring appears in eqn 4 with both $E_s$ and $E_s^2$, denoting an optimal $E_s$ value, which in turn means an optimal $f$. The para substituent in the least substituted – or least lipophilic – of the two rings, raises activity by virtue of the positive algebraic sign of the regressor combined with the negative character of the average alkyl-$E_s$ value so that here, too, an H is the favourite substituent.

In 1975 we reported extended and, in our opinion, essentially improved equations, comprising:

a) recognition of the fact that in the case of an optically active diphenhydramine derivative biological activity largely stems from one of the two antipodes. In a regression study the greater activity contribution of the two is introduced in the computation or, where only racemate activities are available double the antihistamine value of this racemate is taken;
b) derivatives other than those obtained by alkyl substitution (halogen, methoxy) were examined as well;
c) change from the Magnus antihistamine values to the $pA_2$ values determined by Ariëns method (ref. 27).

It was possible to design at least three equations expressing in a reasonably satisfactory manner the relation between structure and antihistamine activity. For the purpose of this presentation, the following will suffice:

$$pA_2 = 0.290(\pm.062)\ E_s^{o,m} + 0.416(\pm.142)\ E_s^{p} - 0.795(\pm.138)\ (E_s^{p'})^2 - 2.275(\pm.689)\ \sigma'_{R(p)} + 4.958 \qquad (5)$$

$$n = 30 \quad r = 0.968 \quad s = 0.274 \quad F = 110.5$$

where

$E_s^{o,m}$ = sum of the steric Taft parameters of <u>all</u> ortho and meta substituents in both rings;

$E_s^{p}$ = steric Taft parameter of the para substituent in the ring supposed to be involved in receptor binding;

$E_s^{p'}$ = steric Taft parameter of the para substituent in the other ring in the case of para-para' disubstitution. If not para-para' disubstituted, the hydrogen $E_s$ value is used;

$\sigma'_{R(p)}$ = a resonance parameter introduced by Taft (ref. 28) and to be regarded as a Hammett $\sigma$ constant corrected for inductive contributions.

The difference with eqn 4 is that all steric parameters for ortho and meta in

*) Strong collinearity is observed between $E_s$ and $f$ in a series of substituents including the halogens and some of the lower alkyl groups; r amounts to 0.931 (ref. 22).

both rings have been introduced or rather that the entire lipophilicity effect in the ortho-meta region has actually been accounted for.

Furthermore, the quadratic appearance of $E_S^{p'}$ combined with a negative regressor value expresses an amplified deterioration caused by a second para substituent.

The final difference with eqn 4 is that eqn 5 contains the $\sigma_R'$ parameter for the introduction of the mesomeric effect of a para substituent; positive mesomeric effects - expressed by negative $\sigma_R'$ values - prove advantageous to antihistamine activity.

In this context, the functional difference between the two rings is rather strongly accentuated. One of them is believed to be receptor-bound, presuming a $\pi - \pi$ mechanism of interaction, and among the functions of the other ring there would be an interactional one with the ether-O, to be regarded as a spatial ring-$\pi$ orbital overlap with the p-orbits of the O atom.

It must be admitted, however, that the ring assignment is no prerequisite and perhaps it might be necessary to change the role of the two rings, while upholding the hypothesis that presumes the non-equivalence of the two aromatic rings. This would mean that the substituted ring in para diphenhydramine derivatives is to be held responsible for the primary receptor interaction, which is the one participating in the $\pi - \pi$ binding mechanism. In this way it would be possible to clear up a discrepancy signalized in a paper by Nauta and Rekker (ref. 29).

## ROLE OF THE ETHER-O ATOM IN THE DIPHENHYDRAMINE STRUCTURE

The ether-O atom plays no specific role in what has been argued about structure and antihistamine activity of diphenhydramines in the previous section. Without ill effects this atom may be replaced by other electronegative groups such as S and N or by a C=C system and even be omitted. In the last case, the fairly reasonably active diarylaminopropanes are obtained.

Our point of view has always been that the ether-O atom, because of its 'through space'-interaction with the ring $\pi$-orbitals, would cause a certain local structure rigidity, comparable to that in the conjugated diaryl-butenes and diaryl-propenes. The fact that the diarylaminopropanes, in which this rigidity plays no role at all, are active prompts us to reconsider our view.

The idea of a spatial overlap of specified orbitals in diphenhydramines or related structures such as benzhydrols and benzylalcohols got a good confirmation by UV spectroscopy (ref. 30) and after that, additional support was obtained from the increased lipophilicities of benzhydrols and benzylalcohols as compared to what may be normally expected. Such higher log P values point to an O less liable to hydration, thus suggesting strongly some sort of interaction process in which the lone electrons of O are significantly involved.

In this connection, the following may be proposed. It is well-known that diphenhydramine, besides exerting antihistamine activity, possesses an anticholinergic activity component. In our opinion, accumulated evidence suggests that the ether-O atom is of eminent importance in that anticholinergic component, probably participating with its lone electron pairs in receptor binding in one way or another.

By implication,

a) if O is replaced by S or by N, the anticholinergic activity component will be retained, because the lone electron pairs remain available; this is exemplified in Table 1;

b) if the ether-O atom is omitted, in other words, if we switch from diphenhydramines to the diarylaminopropanes just mentioned, the anticholinergic activity component will become much smaller, if not disappear altogether. Detailed information is not to be found in the literature but it is worth stating that no diarylaminopropanes with a reasonable activity pattern are referred to in any compilation. Similar considerations apply to diarylpropenes; on these compounds exact information does exist, however. Reference is made to studies by Waringa (ref. 17), who compared both antihistamine and anticholinergic activities of a number of diarylpropenes with those of correspondingly structured diphenhydramines. These studies make it clear that the antagonistic action of diarylpropenes against furthrethonium-induced rat jejunum contractions, besides being rather limited, shows little differentiation. Apparently, the $\pi$ electrons of the C = C bond cannot altogether take over the role of the lone electrons of O, S and N, present in, respectively, ethers, thioethers and ethylenediamines;

c) it must be possible to achieve shifts in the combined antihistamine-anticholinergic activity pattern, provided that the spatial orbital overlap just mentioned can be sufficiently influenced, as can, indeed, be accomplished by a thought-out choice of the para substituent, which may be $CH_3$, OH, $OCH_3$ or halogen. These substituents have a positive mesomeric character, which may be taken to mean that their contributions to the signalized orbital overlap become stronger. Again, there is a good evidence from UV absorption data. The effect in question cannot be expressed in terms of the Hammett $\sigma$ parameter in a regression equation. This is not quite surprising, however, because $\sigma$ also includes a variable negative inductive component so that the actual $\sigma$ values to be used in a regression equation may be either negative or positive. It proved, therefore, advisable to employ the $\sigma_R'$ values (ref. 28), all of which are negative for the substituents just mentioned. We make reference to Table 4, from which it also appears that the $\mathcal{R}$ parameter of Swain and Lupton (ref. 31) or Charton's $\sigma_D$ parameter (ref. 32), too, would lend itself for what is aimed at - namely the exclusive parametrization of a resonance effect.

TABLE 4

Some $\sigma$ and $\sigma$ type parameters for para-substituents in diphenhydramines

| substituent | $\sigma$ (Hammett) | $\sigma'_R$ (Taft) | $\mathcal{R}$ (Swain-Lupton) | $\sigma_D$ (Charton) |
|---|---|---|---|---|
| $CH_3$ | -.17 | -.13 | -.14 | -.15 |
| OH | -.37 | -.61 | -.64 | -.62 |
| $OCH_3$ | -.27 | -.50 | -.43 | -.59 |
| F | .06 | -.44 | -.34 | -.52 |
| Cl | .23 | -.24 | -.16 | -.27 |
| Br | .23 | -.22 | -.18 | -.26 |
| I | .18 | -.19 | -.20 | -.15 |

D = delocalization

Although a satisfactory relation between anticholinergic activity and a given set of structural parameters could not be established yet, the study of the various series of diphenhydramine derivatives has revealed that this anticholinergic activity has a trend to increase as a result of ring substitutions which lower antihistamine activity, while it is decreased by substitutions increasing antihistamine activity. In simplest terms, this phenomenon is visualized in Fig. 6. It must be emphasized that there is no more than just a trend towards complementary coupling of the two activities in which the O, S or N atom with its lone

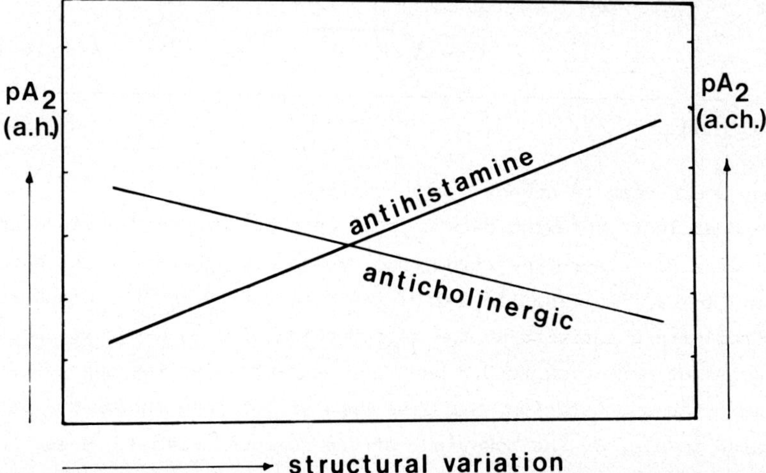


Fig. 6. Simplified visualization of complementary coupling of antihistamine (left-hand vertical axis) and anticholinergic (right -hand vertical axis) activities in diphenhydramine type structures.

TABLE 5

Course of antihistamine and anticholinergic activities in some diphenhydramine analogs

R'

$\alpha \overset{H}{\underset{R}{C}} - O - CH_2 - CH_2 - N(CH_3)_2$

| R | antihistamine activity $pA_2$ | | | | anticholinergic activity (H-fur): $pA_2$ | | | |
|---|---|---|---|---|---|---|---|---|
| | R'= H | R'= o-$CH_3$ | R'= p-$CH_3$ | $\Delta_p$ | R'= H | R'= o-$CH_3$ | R'= p-$CH_3$ | $\Delta_p$ |
| -H | 5.6 | a | 5.2 | (-0.4) | 4.6 | a | 4.8 | (0.2) |
| | 7.0 | 6.5 | 7.8 | 0.8 | 7.2 | 7.5 | 6.2 | -1.0 |
| | 6.9 | 6.2 | 8.0 | 1.1 | 6.7 | 7.2 | 5.9 | -0.8 |
| | 8.0 | 6.2 | 8.7 | 0.7 | 6.7 | 6.8 | 6.1 | -0.6 |
| | 9.1 (with α-H replaced by $CH_3$) | a | 9.3 | (0.2) | a | a | a | |
| | | | Aver.$\Delta_p$ = | 0.9 | | | Aver.$\Delta_p$ = | -0.8 |

[a]) Not available

electrons would seem to occupy a key position.

Table 5 collects relevant data on both antihistamine and anticholinergic activities of a few ether-type structures, which are related to the compounds listed in Table 2. The rises in antihistamine activity and the concurrent drops in anticholinergic activity on the introduction of a para-methyl substituent are fairly constant amounting to 0.9 and 0.8, respectively. The changes in activity, following ortho-substitution, are less regular but they follow the pattern as illustrated in Fig. 6. The behaviour of the compound with R = H is, for hitherto unknown reasons, reverse; a similar reverse behavioural pattern has been observed between N-dimethyl-cinnamylamine and its para-methyl derivative (ref. 17).

Table 6 is of interest as it illustrates nicely how closely an attempt to improve antihistamne activity is linked up with parameter choice. The 4-F derivative of diphenhydramine shows an increase by 0.5 as compared to the unsubstituted compound due to the rather strongly negative $\sigma'_R$ value and the small - but always disadvantageously acting - bulk of F ensuing at the same time. However,

TABLE 6

Influence of para-F substitution on the antihistamine activity of diphenhydramine

| substituents | $pA_2$ |
|---|---|
| none | 8.0 |
| 4-fluoro | 8.5 |
| 4,4'-difluoro | 8.4 |

the F atom is so small in size that a second introduction in para-position does not reduce antihistamine activity so dramatically as is usually the case with second para-substitutions. This is, actually, the reason for the $pA_2$ values of 4-F and 4,4'-diF-diphenhydramine to be nearly identical.

MORE EVIDENCE FOR THE IMPORTANCE OF HYDROPHOBICITY AS A MAJOR FACTOR IN THE ANTIHISTAMINE ACTION OF DIPHENHYDRAMINE AND RELATED STRUCTURES

a) In 1973 Nauta et al. (ref. 15) published a study on the antihistamine action of a series of diphenhydramines with the terminal amino group varying from $-NH_3^+$ to $-NH(C_3H_7)_2^+$. Also, they examined the effect of including the N atom in rings of variable sizes, the best fit being obtained using the equation

$$pA_2 = 1.378(\pm.437)\ D + 2.838(\pm1.086)\ \ell - 0.419(\pm.153)\ \ell^2 - 0.709(\pm.425)\ \pi_{N^+} -1.254(\pm.685)\ \log P - 0.116 \qquad (6)$$

$$n = 27 \quad r = 0.914 \quad s = 0.402 \quad F = 26.4$$

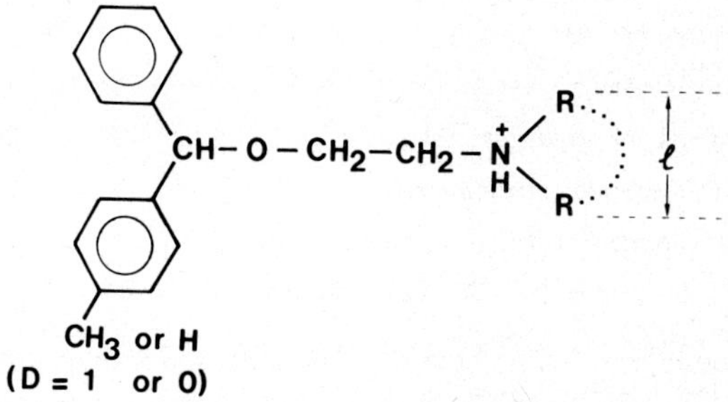


Fig. 7. Structural pattern considered in eqn 6.

In eqn 6 log P represents the octanol-water partition of the HCl salt of the diphenhydramine derivative proper, and $\pi_{N^+}$ is the measured log P value minus the total lipophilicity value of all substituents located on the N atom. In fact, the latter is an $f_{N^+}$ value but at the time that the equation was reported, the $f$ concept was not yet fully operational. The $\ell$ in the equation is the width of the $-NH(RR)^+$ unit with an optimal value of 3.4 Å. D denotes a dummy parameter taken to be 1 if a para-$CH_3$ group is present and 0 if no such group occurs (other types of substitution were not studied in this connection).

Again, the importance of lipophilicity as a descriptive parameter of antihistamine action comes to the fore. It is, however, not easy to establish how lipophilicity operates here in all its aspects. The $pA_2$ value is higher as $\pi_{N^+}$ is more negative, and this in turn is true for cationic heads with a ring structure that is not too small, consisting of, say, 6 - 7 ring partners. Ring sizes as meant here cause the optimal width of the cationic head to be exceeded, however, and, moreover, there is an increase in overall lipophilicity which, although positive itself, forms an unfavourable factor for the $pA_2$ because of its negative regressor value in eqn 6. To complete the picture of complexity, it must be added that $\pi_{N^+}$ and the Taft $\sigma^*$ values of the cationic head show a clear tendency of running parallel.

b) The next equation was first published by Waringa et al. (ref. 18, 29) in 1975 putting the $pA_2$ values of 7 classes of antihistamines together into one category by means of 6 dummy parameters and one hydrophobic fragmental value either belonging to the cis - positioned ring (structures belonging to classes I and II, or to its presumed equivalent as far as the structures from classes III - VII are concerned. The integrated equation (7) is primarily usable in that it clarifies essential lipophilicity relations while helping to establish which of the two rings is capable of functioning in the receptor.

$$pA_2 = 1.243(\pm.133)\, f_{\text{"cis"}} + 5.190 \qquad (7)$$

| | | |
|---|---|---|
| (I) | 1,1-diaryl-3-aminopropenes | $+ 0.000\, D_I$ |
| (II) | 1,1-diaryl-3-N-pyrrolidinopropenes | $+ 1.187(\pm.292)\, D_{II}$ |
| (III) | diphenhydramines | $+ 0.573(\pm.324)\, D_{III}$ |
| (IV) | ethylenediamines | $+ 0.384(\pm.375)\, D_{IV}$ |
| (V) | $\alpha$-methyl-diphenhydramines | $+ 1.346(\pm.362)\, D_V$ |
| (VI) | 1,1-diaryl-3-aminopropanes | $+ 0.932(\pm.357)\, D_{VI}$ |
| (VII) | aza-diphenhydramines | $+ 0.619(\pm.360)\, D_{VII}$ |

$n = 37 \quad r = 0.955 \quad s = 0.364 \quad F = 54.4$

The equation confirms convincingly that diarylaminopropanes have a much greater antihistamine action than diphenhydramines - $\Delta pA_2 = 0.61$ - under the same lipophilic conditions of the cis-ring or its equivalent and permits predictions of the antihistamine effects of a large range of structure types. It must be added, however, that the limitations emerging from the preceding eqations (eqns 4, 5 and 6) remain in full force and by implication, the parametrization of lipophilicity must appear as a quadratic function in the eventually construed regression equation.

TABLE 7

Effect of quaternization on diphenhydramine-type compounds

| compounds | | $pA_2$ antihistamine | $pA_2$ anticholinergic |
|---|---|---|---|
| $BH - O - CH_2 - CH_2 - N(CH_3)_2$ | | | |
| | unsubstituted | 8.0 | 6.7 |
| | 4-methyl | 8.7 | 6.1 |
| $BH - O - CH_2 - CH_2 - N(CH_3)_3^+$ | | | |
| | unsubstituted | 7.3 | 7.4 |
| | 4-methyl | 8.8 | 7.0 |
| BH − O − $CH_2$ − (N-methylpiperidin-yl, N–$CH_3$) | | | |
| | unsubstituted | 7.9 | 7.7 |
| | 4-methyl | 8.9 | 7.2 |
| BH − O − $CH_2$ − (N,N-dimethylpiperidinium-yl, $N^+(CH_3)_2$) | | | |
| | 4-methyl | 9.8 | 7.4 |

BH = benzhydryl moiety

c) It has often been suggested that the presence of a quaternary N atom precludes antihistamine action, even imparting an obviously anticholinergic character to a given compound. Thiazinamium is a good antihistamine, however, despite the undeniable presence of a centrally operating anticholinergic activity component, thus indicating that the concept just outlined lacks general validity. Therefore, quaternary diphenhydramines in priciple have a fairly strong antihistamine action as well, if at least the benzhydryl moiety satisfies requirements.

Some pertinent data about a limited number of structures are to be found in Table 7. Obviously, a quaternary N atom is in no way an obstacle to the development of antihistaminic properties in such structures.

Of two quaternary structures - thiazinamium and pirdonium - the log P values in octanol-water have been determined. These values are, of course, rather low - 0.50 and 0.64, respectively, when measured under comparable conditions - and due to the absence of an appropriately basic species with a much higher log P as is the case in diphenhydramine itself (log P = 3.30), structures with quaternary N of the type mentioned in Table 7 will experience much more difficulty in

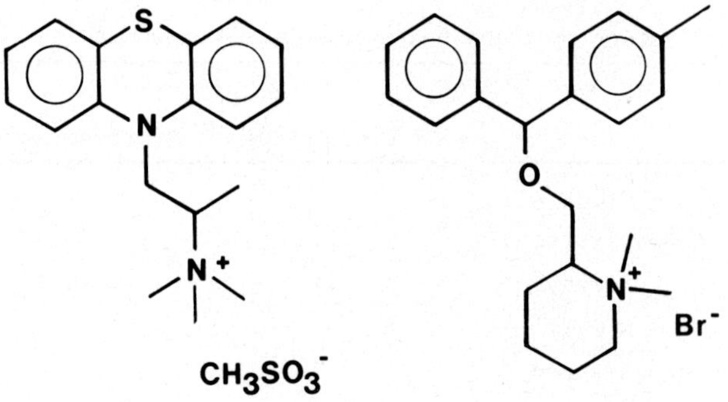

Fig. 8. Examples of quaternary antihistamines.

passing the blood-brain barrier than their tertiary analogues, thus being clearly more peripheral in action.

Conversely, thiazinamium and pirdonium are typical examples of compounds which, although hampered by low log P's, are still lipophilic enough to undergo a low yet significant passage through the blood-brain barrier.

CONCLUSIONS

1) Lipophilicity provides a major parameter in the description of antihistamine behaviour of drugs and a quadratic $f$ (or log P) relationship seems to be involved as well. The importance of this parameter was overlooked in the first stages of antihistamine research so that a complicated set of steric replacements had to be engaged.

2) Even a simple substitution series with alkyl groups would have added strength to the concept based on $f$ and $f^2$ but would also have pointed to the necessity of searching for further parameters, especially for those connected with the dimensions of the 'hydrophobic field'.

3) In the diphenhydramine series the O atom plays a rather remarkable role in so far as it is not required to be present for antihistamine action but if it does occur it incorporates (or fortifies) a clearly anticholinergic activity component. A rational choice of the ring substituents makes it possible to manipulate antihistamine and anticholinergic effects in the series in question.

4) The study of diphenhydramine derivatives with varying cationic heads provided useful information on the effective width of this head, completing the picture given in Fig. 3d to the one given in Fig. 9.

5) A set of dummy parameters satisfies the need of putting several classes of

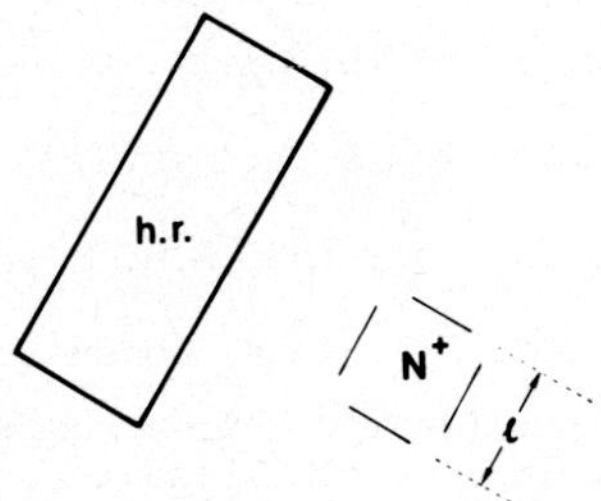


Fig. 9. Schematic structure pattern of an antihistamine; h.r. = hydrophobic region; $N^+$- location designated by a broken square and an optimal width of $\ell$= 3.4 Å.

antihistamines into one category with the application of only one physicochemical parameter - the hydrophobic fragmental constant of one of the two aryl groups. One should bear in mind that this does not necessarily mean a discrepancy with conclusion 1. An extension of the material will definitely require the application of a squared $f$.

6) A basic concept for an adequate handling of lipophilicity data at the onset of antihistamine research in the mid forties would have implied an essential restriction on the material to be synthesized and might have provided the key to a more sophisticated anticholinergic research in an early stage.

## REFERENCES

1 G. Ungar, J.-L. Parrot and D. Bovet, C.R. Soc. Biol. (Paris), 124(1937)445-446.
2 E. Fourneau and D. Bovet, Arch. Int. Pharmacodyn., 46(1933)179-191.
3 D. Bovet and A.-M. Staub, C.R. Soc. Biol. (Paris), 124(1937)547-549.
4 B.N. Halpern, Arch. Int. Pharmacodyn., 68(1942)339-408.
5 G.R. Rieveschl, U.S. Patent 2,421,714 - June 3, 1947; Applic. date April 18,1944; Chem. Abstr. 41(1947)5550h.
6 O. Schaumann, Med. u. Chem., 4(1942)229.
7 B.N. Halpern and R. Ducrot, C.R. Soc. Biol. (Paris), 140(1946)361-363.
8 W.G. Stoll, Ch.J. Morel and Ch. Frey, Helv. Chim. Acta, 33(1950)1194-1207.
9 A.C. White, A.F. Green and A. Hudson, Brit. J. Pharmacol., 6(1951)560-571.
10 W.Th. Nauta, R.F. Rekker and A.F. Harms, Proceedings 3rd Int. Pharmacol. Meeting 1966, Vol.7, Physicochemical aspects of drug actions. Oxford-New York, Pergamon Press 1968.
11 R.F. Rekker, W.Th. Nauta, T. Bultsma and C.G. Waringa, Europ. J. med. Chem., 10(1975)557-562.
12 R.F. Rekker, H. Timmerman, A.F. Harms an W.Th. Nauta, Arzneimittel-Forsch., 21(1971)688-691.
13 R.F. Rekker, H. Timmerman, A.F. Harms and W.Th. Nauta, Chim. Thérap., 7(1972)279-282.
14 A.F. Harms, W. Hespe, W.Th. Nauta, R.F. Rekker, H. Timmerman and J. de Vries, Drug Design VI (Ed. E.J. Ariëns), New York, Academic Press 1975.
15 W.Th. Nauta, T. Bultsma, R.F. Rekker and H. Timmerman, Medicinal Chemistry -Milan 1972, Special contributions (Ed. P. Pratesi), London, Butterworths 1973.
16 A.F. Casy and R.R. Ison, J. Pharm. Pharmacol., 22(1970)270-278.
17 C.G. Waringa, Thesis, Vrije Universiteit, Amsterdam 1974.

18 C.G. Waringa, R.F. Rekker and W.Th. Nauta, Europ. J. med. Chem., 10(1975) 349-352.
19 H. Timmerman, R.F. Rekker and W.Th. Nauta, Arzneimittel-Forsch., 20(1970) 1258-1259.
20 C. van der Stelt, A.F. Harms and W.Th. Nauta, J. Med. & Pharm. Chem., 4(1961) 335-349.
21 C. Hansch, P.P. Maloney, T. Fujita and R.M. Muir, Nature (London), 194(1962) 178-180.
22 R.F. Rekker, The Hydrophobic Fragmental Constant, Elsevier, Amsterdam 1977.
23 W.Th. Nauta and R.F. Rekker (Eds.), Pharmacochemistry Library, Vol. 3: Pharmacochemistry of 1,3-Indandiones, Elsevier, Amsterdam 1981, Appendix A.
24 F. Leonard and Ch.P. Huttrer, Histamine Antagonists, Rev. No 3 Chemical Biological Coordination Center, Nat. Res. C., Washington D.C. 1950.
25 D.T. Witiak, in: A. Burgen Ed.), Medicinal Chemistry, 3rd. Ed. New York Wiley-Interscience 1970.
26 R. Magnus,Arch. Gesamte Physiol. Menschen Tiere 102(1904) 123.
27 E.J. Ariëns and A.M. Simonis, Arch. Int. Pharmacodyn. Ther. 141(1963) 309.
28 R.W. Taft, in "Steric Effects in Organic Chemistry" (Ed.: M.S. Newman), pg 594, Wiley, New York 1956.
29 W.Th. Nauta and R.F. Rekker, in Handbuch der experimentellen Pharmakologie, Vol. XVIII/2 Histamine II and Anti-Histamines (Ed.: M. Rocha e Silva), pg 215, Springer-Verlag, Berlin 1978.
30 R.F. Rekker and W.Th. Nauta, Rec. Trav. Chim. Pays-Bas, 87(1968) 1099-1109.
31 C.G. Swain and E.C. Lupton, J. Amer. Chem. Soc., 90(1968) 4328.
32 M. Charton, personal communication to the author.

J.A. Keverling Buisman (Editor), *Strategy in Drug Research* 


# EXCEPTIONS IN QUANTITATIVE STRUCTURE-ACTIVITY RELATIONSHIPS (QSAR), POSSIBLE REASONS

J.K.SEYDEL and K.-J.SCHAPER
Borstel Research Institute, Biochem.Dept., D-2061 Borstel (G.F.R.)

ABSTRACT

It is one of the advantages of QSAR analysis to detect statistically significant outliers from the general regression established. In many cases compounds are hidden behind these exceptions for which a deviating physicochemical or biological behaviour is operative, thus questioning the underlying correlation model used. A detailed analysis of such compounds may contribute to a better understanding of processes in drug action in general, to the derivation of the mode of action and/or to the development of a new lead. Examples will be presented where the reasons for the obtained deviations are diagnosed. Exceptions in QSAR can possibly be explained by the dependence of the biological response on the observation time, by the presence of two modes of action, which depend on different structural parameters, by a sudden change in metabolic pattern or excretion mechanism, by the use of substituent constants which may not describe the physicochemical properties correctly, by limitation in solubility etc.

---

## INTRODUCTION

From the various approaches used in QSAR analysis the so called extrathermodynamic or linear free energy approach of Hansch and Fujita [1] is still most often applied. The possible relationships between physicochemical properties and biological activities are examined statistically. This is also true for other methods used in QSAR analysis. By the use of statistics it is possible to accept or to reject such relationships and also to detect outliers. Because of the statistic nature of the QSAR analysis we have to expect exceptions in a certain number of cases. This is not limiting the general usefulness of the method, which has been proven in a large number

*References p. 354*

of examples [2-4]. On the contrary the exception can lead to most important informations for the development of new drugs and for the detection of the mechanisms "producing" the exception.

In this paper we shall not discuss examples where the regression equation failed to predict the biological activity of a new analog because 1. the prediction was based on a poorly designed series or an invalid regression equation, 2. the prediction was derived from an extrapolation outside the parameter space presented in the original data set and 3. the condition for biological testing was changing. Rather we would like to present some examples where a deviation from the general regression was found in statistically relevant equations within the parameter space covered. In such a case we cannot explain the deviation by the forementioned possibilities rather we have to analyze our biological and physicochemical parameters and the possible involved mechanism which may hint to a change in the rate determining step.

## RESULTS

### Time dependence of the biological response

Despite the fact that in cell-free enzyme systems permeation of ionized drugs to the receptor should not become the rate determining step, we have observed the deviation of more ionized drugs from the linear regression found between cell-free folate inhibitory activity, $i_{50}$, of sulfonamides (SA) and the corresponding electronic substituent parameters (pKa, ppm) [5-6]. Compounds with a pKa lower than 7 were found to be highly active in the cell-free system, nevertheless they are less active than expected from the prediction (eq 1) (Fig. 1, no. 44, 47). These inhibitory activities have been determined by a single point method, i.e. the inhibition of folate synthesis was determined after a fixed time interval of incubation (5 hrs) of the enzymatic reaction mixture. These derivatives do even more deviate from the regression found between whole cell inhibitory activity (E.coli, MIC) and the pKa of the SA (Fig.1, upper part) or ppm of the amino group of corresponding precursor amines. For this system a limitation in the permeability of the bacterial cell wall could be assumed. The deviation from the regression found in the cell-free system, however, seems not explainable by this argument.

Instead of neglecting the small but statistically significant deviation we have repeated the determination of the cell-free inhibitory activities of the SA using a kinetic method.

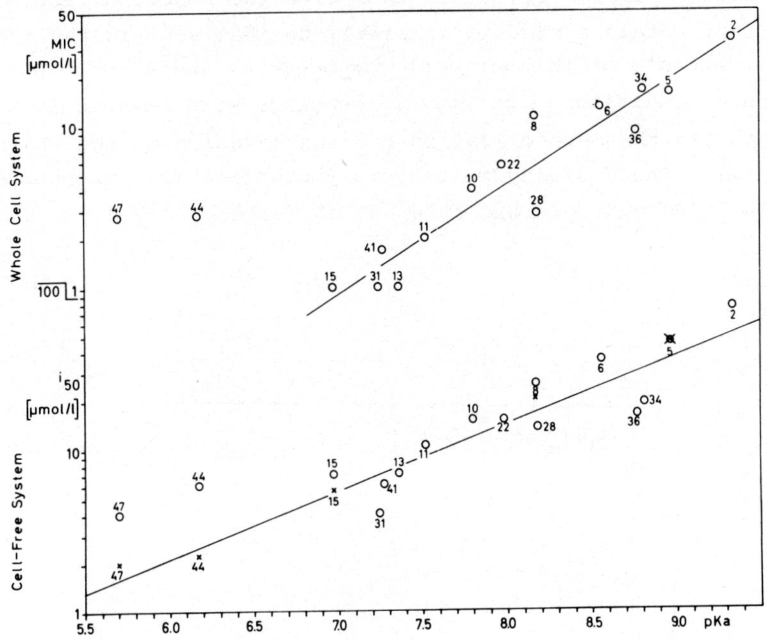


Fig. 1. The relationship of whole cell (MIC, E.coli) and cell-free ($i_{50}$, $k_{50}$) inhibitory activities to pKa values of substituted $N^1$-phenylsulfanilamides. Cell-free inhibitory activities have been determined after a fixed time interval (5 hrs, o) or by the kinetic method (x) [6, 8].

Figure 2 shows a typical experiment in which the amount of folate like material produced in the reaction mixtures as a function of time was determined for several SA concentrations. The concentration of SA causing a 50 % inhibition in the rate of folate synthesis, $k_{50}$, has been derived from such plots. It became obvious that the activities ($k_{50}$) of all but the very highly active derivatives (44,47; which deviate from the line) are the same as those obtained with the single point method ($i_{50}$). An explanation was found when the kinetics of inhibition was studied for the length of time involved in the single point method experiments (5 hrs). In case of a highly active SA, 2-bromo-4-nitro-$N^1$-phenylsulfonamide, the reaction under the conditions of the experiment is of pseudo-zero-order, i.e. linear only during the initial time period of approximately 2-3 hrs

*References p. 354*

(Fig. 3, lower part) [7,8]. After this time the reaction returned to a rate of folate synthesis similarly to that seen in the control reaction. Because of this effect, compounds 44 and 47 were underestimated in their inhibitory activity if readings were taken only after 5 hr. The reason was the metabolization and inactivation of the SA in a reaction with the 7,8-dihydro-6-hydroxymethylpterinylpyrophosphate to form a 7,8-dihydropteroic acid analog (Scheme 1) [7,8].

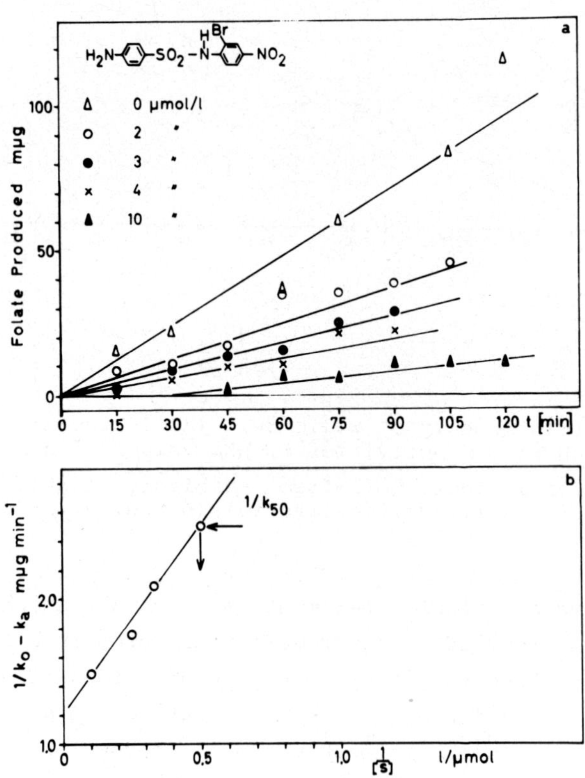


Fig. 2. Determination of the inhibitory activity by the kinetic method. Rate constants for folate synthesis in the presence of several SA concentrations (comp. 47, Fig.1) were obtained (upper part) and used in Lineweaver Burk type plots (below) to obtain estimates of $k_{50}$ [6,8].

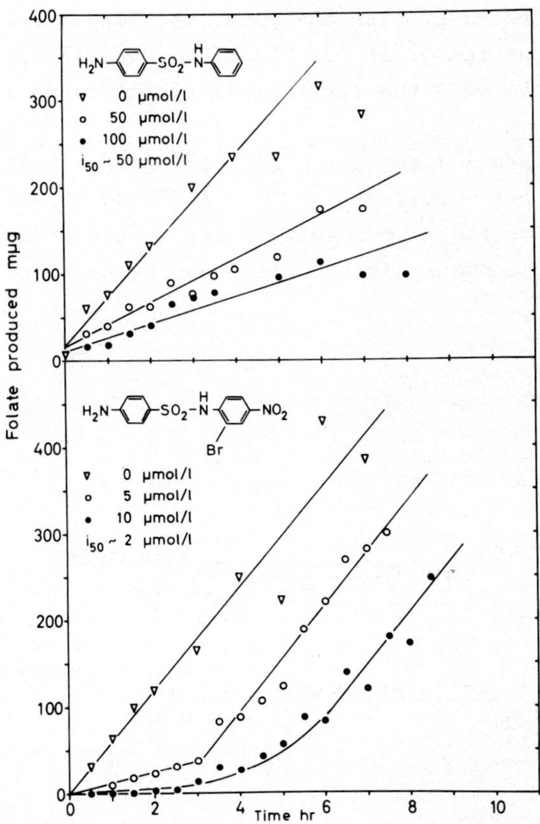


Fig.3. The kinetics of inhibition of folate synthesis (comp. 47, Fig.1) by $N^1$-phenylsulfonamide and by 2-bromo-4-nitro-$N^1$-phenylsulfonamide. The kinetics of inhibition exhibited by $N^1$-phenylsulfonamide were found to be pseudo-zero-order throughout the experiment time. In contrast, the highly active compound, 2-bromo-4-nitro-$N^1$-phenylsulfonamide, exhibited pseudo-zero-order kinetics only for a short initial time. After this time the rate of folate synthesis is similar to that seen in the control [7].

The observed deviation for some of the SA was therefore caused by a time dependence of the biological response on the metabolic reaction. This became the decisive step if highly active SA were tested because the small amounts of drugs present in the reaction mixture became inactivated during the experimental time interval used.

This effect detected by QSAR analysis, was leading to the exploration of the mode of action of SA [7, 8]. If $k_{50}$ values are introduced for these SA into eq 1 the statistical significance is improving (eq 2).

| | n | r | s | |
|---|---|---|---|---|
| $\log i_{50} = 0.32\ \mathrm{pKa} - 1.40$ | 16 | 0.88 | 0.18 | (1) |
| $\log k_{50} = 0.41\ \mathrm{pKa} - 2.14$ | 16 | 0.94 | 0.15 | (2) |

The importance of the time interval used in the biological experiment for transport phenomena has been stressed by Dearden [9].

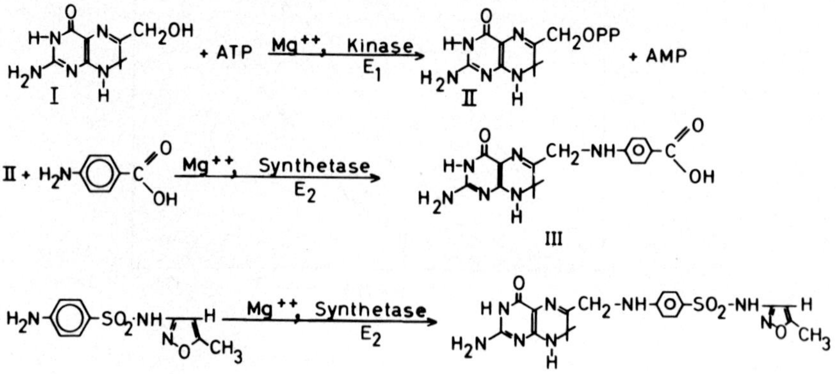

I + ATP —(Mg++, Kinase, E1)→ II + AMP

II + $H_2N$-C6H4-COOH —(Mg++, Synthetase, E2)→ III

II + $H_2N$-C6H4-$SO_2$-NH-(5-methylisoxazol-3-yl) —(Mg++, Synthetase, E2)→ product

Scheme 1. Reaction scheme for the biosynthesis of 7,8-dihydropteroic acid analog in the presence of SA (3-sulfa-5-methylisoxazole).

## Change in mode of action or dual mode of action

Experiments were performed to determine the inhibitory activity of a series of derivatives of diaminodiphenylsulfone (DDS) where one of the amino groups was replaced by other substituents [10].

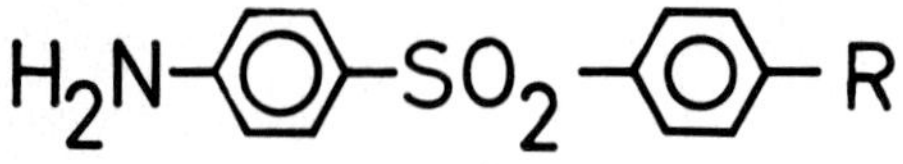

$$H_2N-C_6H_4-SO_2-C_6H_4-R$$

The biological activity was determined using E.coli as test organisms and bacterial growth kinetic techniques to follow the decrease in pseudo-first-order generation rates of the cultures in the absence and presence of graded inhibitor concentrations.

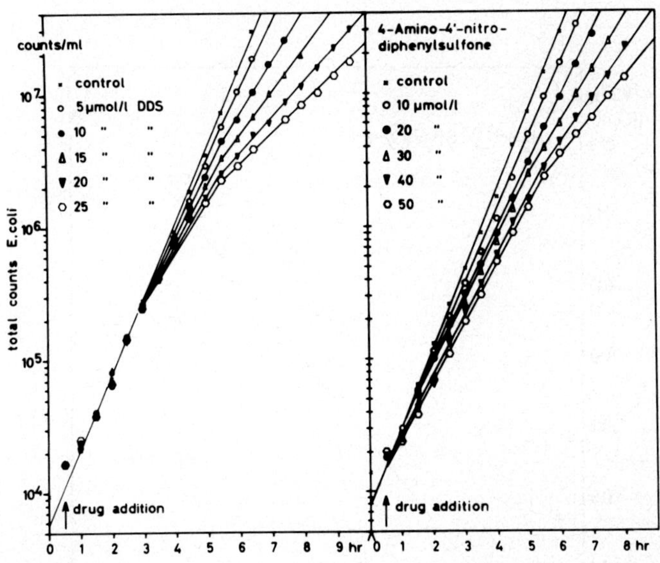


Fig. 4. Typical generation rate curves of E.coli (mutaflor) at 37°C in the presence of various concentrations of sulfones. Left: 4,4'-diaminodiphenylsulfone; right: 4-amino-4'-nitrodiphenylsulfone.

Figure 4 (left part) shows a typical curve where the logarithm of the number of bacteria present in a certain culture volume (during the logarithmic growth phase) is plotted against time at various drug (DDS) concentrations. From such plots the $i_{10}$ values are calculated using a computer program for nonlinear regression analysis. $i_{10}$ values were determined because of the low solubility of some of the derivatives. The observed variance in the concentration necessary to reduce the bacterial generation rate constant by 10 % was explainable by the corresponding changes in the lipophilicity of the derivatives. The lipophilicity is expressed as retention time ($\log k'_r$) obtained by reversed phase high pressure liquid chromatography (HPLC)(eq 3).

| | n | r | s | |
|---|---|---|---|---|
| $\log i_{10} = 0.938 \log k'_r + 0.59$ | 8 | 0.88 | 0.16 | (3) |
| $\log i_{10} = 1.10 \log k'_r + 0.599$ | 7 | 0.96 | 0.10 | (4) |

The linear correlation is also shown in Fig. 5.

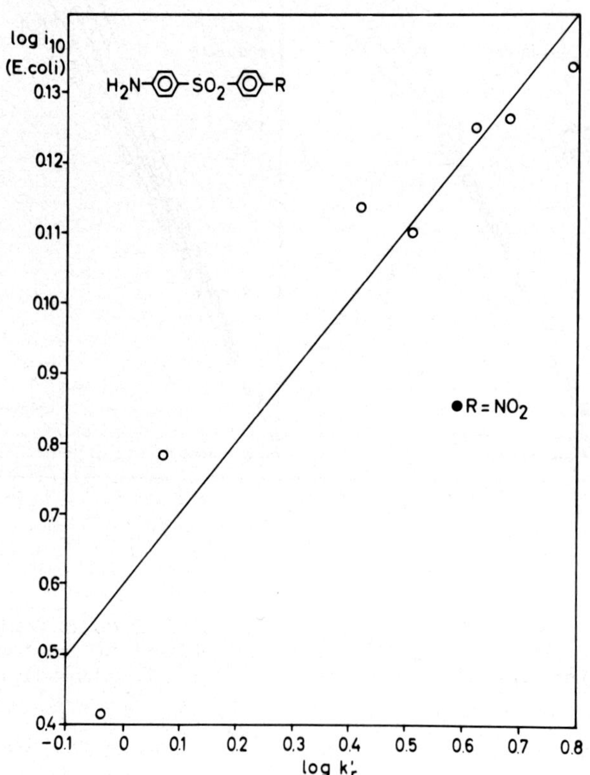


Fig. 5. Relation of inhibitory activities, $i_{10}$, (whole cells, E.coli) to the lipophilicity, $\log k'_r$ (retention time, reversed phase, HPLC) of the 4'-substituted diphenylsulfones.

Again an exception can easily be detected, which deviates from the regression significantly, it is the 4-amino-4'-nitrodiphenylsulfone. One is inclined to assume an additional activity of the nitro group as shown in many other examples from the literature. Fortunately the biological test method used was a kinetic approach so that this assumption could be verified easily. For all 7,8-dihydropteroic acid synthetase inhibitors a lag phase of about 5 generation times has been observed [11, 12] due to a pool of 7,8-dihydrofolic acid within the bacteria. This holds also for all other sulfones tested (Fig.4, left part). In the case of the 4'-nitro derivative, however, the onset of action is almost immediately (Fig. 4, right part), indicating an additional mode of action and explaining its deviation from the general regression line. If the outlier is omitted from the regression analysis eq 4 is obtained.

A similar reason holds for the exceptionally high activity of $N^1$-4-amino-phenylsulfanilamide (pKa 9.5) where a too strong inhibitory potency has been found (MIC = 11.25 μmol/l) whereas according to the general regression equation [4, 8] a MIC value of 43 μmol/l is calculated.

$$\log MIC = 0.67\ pKa - 4.74 \qquad n = 18 \quad r = 0.95 \quad s = 0.14 \qquad (5)$$

In a cell-free folate synthesizing enzyme system, however, the $i_{50}$ was determined to be $i_{50}$ = 70 μM, that means the activity in the cell-free system is as low as expected.
If this $i_{50}$ value is inserted into the general equation (eq 6) which describes the correlation between log MIC and log $i_{50}$ for all other SA studied, a MIC value of 40 μmol/l is calculated [6, 8].

$$\log MIC = 1.39 \log i_{50} - 0.96 \qquad n = 21 \quad r = 0.96 \quad s = 0.166 \qquad (6)$$

which is in agreement with the calculated MIC using eq 5. This result indicates that an additional inhibitory effect of $N^1$-4-amino-phenylsulfanilamide is operative outside the folate synthesizing enzyme system thus increasing the total inhibitory potency of this SA derivative.

## Activity resulting from a combination of specific and unspecific effects

An example for a class of compounds where the activity results from a combination of specific and unspecific effects - the latter giving rise to exceptions in QSAR analysis - is the class of antitubercularly acting (H37Rv) derivatives of isoniazid.

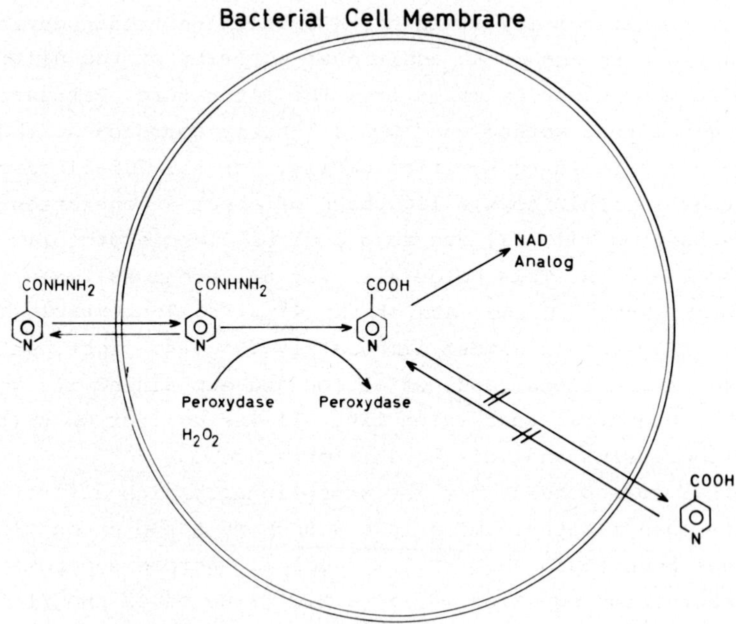


Scheme 2. Schematic drawing of the "isonicotinic acid" mode of action hypothesis in isonicotinic acid hydrazide (isoniazid) action[13].

There is some evidence [4, 13, 14] that isoniazid once inside the bacterial cell is enzymatically oxidized to isonicotinic acid (INA) and subsequently incorporated into an analog of nicotinamide adenine dinucleotide (NAD) instead of nicotinic acid (Scheme 2) by a glycosidation at the pyridine nitrogen. This quaternization reaction is supposed to be the origin of the specific effect whereas the oxidative degradation of the hydrazide moiety gives rise to the unspecific effect.

The influence of substituents on the activity has been analyzed by simulating the physiological quaternization of 2-substituted INA derivatives by an in vitro quaternization of 2-substituted pyridines by methyliodide in methanol.

When plotting the biological activity, log (1/MIC), against the chemical reactivity, log $k_{rel.}$, an excellent linear correlation is found for those compounds where $k_{rel.}$ is at least about 2 % of the rate of the unsubstituted pyridine (Fig. 6).

$$\log (1/MIC) = 1.778 \log k_{rel.} - 0.3 \qquad n = 11 \quad r = 0.93 \quad s = 0.38 \qquad (7)$$

Five derivatives with a rather low chemical reactivity show antibacterial activities which although being quite low are significantly larger than predicted by the regression line.

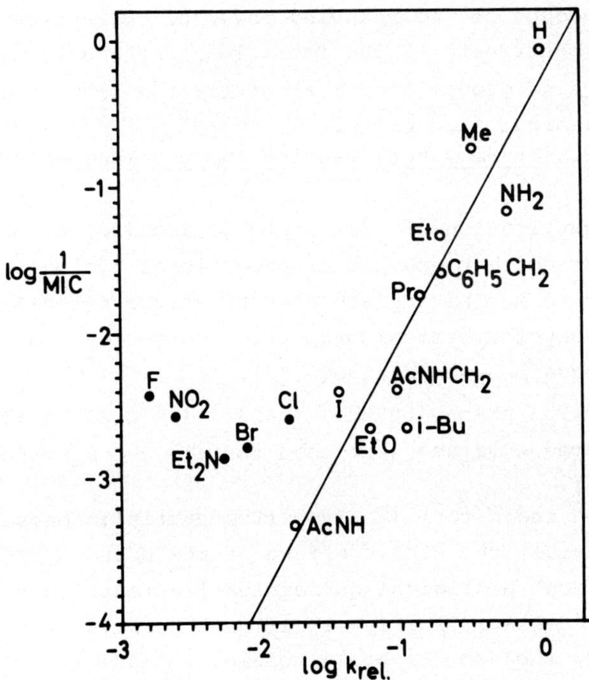


Fig. 6. Relation of inhibitory activities, MIC (H37Rv), of 2-substituted isonicotinic acid hydrazides to the rate constant ($k_{rel.}$) for quaternization by methyliodide (in methanol) of the corresponding 2-substituted pyridines.

For these 5 compounds we assume the disturbance of bacterial oxidases by the hydrazide group - an unspecific effect connected with all derivatives - to become perceptible. For the more reactive

*References p. 354*

derivatives towards quaternizing agents this additional unspecific inhibitory effect (which is comparable with the activity of benzoic acid hydrazide) is largely exceeded by the specific effect.

It has been found that the reactivity of isonicotinic acid hydrazides substituted in 2-position towards oxidation by iron(III)-salts shows a V-shaped Hammett- or Brønsted plot [15]. As may be expected, the oxidizability of the hydrazide group mainly decreases with increasing electron attracting properties of the substituents. But for derivatives with very high electron attracting power (like Cl or $NO_2$) the rate of oxidation increases again. Perhaps this nonlinear dependence of the reducing power of the hydrazides on $\sigma$(Hammett) may contribute to the deviation of the derivatives with electron attracting groups from the correlation between biological activity and chemical reactivity.

<u>Substituent constants may not describe the physicochemical properties correctly</u>

From our investigation of 2-substituted isonicotinic acid hydrazides (INH) another example of exceptional biological activity was obtained which may be explained by substituent constants not describing the physicochemical properties correctly. For 19 derivatives the following equation was derived [13]:

$$\log(1/MIC) = 0.232\ pKa - 1.073\pi - 1.454 \qquad n = 19 \quad r = 0.88 \quad s = 0.41 \qquad (8)$$

In eq 8 calculated $\pi$ values were used for the 2-$C_6H_5$- and 2-vinyl-INH (see text below).

In this equation the $\pi$-term (derived from partition measurements) is expressing mainly the steric effect of the ortho-substituents on the hypothetical biological quaternization reaction to the NAD-analogs. We found statistically significant correlations of $\pi$(obs.) with $E_s$(Taft) or the Van der Waals volume, $V_w$ [13].

When analyzing the activity data we got the impression that the steric effect of all but two of the derivatives was described fairly well by $\pi$(obs.)(excluding compounds containing amino substituents). For 2-phenyl- and 2-vinyl-INH the steric effect exerted on the nucleophilic pyridine nitrogen seemed to be much lower than indicated by the two $\pi$(obs.) values which correspond to substituents coplanar to the pyridine ring or to freely rotating groups. In enzyme catalyzed reactions such as the quaternization of INA derivatives by the ribosyl moiety, the possibility has to be considered that the phenyl ring in the 2-position is perpendicular to the reaction centre and has a lower steric effect in the transition state. Thus the effective $\pi$ value should be much lower. Kutter and Hansch [16] published the $E_s$ value for a phenyl group perpendicular to a reaction centre. By introducing this value into an equation correlation π with $E_s$, a new "steric" π value of $C_6H_5$ was obtained (π = 1.13) which better reflects the effective steric effect than π(obs.) = 2.49. As it can be assumed that the steric effect of a perpendicular vinyl group is very similar to the effect of a perpendicular phenyl group, the same π(calc.) value was used for this group to give the above relation between activity and pKa and π (eq 8). By this equation the activity of both derivatives (phenyl and vinyl) is described very well when the calculated π value is introduced whereas π(obs.) results in MIC values deviating very much from observed MIC values.

TABLE 1
Observed and calculated MIC values of 2-phenyl- and 2-vinyl-INH using π observed and π calculated values and eq 8.

| | MIC obs. [μM/l] | MIC with π(obs.) | MIC calc.with π(calc.) |
|---|---|---|---|
| $C_6H_5$ | 50 | 1226 | 42.4 |
| Vinyl | 35 | 87.2 | 32.4 |

This example may indicate that substituent constants derived from chemical reactions may not always be suitable to simulate the conditions in biochemical reactions.

Change in excretion mechanism

Another example is derived from studies done in quantitative structure-pharmacokinetics relationship (QSPR) analysis. For this type of relationships only few quantitative examples are known and the scatter of the data is normally larger than for instance for the evaluation of enzyme inhibitory activities. This is due to the nature of the pharmacokinetic parameters. Nevertheless successful correlations have been described by Lien, Seydel, Martin and also been reviewed [17-20].

The example for an explainable outlier is derived from QSPR analysis of the rate of elimination, $k_{el}$, of sulfapyrimidines in rats after i.v. administration. SA are in general excreted via urine by glomerular filtration, this applies also to the main metabolites $N^4$-acetyl- and $N^4$-glucuronyl-SA.

The elimination rate constant for a series of substituted 4-sulfa-

*References p. 354*

pyrimidines was linearly related to the lipophilicity expressed as retention time $k'_r$ from reversed phase HPLC (eq 9).

$$\log k_{el} = -1.19 \log k'_r + 0.94 \qquad n = 8 \quad r = 0.75 \quad s = 0.33 \tag{9}$$

The derivative which deviates most from the regression line was the 2-phenyl-4-sulfapyrimidine. An analysis of the clearance of this drug resulted in the observation that the clearance determined as the product of elimination rate and volume of distribution was 5.9 ml $min^{-1}$. The glomerular filtration rate (GFR) is, however, only 2-3 ml $min^{-1}$ in rats. This was not exceeded by all other SA. This means that by substitution with a phenyl ring in o-position the excretion mechanism has changed, an additional tubular secretion occurs. This explains the exceptionally high elimination rate of 2-phenyl-4-sulfapyrimidine. If this derivative is therefore omitted from the regression analysis eq 10 is obtained.

$$\log k_{el} = -1.37 \log k'_r + 1.13 \qquad n = 7 \quad r = 0.90 \quad s = 0.22 \tag{10}$$

## Competition for protein binding sites; change in protein structure

Binding of drugs to plasma protein may decrease the protein binding capacity for other exogenous or endogenous compounds. Especially for drugs with high affinity to serum protein a competitive displacement from binding sites can be expected and has often been observed especially in case of acidic compounds. In some cases it was possible to quantitatively correlate the degree of displacement of a bound reference molecule by competitor molecules with the lipophilic and electronic properties and the concentration of the drugs [20, 22]. Usually the displacement increases with increasing lipophilicity of the competitor. For example Pitkin et al. [23] recently investigated the binding difference of acidic cephalosporins with and without fatty acids of different chain lengths (Table 2). Up to a chain length of 10 carbons of the competitor, displacement of cephalothin increases but at longer chain lengths it decreases again. If a restricted area for hydrophobic binding at the binding site is assumed, a constant degree of displacement should be expected in case the lipophilic moiety of the competitor exceeds this area. From this viewpoint the decreasing displacement at very long chain lengths has to be considered as an exception which may be explained by steric effects.

TABLE 2

Effect of fatty acid chain length on protein binding of cephalothin (molar ratio of acid to cephalothin 10:1)

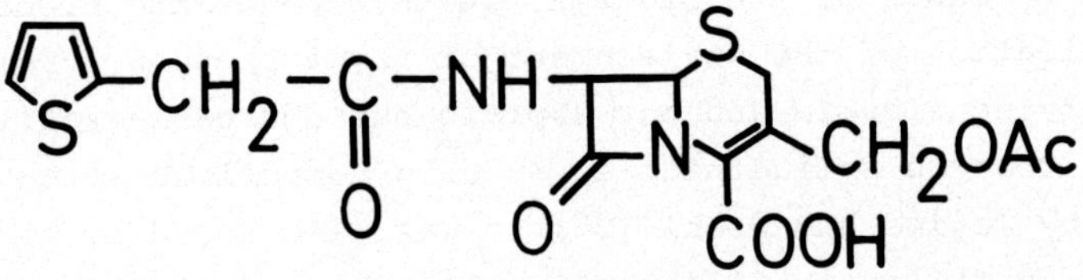

| Fatty acid chain length | Binding difference (%) |
|---|---|
| 6 | 0 |
| 8 | 32 |
| 10 | 45 |
| 12 | 37 |
| 14 | 22 |
| 16 | 2 |
| 18 | 1 |

Another example for an increase of displacement followed by a decrease at increasing chain length of competitor has been presented by Perrin and Nelson [24], who investigated the displacement of sulfaethidole from bovine serum protein (BSA) by alkyldimethylbenzylammonium chlorides (Table 3) and found some evidence that these different classes of compounds share the same binding site of bovine serum albumin.

TABLE 3

Displacement of sulfaethidole (SETD) from protein binding by alkyldimethylbenzylammonium chlorides ($N^+$) at [BSA] = 14.5 μM, [SETD] = 25.2 μM, $[N^+] \sim 260$ μM.

| alkyl chain length of competitor | % displacement of SETD |
|---|---|
| 8 | ~ 4 |
| 10 | 5 |
| 11 | 13 |
| 12 | 35 |
| 13 | 72 |
| 14 | 88 |
| 15 | 85 |
| 16 | 76 |
| 17 | 67 |
| 18 | 62 |
| 19 | 52 |

Perrin and Nelson [24] also investigated the circular dichroism (CD) curve of BSA in presence of the alkylammonium chlorides. Alkyl-chain lengths below $C_{13}$ did not modify the spectrum, but higher analogs changed the curve in the region associated with the aromatic amino acid residues of the protein. These changes are probably due to a modification of the environment of tryptophan or tyrosine residues of the albumin and may explain the decreasing affinity of albumin towards sulfaethidole. In drug competition studies performed by Tejima and Ozeki [25] it was also found by CD measurements that fatty acids induce different conformational states of the albumin molecule. This may also be the explanation for the results of Pitkin et al. [23]. Another explanation presented by Perrin and Nelson [24] may be micelle formation as a competition phenomenon to binding. In the case of sulfaethidole/alkylammonium competition micelle formation can be expected to be competitive to binding of $C_{16}$ and longer chain homologues.

Limitation in solubility

The last example considers the limitation in solubility as an explanation for outlayers. Limitation in solubility may often be the explanation for exceptionally low activities obtained especially from in vivo experiments. Ferguson [26] has already stressed the possibility that the decrease in water solubility can be faster than the increase in lipid solubility and that this phenomenon can explain the observed nonlinearities in the relation between biological response and lipophilicity.

The tumor inhibitory potency of a homologous series of triazenes has been evaluated by Wilman and Goddard [27] in mice. For increasing chain lengths of the substituents from methyl to hexyl, including propinyl, allyl, and 2-methyl-butyl, no dependence of the activity on increasing lipophilicity was observed, i.e. the log $ED_{50}$ values remained constant. If, however, R becomes $C_7$ or $C_8$ a sudden inactivity of the compounds was observed. The solubilities (S) of the studied compounds have also been determined. A plot of log S versus log P is linear. At the log P value obtained for the triazene derivative with R = $C_7$ or $C_8$ the two lines log $ED_{50}$/log P and log S/log P intersect (Fig. 7). The observed break point in activity for the derivatives with substituents $C_7$ and $C_8$ is therefore very probably due to their insolubility, i.e. these derivatives do not achieve the necessary concentration especially if the receptor is in a polar region. An exception in this data set which remains unexplained is the observed inactivity of the benzyl derivative. One may speculate that this is due to the different type of substituent and a possible different metabolism.

Other examples on the influence of the solubility on the decrease of activity with lipophilicity at high values for log P have been discussed by Flynn and Yalkowski [28] and by Yalkowski and Morozowich [29].

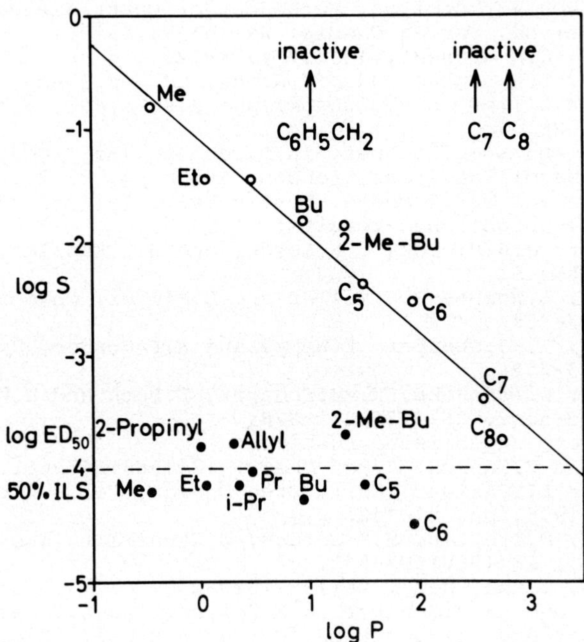


Fig.7. Relation between the logarithm of the antitumor activity of triazene derivatives (log $ED_{50}$, $ED_{50}$ = effective dose for 50 % increase in life span, ILS) and log P (--●--) and between the logarithm of the water solubility (log S) and log P (—o—). Data from Wilman and Goddard [27].

In conclusion:

The examples listed discuss a small selection of reasons which may lead to exceptions in the prediction of QSAR. It is obvious that one should evaluate very carefully the possible reason for such exceptions as they can lead to most valuable informations. A necessary precondition is that the QSAR analyzer has a broad insight into the biological test systems applied.

## REFERENCES


1 C.Hansch and T.Fujita, J.Am.Chem.Soc., 86(1964)1616-1626.
2 C.Hansch, in J.A.Keverling Buisman (Ed.), Biological Activity and Chemical Structure, Elsevier, Amsterdam, 1977.
3 Y.C.Martin, Quantitative Drug Design, Marcel Dekker, New York, 197[illegible]
4 J.K.Seydel and K.-J.Schaper, Chemische Struktur und biologische Aktivität von Wirkstoffen. Methoden der Quantitativen Struktur-Wirkung-Analyse, Verlag Chemie, Weinheim, 1979.
5 J.K.Seydel, J.Med.Chem., 14(1971)724-729.
6 G.H.Miller, P.H.Doukas and J.K.Seydel, J.Med.Chem., 15(1972)700-70[illegible]
7 L.Bock, G.H.Miller, K.-J.Schaper and J.K.Seydel, J.Med.Chem., 17(1974)23-28.
8 J.K.Seydel and K.-J.Schaper, in M.Sandler (Ed.), Enzyme Inhibitors as Drugs, Macmillan Press, London, 1980, pp. 53-71.
9 J.C.Dearden and M.S.Townend, Pestic.Sci., 10(1979)87-89.
10 J.K.Seydel, unpublished results.
11 E.R.Garrett, J.B.Mielck, J.K.Seydel and H.J.Kessler, J.Med.Chem., 12(1969)740-745.
12 J.K.Seydel, E.Wempe, G.H.Miller and L.Miller, Chemotherapy, 17(1972)217-258.
13 J.K.Seydel, K.-J.Schaper, E.Wempe and H.P.Cordes, J.Med.Chem., 19(1976)483-492.
14 J.K.Seydel, S.Tono-oka, K.-J.Schaper, L.Bock and M.Wiencke, Arzneim.-Forsch., 26(1976)477-478.
15 K.-J.Schaper, unpublished results.
16 E.Kutter and C.Hansch, J.Med.Chem., 12(1969)647-652.
17 E.J.Lien in E.J.Ariens (Ed.), Drug Design, Vol.5, Academic Press, New York, 1975, pp. 81-132.
18 J.K.Seydel, D.Trettin, H.P.Cordes, O.Wassermann and M.Malyusz, J.Med.Chem., 23(1980)607-613.
19 Y.C.Martin, J.Med.Chem., 24(1981)229-237.
20 J.K.Seydel and K.-J.Schaper in M.Rowland and G.Tucker (Eds.), Pharmacology and Therapeutics, Pergamon Press, Oxford, 1982.
21 H.Körner and J.K.Seydel, unpublished results.
22 K.-J.Schaper and J.K.Seydel, poster presentation at this symposium.
23 D.H.Pitkin, P.Actor and J.A.Weisbach, J.Pharm.Sci., 69(1980) 354-358.
24 J.H.Perrin and D.A.Nelson, Biochem.Pharmacol., 23(1974)3139-3145.
25 K.Tejima and S.Ozeki, Chem.Pharm.Bull., 28(1980)585-593.
26 J.Ferguson, Proc.Roy.Soc.(London) 127B(1939)387-404.
27 D.E.V.Wilman and P.M.Goddard, J.Med.Chem., 23(1980)1052-1054.
28 G.L.Flynn and S.H.Yalkowsky, J.Pharm.Sci., 61(1972)838-852.
29 S.H.Yalkowsky and W.Morozowich, in E.J.Ariens (Ed.), Drug Design, Vol. 9, Academic Press, New York, 1980, pp. 127-130.

J.A. Keverling Buisman (Editor), *Strategy in Drug Research*



# SOME PREREQUISITES AND TECHNIQUES TO MAKE QSARs PREDICTIVE

R. FRANKE

Akademie der Wissenschaften der DDR, Forschungszentrum für Molekularbiologie und Medizin, Institut für Wirkstofforschung, Berlin (DDR)

## ABSTRACT

Prediction is the final goal and the ultimate measure of success of any QSAR approach. Not only does it imply the forecasting of biological activities for as yet uninvestigated compounds but also such qualitative aspects as, for instance, the selection of the most promising directions for further synthesis, hypotheses on mechanisms of action or the preselection of compounds for a screening program, etc. Quite a number of conditions must be fulfilled in order to render a QSAR truly predictive; a.o. properties of biological data and training series must be known, and there must be the correct choice, application and interpretation of QSAR methods. These topics will be discussed together with possible strategies to avoid the evaluation of QSARs without predictive power. Examples of successful predictions will be presented.

## INTRODUCTION

The basic objective of QSAR work is to produce new knowledge by correlating known facts. As far as this knowledge extends beyond a mere description it is called a prediction. There are several levels of prediction corresponding to the different stages and purposes of drug research, i.e. lead generation, lead optimization, preselection of compounds for biological screening programs and mechanisms of action. The "classical" aim of QSAR investigations is that of lead optimization which will, therefore, be the main topic of this presentation.

It is relatively easy to derive QSARs which yield a good description of biological potency in terms of drug properties <u>within</u> a training series. High descriptive power, however, does by no means automatically guarantee predictive power, and to make QSARs really predictive is not an easy task. The predictive power of a QSAR depends on the amount of information extractable from the data of the training series. Since even the most sophisticated QSAR method cannot extract more information than is really present, the information content of data is one of the most crucial factors for the validity of predictions.

For a high information content the data must reflect the true relationship between biological potency and chemical structure completely, straightforwardly, and

*References p. 379*

unambiguously. Therefore, the selection of representative congeners for training series as well as the design and interpretation of biological experiments are of primary importance for successful QSAR predictions. Another important aspect is the choice of appropriate QSAR methods according to the properties of the data and their skilful application strictly within their limits. This implies, of course, that physically meaningful molecule parameters and models are used and that the rules of statistics are not violated; these topics, however, will not be discussed in this presentation. For practical work stepwise strategies starting with simple models which are then refined during the course of a study are always to be recommended.

## CHEMICAL DATA SPACE

### Completeness

To derive a meaningful QSAR requires, first of all, that the congeners compromisin the training series span a sufficiently large range of all properties governing biological potency. The influence of properties not sufficiently represented cannot be detected and the resulting QSAR would consequently lead to false predictions for all compounds which differ in these properties from those in the training series. An example of this type has recently been reported by Lambrecht et al. (ref.1) who showe that a QSAR prediction made by Lien et al. (ref.2) of the affinity of two quaternary esters for the muscarinic receptor was not correct. The reason was that certain steri effects, not varied within the training series considered by Lien et al. and, therefore, not reflected in the resulting QSAR, became a dominant factor in the new analogs

It is, of course, not always easy to hypothesize in an a priori QSAR analysis which properties will be important for biological potency. A good strategy to apply in such cases is always to begin with pilot studies of small sets of compounds in an attempt to derive very simple models in a first step. These models can then aid in directing further studies during which they are refined until, eventually, a "fine-tuned" QSAR is obtained and the search space exhausted. Existing QSARs which were evaluated for a similar biological effect may be quite helpful here. It is not the prediction of a supercompound in a dramatic overnight discovery but rather the systematic application of such stepwise strategies which will best utilize the power of QSAR as a tool for the rational design of better new drugs. This has been well recognized by many people, especially those in the pharmaceutical industry. In order to illustrate this important point I should like to quote three recent examples.

The first example concerns the work of Unger and colleagues (refs. 3, 4) on alkyl carbamoyl β-blockers. In a first step, plots of the activity of a small number of analogs in the adenylate cyclase system from heart and lung versus lipophilicity led to a simple model of $\beta_1$- and $\beta_2$-exoreceptors predicting high $\beta_1$- and low $\beta_2$-blocking activity (high selectivity) for short, bulky and lipophilic substituents. Such substituents could bind very well to the $\beta_1$-exoreceptor but would fall into an exoreceptor cleft at the lung-$\beta_2$-receptor. Bulky substituents were also thought to be less depressive since depressivity probably is related to membrane binding. Further experiments showed that this hypothesis was, in principle, correct but that the lipophilicity of substituents should not be too high in order to maintain efficient transport in vivo. This "short-bulky-moderately lipophilic" hypothesis together with results from a few substituents eventually gave rise to the endobicyclo (3.1.0)-hexylethyl (EBHE) side chain which proved to be quite exceptional and led to a highly active, cardioselective and nondepressive β-blocker which was selected for clinical evaluation. In the course of this study it became apparent that, within the framework of the starting hypothesis, subtle steric effects are of great importance. Taking the EBHE side chain as reference, steric properties of 40 substituents were parameterized by a special set of geometric and topological descriptors, and these descriptors together with hydrophobicity parameters finally led to very satisfactory QSARs for activity at the heart and lung β-receptors as well as for the depressivity providing considerable understanding of the nature of β-adrenergic receptors and confirming the receptor model used in the design of the new side chain. The EBHE side chain appears to be nearly optimal and can be transferred to other aromatic nuclei while maintaining cardioselectivity and low depressivity.

The second example I want to discuss here is provided by the work of Zeelen and colleagues (refs. 5-7) on progestational steroids. Starting with a pilot series of only four derivatives of lynestrenol (substituted at the 11 β-position), selected as they differed in lipophilicity, size and electronic effect, a simple correlation with $E_S$ was obtained indicating a steric effect on progestational potency. Next the question was raised whether this steric effect operates directly at the substituent or indirectly via a distortion of the molecules leading to a change in the shape of the steroid skeleton. Synthesis and testing of only one carefully selected analog was sufficient to indicate that the latter was the case. In the next step the influence of hydrophobicity and of substituent shape was examined by including four additional derivatives in the series. Hydrophobicity showed no effect, but the bulkiness of substituents turned out to be of importance in that substituents which stick out too far at the 11 β-position interfere with receptor binding. Thus, quite a clear picture of the factors governing activity was obtained after studying a very small set of cleverly selected compounds. It was concluded that potent derivatives of lynestrenol will result with substituents inducing a certain amount of bending of the steroid skeleton without increasing the bulk of the molecule too much. This prediction could be verified experimentally and led to a very promising compound as a new contraceptive progestagen.

The last example to be mentioned in the context of stepwise QSAR supported strategies concerns the work of Cramer and colleagues (ref. 8) on pyranenamine antiallergy compounds. After some pilot investigations a simple graphical analysis suggested the synthesis of more hydrophilic and electronically neutral analogues. In following up this concept some other aspects, such as bulk effects, hydrogen bonding, and stability were also considered. In a final stage, fine tuning of the QSAR was achieved by directed synthesis leading to a new compound with a unique structure and very high activity.

These and many other examples demonstrate that during the testing of QSAR-based interactive hypotheses, a space of relevant and important properties can be systematically filled and explored.

## Design of training series

A complete property space which manifests itself in large variances of the corresponding molecule parameters is a necessary condition but not sufficient to obtain a data set optimally suited for the evaluation of a QSAR. Another important requirement is that all properties are varied independently so that no collinearities (correlations) exist between the corresponding molecule parameters. This is a very important point since such collinearities have two serious consequences:

1. The influence of different properties on biological potency can no longer be separated so that an interpretation of QSAR results becomes impossible and false predictions may result. For the virostatic potency of 1-amino-3-nitrilo-4-p-aminophenylpyrazoles substituted in position 3 of the heterocyclic ring ($R_1$) and in the p-amino group of the phenyl ring ($R_2$), for example, the following two equations were obtained from a Hansch analysis (ref. 9) where the suffixes refer to $R_1$ and $R_2$ respectively:

$$\log BR = 0.11\,\pi_1 - 0.79\,\pi_1\,\sigma_1 - 2.04\,E_{S,2} + 0.78\,\sigma_2^* - 1.70 \qquad (1)$$

$$n = 19 \qquad r = 0.915 \qquad s = 0.181$$

$$\log BR = 0.10\,\pi_1 - 0.51\,\pi_1\sigma_1 + 0.46\pi_2 - 1.88$$

$$n = 19 \qquad r = 0.749 \qquad s = 0.289 \qquad (2)$$

The $\pi_1\sigma_1$ -term is an electronic correction which accounts for electronic differences between the pyrazoles and the standard series of monosubstituted benzenes from which the $\pi$ values were taken. According to eq.(1) virostatic potency increases with the hydrophobicity of substituents in $R_1$ and with size and electron attracting power of substituents in $R_2$. Eq.(2), however, tells a completely different story regarding substituents in $R_2$: only the hydrophobicity of these substituents should be important whereas steric and electronic effects are absent. The reason for this apparent discrepancy is a high multiple collinearity between $\pi_2$, $E_{S,2}$, and $\sigma_2^*$ allowing replacement of the linear combination of $E_{S,2}$ and $\sigma_2^*$ in eq. (1) by a simple $\pi_2$-term in eq. (2):

$$\pi_2 = -\,3.30\,E_{S,2} + 0.96\,\sigma_2^* + 0.81 \qquad (3)$$

$$n = 19 \qquad r = 0.827 \qquad s = 0.387$$

Fortunately, statistics clearly show here (which will not always be the case) that eq. (1) is to be preferred. This equation showed high predictive power and led to several potent new analogs; predicted potencies agreed with experimental values within the error of the bioassay.

2. The presence of collinear variables in a regression model will increase the confidence intervals of the regression coefficients and, hence, of predicted values. In an extreme case, a regression equation may primarily reflect collinearities and not a relationship between dependent and independent variables. Clearly, such equations are completely useless and of no predictive value even though they may show quite good F- and t-statistics (danger!). A useful method which can be applie here as a data pre-processing step is factor analysis (refs. 10-13). With the help of this method which will be discussed in the next section it is possible to recognize collinearities (see also ref. 14) and to select combinations of variables in such a way that collinearities are avoided. This eliminates the mathematical problem but does not, of course, solve the problem of non-separability of different effects on biological potency.

In the multi-parameter case it is not an easy task to select analogs in such a way that an optimal training series is obtained since, according to the above discussion, all of the following conditions must be fulfilled simultaneously:

- a smallest possible number of analogs
- large variance of all molecule parameters important for biological activity
- systematic exploration of the whole parameter space
- absence of collinearities

Therefore, special computerized methods for series design have been developed. All of these methods begin with a presentation of all accessible analogs or substituents (starting set) within the parameter space (Cartesian coordinate system with the molecule parameters as axes). Usually, the molecule parameters (variables) are applied in a normalized form (mean of zero and standard deviation of unity) in order to eliminate the effects of different scales. Then the task is to select the analogs in such a way that the distance between the points corresponding to them is sufficiently large and that the whole space is covered in nearly equal steps. Such a selection is then thought to fulfill the requirements mentioned above sufficiently well. As will be seen, however, this is not generally true, and the quality of the resulting training series depends on the method used. Several quality criteria may be used to judge the optimality of the training series (refs. 4, 15). We have found it convenient to use the determinant of the correlation matrix, $D_S$, as a measure for multiple **collinearities** and the "variance coefficient" $V_S$ as the measure of data variance. The latter is defined as:

$$V_S = 1/m \sum_{i=1}^{m} s_{is}^2/s_{ip}^2 \qquad (4)$$

$m$ = number of variables considered

$s_{is}^2$ = variance of the i-th variable within the training series

$s_{ip}^2$ = variance of the i-th variable in the starting set

and represents an average of the training series variance as compared with the variance in the starting set; it becomes unity if both variances are equal. The determinant $D_S$ becomes unity if collinearities are completely absent (for standardized data) and converges to zero as collinearities increase. Good training series should thus have high values of $D_S$ and $V_S$.

Since $D_S$ is a measure for collinearities and is also connected with Euclidean distances between the analogs in parameter space, maximizing $D_S$ is a possible approach to optimal training series. This technique is called D-optimal design (see e.g. ref. 4, 16-18) and is very effective in avoiding collinearities. It tends, however, to select mainly analogs representing the extremes of variables or, in other words, analogs from the boundary region of parameter space. As a consequence, the exploration of parameter space may not always be as systematic as one would like it. The maximization of $D_S$ involves an enormous amount of calculations for any ab initio design so that this technique cannot be recommended for that purpose. For "constrained" design problems (for instance, extension of an already existing set of analogs by a limited number of additional compounds), however, stepwise procedures are available (ref. 4) which seem to be quite effective.

Another possibility for series selection is to consider directly Euclidean distances in parameter space, using, for example, the methods proposed by Hansch and co-workers (ref. 19) and by Wootton et al. (ref. 20). The method of Hansch and co-workers is based on cluster analysis. Clusters of substituents (points) are found so that the similarity of substituents with respect to all molecule parameters considered is maximal within each cluster and minimal among the clusters. A good selection of substituents (analogs) will result if substituents from different clusters are chosen.

The method of Wootton et al. (ref. 20) is a stepwise multidimensional mapping technique. In each step the substituent is selected which is closest to the center of gravity of all hitherto selected points in parameter space but further apart than a pre-set minimal Euclidean distance, $D_{Min}$. The first step is to choose a suitable starting substituent (for instance, hydrogen). Next, the Euclidean distances from the corresponding point in parameter space to all other substituent points are computed, and the second substituent is selected as that one closest in space after deleting all points falling into the distance range defined by $D_{Min}$. The third substituent is found as the one closest to the center of gravity of the two points already selected while ensuring that the distance to either is larger than $D_{Min}$. The procedure is continued until the whole parameter space is explored and the desired number of analogs found; this number is adjusted by choosing an appropriate value of $D_{Min}$.

Both methods will yield training series with large variances of molecule parameters (high $V_S$ values; see Table 1) and have proven to be of practical value (see e.g. refs. 21-25). Collinearities, however, are not necessarily minimized (see Table 1). This led us to develop what we have called the PCMM technique (refs. 15, 26). PCMM is a combination of principal component analysis and multidimensional mapping and starts from the fact that a hyperplane can be fitted to the points corresponding to the analogs if collinearities are present. It is obvious that the collinearities are due mainly to those points which are close to this hyperplane and could thus be eliminated by deleting such points. In order to do that without losing too much of the information contained in the corresponding region of parameter space the substituents are divided into two sets in a first step. Set 1 contains the points close to, and set 2 those points distant from the hyperplane as judged from Euclidean distances between the points and the plane; these distances are computed with the help of principal component analysis. To each of the two sets the multidimensional mapping technique of Wootton et al. (ref. 20) is now applied separately in such a way that a higher percentage of analogs is selected from set 2. In so doing one must allow for a change in the position of the hyperplane during the selection of analogs. In order to account for this behaviour an automatic stepwise iteration procedure is used where the position of the hyperplane is adjusted after each step.

Table 1 compares the mean values of $D_S$ and $V_S$ for a training series selected from a starting set of 90 substituents (ref. 19) in the parameter space spanned by $\pi$, R, F, and MR with four different techniques:

- random selection
- stochastic selection from the clusters presented in (ref. 19)
- multidimensional mapping according to Wootton et al. (ref. 20)
- PCMM method (ref. 15).

TABLE 1

Values of $D_S$ and $V_S$ for training series[a] selected from a starting set of 90 substituents (parameter space: $\pi$, F, R, MR) by different methods (see text)

| Selection method | $D_S$ [b] | $V_S$ [b] |
|---|---|---|
| Random | 0.434 | 0.833 |
| From clusters | 0.370 | 1.668 |
| Multidimensional mapping | 0.613 | 2.146 |
| PCMM method | 0.825 | 1.750 |

[a] ten analogs

[b] mean values from ten selections

All three design techniques yield series with a large data variance ($V_S$ values), but only the PCMM method effectively minimizes collinearities as can be seen from the $D_S$ values. Randomly selected series are - as was to be expected - very far from being optimal (they have a small data variance and many collinearities) and cannot be considered representative. Clearly, a careful selection of training series by an appropriate series design method is indispensable.

The PCMM technique seems to be the method of choice, but for small starting sets (less than 50 substituents) a much simpler method has turned out to have specific advantages. This method is based on the two-dimensional mapping of intraclass correlation matrices and is called TMIC method (refs. 26-28). The intraclass correlation coefficient characterizes the relatedness of pairs of substituents with respect to a set of variables. Computation of the intraclass correlation coefficients for all pairs of substituents yields an intraclass correlation matrix which can be decomposed by principal component method (ref. 31). All substituents of the starting set are then presented in the two-dimensional Cartesian space spanned by the first two principal components as axes. As a result a two-dimensional map is obtained from which a training series can be selected by a simple inspection. Substituents similar with respect to the molecule parameters considered are clustered together so that a good training series with a large data variance and few collinearities will be obtained if substituents distant from each other are selected in such a way that the whole space is systematically covered. The advantage of the TMIC method is not only its simplicity but also a very clear presentation of the full picture of data structure in a way which is close to the usual way of thinking of organic chemists.

All series design methods can adequately take into account synthetic feasibility since different training series can easily be derived from the same starting set. A proper series design is not only important for QSAR work but also has a direct economical impact in that it can save the synthesis of compounds which do not add information. In many examples of the past the number of such compounds is very large (see e.g. refs. 29, 30). According to an estimate made by Martin (ref. 25) the use of series design strategies leads to a 2.75-fold increase (on an average) in the information gained per compound synthesized.

If the parameter space to be considered is not known and hard to postulate, stepwise strategies as outlined in the preceding paragraph can be applied. A small pilot series can be designed using a standard set of molecule parameters from which, after synthesis and biological testing, a tentative QSAR is evaluated (see e.g. ref. 21). This QSAR can then aid in the design of the final training series.

Factor analysis of data preprocessing step

The objective of factor analysis (see e.g. refs. 10-13, 31) is to decipher the number and nature of basic descriptors behind a data matrix. These basic descriptors, which may be regarded as representing fundamental influences responsible for the data structure as a whole, are called "common factors" and are calculated by standard procedures (ref. 31). They account for the variance which is common to all variables. The correlations between the variables of the data matrix and the factors are characterized by the so-called factor loadings which form a matrix (one loading for each possible pair of variable and factor) called a factor pattern. From this pattern the following information can be obtained (after transforming the factor pattern matrix to give the simplest possible structure):

1. Variables with non-zero loadings in the same factor are correlated. The higher the loadings the higher the correlation.
2. Variables which have non-zero loadings only in different factors are not correlated.

If the data matrix to be factor analyzed contains the biological response and molecule parameters for the compounds of a training series as variables the resulting factor pattern will allow a rational selection of variables for regression analysis according to the following criteria:

1. The number of terms in the regression equation(s) is equal to the number of factors in which the variable "biological response" has a non-zero loading.
2. Only those molecule parameters are important which also have non-zero loadings in these factors.
3. Molecule parameters having high loadings in the same factor are collinear and are, therefore, not to be combined in the same regression equation.

The first two criteria reduce the number of regression equations to be computed, and the last one eliminates collinearities.

As an example I should like to discuss some results on the inhibition of the NADH-oxidase system from ETP by substituted phenoxyacetic acids (ref. 11). The variables considered are summarized in Table 2 together with the factor pattern obtained from factor analysis (factor loadings in the three significant common factors).

TABLE 2

Factor pattern (simple structure) obtained for the inhibition of NADH-oxidase by substituted phenoxyacetic acids (only the significant non-zero loadings are listed)

| Variable | Factor pattern | | |
|---|---|---|---|
| | First factor | Second factor | Third factor |
| log BR | 0.77 | | 0.54 |
| $\pi$ | | 0.76 | |
| $\pi^2$ | | 0.70 | |
| $\sigma$ | 0.92 | | |
| $\sigma^2$ | 0.82 | | |
| $\sigma^-$ | 0.93 | | |
| $\sigma^{-2}$ | 0.83 | | |
| S | 0.78 | | |
| P | | -0.76 | |
| $E_S$ | | | -0.86 |
| $E_S^2$ | | | -0.87 |

According to the factor pattern, regression equations describing log BR in the parameter space considered should have two terms since log BR has non-zero loadings in only two factors (first and third factor). Inhibitory potency obviously depends on electronic (first factor) and steric (third factor) properties; hydrophobic effects are absent since log BR has a zero-loading in the second factor. The expected interrelations between the electronic substituent constants $\sigma$, $\sigma^-$ and S are shown in the first factor. Quite surprising is the correlation between $\pi$ and P indicated by the second factor.

In regression analysis one of the electronic substituent constants with a high loading in the first factor should be combined with $E_S$ according to

$$\begin{aligned} \log BR &= f(\sigma , E_S) \\ &= f(\sigma , E_S) \\ &= f(S , E_S) \end{aligned} \qquad (5)$$

Equations with $\sigma^2$, $\sigma^{-2}$ and $E_S^2$ must not be considered because of the high correlations between the respective linear terms (this does not completely rule out, however, the possibility that the true relationship between log BR and these variables may be parabolic).

All these conclusions were fully confirmed by the results of regression analysis (as a control, regression equations for all possible combinations of variables were calculated). The best equation which could be obtained reads:

$$\log BR = 0.75\ \sigma^- - 0.23\ E_S + 3.34$$

$$n = 17 \qquad r = 0.923 \qquad s = 0.249$$

Addition of a third term does not improve the results, and there is no relationship in which $\pi$ or $\pi^2$ are statistically significant.

## BIOLOGICAL RESPONSE DATA

The properties of biological response data are key factors for the quality and predictive power of QSARs. Many problems arise in designing and performing biological experiments (see e.g. ref. 32). Only some selected aspects will be outlined here since a more detailed discussion would be far beyond the scope of this presentation.

### Complex responses

Many biological response data are a composite of different components. For a real understanding and a meaningful QSAR analysis it may be necessary to consider these components separately. In the field of phytopharmacology, for example, we have noticed that sometimes only poor QSARs could be obtained with conventional response parameters (e.g., $pI_{50}$, etc.). Therefore, a more complex model to fit dose-response curves was derived allowing for the presence of drug-receptor complexes of different composition all contributing to the overall biological response BR in an additive manner (refs. 33-35):

$$BR = \Sigma [D]^i \Psi_i \Pi K_i / (1 + [D]^i \underset{i}{\Pi} K_i) \tag{7}$$

[D] concentration of free drug in the vicinity of the receptor

$K_1$ apparent equilibrium constant for the formation of the i-th drug-receptor complex

$\Psi_i$ apparent intrinsic activity of the i-th drug-receptor complex

This model turned out to be quite useful in a number of cases (refs. 33, 34, 36-39). An acceptable QSAR for the plant growth inhibiting potency of substituted piperidinoacetanilides, for example, could only be obtained with response parameters derived from eq. (7) but not with conventional $pI_{50}$ values ($\delta_{NH}$: chemical shift of the amide proton; $pI^*_{50}$: corrected $pI_{50}$ derived from eq. (7); $\Psi_1$: apparent intrinsic activity related to the first drug-receptor complex):

for meta- and para-substituted compounds

$$pI^*_{50} = 0.85\pi + 0.66\ \delta_{NH} \tag{8}$$

$$n = 13 \qquad r = 0.920 \qquad s = 0.180$$

for ortho-substituted compounds

$$\log \Psi_1 = 0.12\ E_S - 0.20 \tag{9}$$

$$n = 6 \qquad r = 0.900 \qquad s = 0.195$$

Eq. (9) indicates a particular behaviour of the ortho-substituted compounds influencing the intrinsic activity of the first drug-receptor complex via a steric effect.

There are many cases where overall biological response data may lead to incomplete or even erroneous answers which cannot be discussed here in detail. Reference should only be made to the problems of separating intrinsic activity and affinity and of pharmacodynamic and pharmacokinetic effects in pharmacological experiments (see e.g. ref. 11) and also to the importance of microscopic kinetic constants when endeavouring to understand enzymatic reactions and their dependence upon the structure of substrates and inhibitors. A special situation (to be discussed in a later section) arises if an observable biological response is due to the interaction of drugs with more than one receptor.

## Data precision and the choice of QSAR methods

The precision of biological data is always of primary importance. For a Hansch type analysis the data must be real continuous quantities spanning a sufficient range and of a sufficiently high sample-to - error variance ratio. Even for parameters derived from dose-response curves these conditions are frequently not fulfilled (see also ref. 32), and caution is required when applying regression analysis to data of the fixed dose screening type.

In many cases the biological data are so imprecise that potency can only be expressed on a discrete scale in the form of a classification (for instance, very active / active / weakly active / inactive compounds). Classification methods (eg. discriminant analysis, SIMCA, linear learning machine, KNN-method, etc.) must then be applied in QSAR studies (for reviews, see e.g. refs. 12, 13, 40, 41). The resulting QSARs have the form of a classificator allowing the classification of as yet uninvestigated compounds. To a certain extent conclusions as to which molecular properties or structural features are important for biological potency may also be drawn.

Classification methods are also required if effects of different quality are to be considered (for instance, when comparing agonists with antagonists). A case in point is the discriminant analytical investigation of the blood sugar influencing activity of sulphonamides (ref. 42) of the general structure

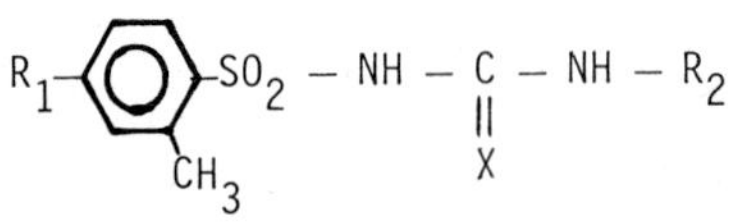

$$R_1-C_6H_3(CH_3)-SO_2-NH-C(=X)-NH-R_2$$

In this example the different quality is the direction of effect; some of the compounds increase the blood sugar level (class 1), some are inactive (class 2), and some show a decreasing effect (class 3). The following non-elementary discriminant functions were obtained:*

* I = indicator variable; I = 1 for x = S and I = 0 for x = 0
w = non-elementary discriminant function
$MR_2$ = molar refractivity of substituents $R_2$
$R_M$ = chromatographic $R_M$-value reflecting, in this case, hydrophilicity

<u>Separation of class 1 from class 2</u>

$$w = 0.143\ MR_2 \tag{10}$$

with the class means

$w_1 = 1.474$

$w_2 = 2.740$

<u>Separation of class 3 from class 2</u>

$$w = 0.15\ MR_2 + 2.82\ I + 8.53\ R_M \tag{11}$$

with the class means

$w_2 = 5.399$

$w_3 = 8.092$

From these results the following conclusions may be drawn:

- Since different sets of molecule parameters are required for the separation of classes 1 and 3 from class 2 (only a poor simultaneous separation of all three classes was achieved) it may be concluded that two different mechanisms operate in steering hyper- and hypoglycemic activity. These mechanisms may well be the interaction of the sulfonamides with β-cells on the one hand and the influence of these compounds on the adrenalin level on the other. Substituent effects on these two opposite processes are different so that it is easy to understand why such closely related compounds influence blood sugar in different ways.
- Most important for hyperglycemic activity are the substituents in $R_2$. Since $MR_2$ is highly correlated with $\pi_2$ eq.(10) indicates that either small and/or hydrophilic substituents will favour hyperglycemic activity whereas larger and hydrophobic substituents will lead to hypoglycemic compounds (see also eq.(11)). This is in agreement with, for example, results of Ruschig et al. (refs. 43, 44) who showed that hypoglycemic activity in N-alkyl substituted sulfonylureas requires substituents with at least three C-atoms.
- The simultaneous occurrence of $R_M$ and $MR_2$ might be indicative of an optimum in hydrophobicity with respect to hypoglycemic activity (because of the solvent system used in TLC, $R_M$ decreases as hydrophobicity increases). The MR term might also reflect polar effects.
- As follows from the I-term in eq. (11) the thioamide group is more favourable for hypoglycemic activity than the amide group.

Selection of the various classification methods to be used for a particular problem depends not only on the biological data but also on the variation of chemical structure within the training series. Especially in retrospective analyses of larger data sets from mass screening, this variation is frequently so wide that the properties of compounds can no longer be parameterized by substituent constants or similar quantities. Descriptors directly derived from the chemical structure are to be used here indicating, for example, the absence or presence of certain structural features. Since these descriptors are discrete variables, heuristic pattern recognition methods (e.g. linear learning machine) which do not depend on assumptions concerning data distribution must be applied. Analyses of this type are very sensitive to the definition and selection of descriptors and have not always led to convincing results. I feel, however, that they do have their place in QSAR work since they allow the extraction of information from the huge data bases which have accumulated during many years of testing. If it is possible to increase the number of positives in screening programs with the help of such methods (see e.g. refs. 45, 46) I would also call that a successful prediction. In the course of such work, furthermore, preliminary information on pharmacophores may also be obtained (see e.g. refs. 46-48). A warning seems to be in order, however, if such approaches are applied to develop general models for toxicity, carcinogenicity or mutagenicity (refs. 49-51). One should be very careful never to replace experimentally determined data by estimates from such models and to keep such estimates far away from files and registers (ref. 52). Although QSAR investigations in the fields of toxicity, carcinogenicity and mutagenicity have yielded valid information, one should be well aware of all limitations if predictions are to be made.

## RESPONSE PROFILES

A useful new drug usually has to be optimal (or at least acceptable) with respect to a certain profile of biological activities. That means that drug design actually implies optimization of a response profile resulting from a battery of biological tests. Methods to integrate such multiple biological data into one multivariate QSAR analysis are available and have been shown to be of great practical importance (for reviews see e.g. refs. 12, 13, 53, 54). Rather than these methods I shall discuss here some specific aspects of multiple data structure important for QSAR predictions.

### Continuous data

The first question to be asked for a battery of tests is what information can be gained or, in other words, whether these tests are unique or some redundant (see also ref. 4). For continuous data this question can be answered by applying the multivariate methods of factor analysis or of principal component analysis (refs. 11-13, 31) (for factor analysis see pertinent chapter above). As an example Table 3 summarizes factor analytical results obtained from multiple biological data of a series of piperidinoacetanilides investigated in eight biological tests (ref. 55). The first factor indicates a relationship between the results from tests 1 and 3 which was, of course, to be expected. Both tests are related to test 8 which may indicate that growth inhibition is connected with the inhibition of protein synthesis (at least for the piperidinoacetanilides). The second factor reveals that tests 2 and 4 are related which again is biologically meaningful. Rather surprising is the relationship between tests 5 and 6 indicated by the third factor. Test 7 shows a completely unique behaviour and is not related to any other test.

TABLE 3
Factor pattern (simple structure ; three significant common factors) obtained from multiple biological response data of a series of piperidinoacetanilides investigated in eight biological tests. Significant non-zero loadings are indicated by a cross.

| No. | Biological test | Factor pattern | | |
|---|---|---|---|---|
| | | First factor | Second factor | Third factor |
| 1 | Growth inhibition in S.alba seedlings | + | | |
| 2 | Amylase activity in Triticum aleurone cells | | + | |
| 3 | Growth inhibition in S.alba hypocotyl | + | | |
| 4 | Dry weight of seedlings | | + | |
| 5 | Anthelmintic activity | | | + |
| 6 | Antifungal activity | | | + |
| 7 | Antibacterial activity | | | |
| 8 | Inhibition of ribosomal protein synthesis | + | | |

This and other selected examples summarized in Table 4 show the many similarities of the respective biological tests and, consequently, point out the redundancy of the corresponding test batteries. Obviously, a definite pattern exists in such data which, in principle, allows the prediction of potencies in one bioassay from the multiple results in the other bioassays. For example, the biological potency of benzodiazepines in the foot-shock test can be calculated from principal components (PC) obtained from a data matrix containing the results from the other four bioassays listed in Table 4 as variables according to ref. 56:

$$\log BR = 0.39\ PC_1 + 0.65\ PC_3 + 0.42 \qquad (12)$$

$$n = 22 \quad r = 0.955 \quad s = 0.21$$

and this equation shows better statistics than two-term equations with molecule parameters as independent variables. Multiple data patterns can also be used to classify compounds with respect to different biological effects (refs. 4, 57-60) and QSAR predictions can be controlled by checking whether they fit into a corresponding pattern; if they do, their reliability can be considered fairly high, if they do not,care should be taken. Finally, QSAR and potency patterns in multiple biological data can be directly compared; they should always be consistent (see next section).

TABLE 4

Interrelated biological tests investigated by factor or principal component analysis

| Type of compounds | Biological test | Number of relevant factors or principal components | Ref. |
|---|---|---|---|
| Non-hormonal anti-inflammatories | Mouse phenylquinone writhing<br>Rat carageenan paw<br>Inhibition of human platelet cyclooxygenase<br>Inhibibition of bull seminal vesicle $PGE_2$<br>Inhibition of collagen-induced platelet aggregation | 2 | (4) |
| Benzodiazepines | Incl.screen<br>Foot-shock<br>Pentylene-tetrazole<br>Electroshock max.<br>Electroshock min. | 2 | (56) |
| 8-Quinolinoles | A.niger<br>A.oryzae<br>Trichoderma viride<br>Trichophyton mentagrophytes<br>M.verrucaria | 2 | (56) |
| Rifamycin B amides | M.aureus<br>S.faecalis<br>S.hemolyticus<br>S.subtilis | 2 | (12, 13, 56) |
| Standard compounds | 36 tests; mouse behaviour and symptomatology screen | 11 | (4) |

Of special interest is a situation where an observable biological response results from reactions with more than one receptor (see e.g. refs. 61, 62) according to

$$\begin{matrix} R_1 & & & \longrightarrow & BR_1 & \searrow & \\ \vdots & & & & \vdots & & \\ R_i & + & D & \longrightarrow & BR_i & \longrightarrow & BR \\ \vdots & & & & \vdots & & \\ R_n & & & \longrightarrow & BR_n & \nearrow & \end{matrix} \qquad (13)$$

$R_i$ = i-th receptor
D = drug
$BR_i$ = partial response produced at the i-th receptor
BR = observable total response

Such response data are not suitable for a normal univariate QSAR investigation. It seems possible, however, to "extract" the components $BR_i$ from a response profile evaluated from a battery of well-selected tests provided that the overall response in each test can be described as a linear combination of the $BR_i$ according to

$$BR\ (T_j) = \sum_i a_{ij}\ BR_i \quad (14)$$

BR (Tj) = observable total response from the j-th test
$a_{ij}$ = weight coefficients

If eq. (14) holds, then a principal component analysis can be applied to evaluate the $BR_i$.

To summarize, the investigation of data structure in multiple bioassays can lead to

- multivariate QSARs,
- recognition of redundant and of unique tests,
- prediction of potencies directly from the biological data,
- control of predictions made from QSARs,
- differentiations of biological effects and separation of partial effects,

and thus it is of great practical importance. This is true, of course, also for discrete data which, however, must be handled in a different manner, which will be discussed in the next section.

Discrete data

As already mentioned many biological potency data are discrete and not continuous, representing potency in terms of a classification. For such data factor or principal component analysis cannot be applied. A convenient method to investigate multiple data structure in such cases can be derived from information theory using Shannon's entropy as a measure of information content (refs. 63, 64).

The information $I(T_i, T(k))$ contained in a set of k tests, T(k), about a given test $T_i$ can be calculated according to

$$I(T_i, T(k)) = H(T_i) - H_{T(k)}(T_i) \quad (15)$$

$H(T_i)$ = Shannon's entropy of test $T_i$
$H_{T(k)}(T_i)$ = Shannon's entropy of test $T_i$ conditional to the set of tests T(k)

References p. 379

The entropies can easily be calculated from the test results of a series of compounds. $H(T_i)$ characterizes the indetermination of $T_i$ and $H_{T(k)}(T_i)$ the remaining indetermination of $T_i$ if the results from T(k) are known. Hence, the quantity

$$I_q = [I(T_i,T(k))/_{H(T_i)}]\ 100\% \qquad (16)$$

represents the gain in information (or decrease in indetermination) of $T_i$ if the results from T(k) are known, in percent of the original indetermination of $T_i$. A high value of $I_q$ indicates that T(k) yields much information about $T_i$ and that $T_i$ and the tests contained in T(k) are closely interrelated.

Such an analysis was performed, for example, with antifungal potencies (expressed as "active" or "inactive") of a series of thioureas against the fungi Aspergillus niger (AN), Botrytis cinerea (BC), Sclerotinia fructigena (SF), Fusarium nivale (FN) and Alternaria solani (AS) (for details see ref. 63). Table 5 presents the stepwise development of $I_q$ for SF as test $T_i$ and all possible combinations of the other four tests as T(k). As can be seen BC shows the highest information about SF followed by AN and AS. The best combination of two tests is that of AN and BC, and the most information is obtained from the set AN, BC and AS (the small increase in $I_q$ after adding FN to T(k) is to be considered insignificant). The results for all five tests are summarized in Table 6. Quite obviously there is some redundancy in this system of tests since high information on AN, BC and SF can be obtained from other tests. Only AS and FN show a unique behaviour (high information content). This pattern should be reflected by the pattern of QSARs describing antifungal activity in terms of molecule parameters. When comparing Table 6 with results from non-elementary discriminant analysis performed with the same data (ref. 65) it turns out that this is indeed the case. Since, for example, the set AN, SF provides high information about BC, the discriminant function describing antifungal activity against BC should be more or less a composite of the discriminant functions obtained for AN and SF. Table 7 shows that this prediction is surprisingly well fulfilled. The consistency of the QSAR and multiple data pattern is very satisfactory and a good indication of the validity of the QSARs; it was helpful for further work.

TABLE 5

Stepwise development of $I_q$ for Sclerotinia fructigena as test $T_i$ and all possible combinations (indicated by a cross) of AN, BC, AS and FN as T(k)[a]

| T(k) | | | | $I_q$ (%) |
|---|---|---|---|---|
| AN | BC | AS | FN | |
| | + | | | 23.4 |
| + | | | | 14.5 |
| | | + | | 12.0 |
| | | | + | 0.1 |
| + | + | | | 40.8 |
| | + | + | | 34.6 |
| | + | | + | 26.9 |
| + | | + | | 24.6 |
| + | | | + | 16.8 |
| | | + | + | 12.4 |
| + | + | + | | 57.7[b] |
| + | + | | + | 43.6 |
| | + | + | + | 39.3 |
| + | | + | + | 30.6 |
| + | + | + | + | 61.2 |

[a] AN: Aspergillus niger
BC: Botrytis cinerea
AS: Alternaria solani
FN: Fusarium nivale

[b] optimal combination of tests

TABLE 6

Optimal sets of tests (T(k)) and the corresponding $I_q$ values for all five fungi

| Test $T_i$ | Set T(k) | $I_q$ (%) |
|---|---|---|
| AN | BC, SF | 46.4 |
| BC | AN, SF | 53.5 |
| SF | AN, BC, AS | 57.7 |
| AS | SF | 11.9 |
| FN | - | - |

References p. 379

TABLE 7

Molecule parameters appearing in the discriminant function describing the antifungal potency of thioureas ($R_1$-NH-CS-NH-$R_2$) against AN, in comparison to the occurrence of the same parameters in the discriminant functions obtained for BC and SF. The sign of the corresponding weight coefficients is indicated by "+" or "-". Superimposition of of the columns for BC and SF exactly yields the column for AN (compare with Table 6)

$\Sigma\sigma$ : sum of Hammett $\sigma$ for aromatic substituents in phenylthioureas (in phenyl- : ring at $R_1$)

$E_s$ (para): steric substituent constant for para-substituents in phenylthioureas (in phenylring at $R_1$)

$I_3$ : indicator variable ($I_3$ = 1 for 2,5-dichlorosubstitution in phenylring at $R_1$)

$\Sigma\pi$ : sum of $\pi$-values of aromatic substituents (in phenylring at $R_2$)

$\Sigma E_s$ : sum of $E_s$ values of aromatic substituents (in phenylring at $R_2$)

$I_1$ : indicator variable ($I_1$ = 1 if phenylring at $R_2$)

| Part of the molecule | Molecule parameters | Discriminant function for | | |
|---|---|---|---|---|
| | | BC | SF | AN |
| $R_1$ | $\Sigma\sigma$ | n.s.* | - | - |
| | $E_s$ (para) | n.s.* | + | + |
| | $I_3$** | n.s.* | - | - |
| $R_2$ | $\Sigma\pi$ | n.s.* | - | - |
| | $\Sigma E_s$ | - | - | - |
| | $I_1$** | + | n.s.* | + |
| | MW | n.s.* | - | - |

* corresponding term not significant (n.s.)

** indicator variables

Data structures of the type presented above are not limited to homologous series as indicated by recent results from our laboratory. They also exist in very large and quite inhomogeneous data sets.

DERIVING PREDICTIONS FROM QSARs

Predictions can be made only within "spanned substituent (or property) space" (SSS) (ref. 66). That means that predictions from QSARs are mainly interpolations, at least as far as lead optimization in the classical sense is concerned. At first glance this might be considered a serious limitation, but one must not forget that interpolation in a multi-parameter space is a very complicated matter and can result in a substantial increase in biological potency. Outside SSS (un-SSS), extrapolations are only possible within a small range. Hansch (ref. 66) has compared a QSAR with a contour map of a certain area (SSS). Conclusions on the contours outside this map (un-SSS) will be possible for the immediate surroundings but virtually impossible for distant areas. An example of a successful prediction in un-SSS comes from an investigation of the hydrolysis of esters of the types $R\text{-}C_6H_4\text{-}OCOCH_2NHCO\text{-}C_6H_5$ (I) and $R\text{-}C_6H_4\text{-}OCOCH_2NHSO_2CH_3$ (II) by papain (refs. 66-68) yielding eq. (17):

$$\log 1/K_m = 0.57\ MR + 0.56\ \sigma - 1.92\ I + 3.74 \qquad (17)$$

$$n = 20 \qquad r = 0{,}990 \qquad s = 0.148$$

I = 1 for type I and 0 for type II compounds

X-ray data of papain led to the hypothesis that the amide moiety of both sets of congeners would fall into a hydrophobic crevice. If so the difference between the two sets expressed by the indicator variable term in eq. (17) should reflect the difference in hydrophobic binding which must then be related to the difference of $\pi$ values of the two amide moieties. From this difference amounting to

$$\begin{aligned} \Delta\pi &= \pi\ (NHCOC_6H_5) - \pi\ (NHSO_2CH_3) \\ &= 0.49 - 1.92 \\ &= -1.67 \end{aligned} \qquad (18)$$

and the coefficient of the I-term in eq. (17), a slope of 1.15 can be estimated from

$$-1.92\ /\ -1.67 = 1.15 \qquad (19)$$

for a $\pi$-term describing hydrophobic binding of the amide moiety to the crevice of the enzyme. The predicted slope of about unity could be fully confirmed after synthesizing and analyzing a set of esters in which the amide moiety was varied ($CH_3OCOCH_2NHCOC_6H_4\text{-}R'$):

$$\log 1/K_m = 1.01\ \pi + 1.46 \qquad (20)$$

$$n = 16 \qquad r = 0.981 \qquad s = 0.165$$

This example nicely shows how predictions in near un-SSS should be combined with a subsequent extension of SSS.

Even within SSS predictions may be wrong. An example has already been discussed at the beginning of this presentation demonstrating that false predictions will always result when new compounds show new properties not accounted for in the training series. This may happen even with quite simple substituents, such as the example discussed by Unger (ref. 4). A QSAR investigation led to the suggestion that hydrophilic, electron-withdrawing substituents should enhance the desired biological activity in a series of antidepressive imidazoline alkyl carbamates. Biological testing however, showed the substituents selected to have a very low activity. The reason was that these substituents were the first in the series capable of hydrogen-bonding. This finally led to an extension of the QSAR with satisfactory results.

Sometimes non-relevant molecule parameters may occur in QSARs as substitutes for the really important variables without effecting the descriptive power of the resulting QSAR. The predictive capacity, however, will break down completely for all compounds where such a substitution is not possible. In addition, the QSAR will lead to erroneous conclusions. Two examples may suffice to demonstrate this point:

1. Activity of hydroxytryptamines at the LSD receptor (from ref. 69): (suffixes refer to carbon atom numbering)

$$\log BR = 18.09\, f_1 - 74.77\, q_1 + 1.182\, \pi_7 - 13.06 \qquad (21)$$
$$n = 15 \qquad r = 0.962 \qquad s = 0.288$$

$$\log BR = -128.4\, q_7^2 + 13.07\, q_7 - 0.462 \qquad (22)$$
$$n = 15 \qquad r = 0.924 \qquad s = 0.337$$

The dominating term in eq. (21) is the $\pi_7$-term indicating hydrophobic interactions of substituents in position 7; in addition electronic properties ($q$ = charge; $f$ = frontier electron density) are also important. According to eq. (22), however, there is no influence of hydrophobicity, and biological potency depends on the charge at C-atom 7. The parabolic dependence on $q_7$ has its maximum at about $q_7 = 0$ which is surprising at a first glance. The background for this peculiar finding simply is that at zero charge hydrophobic interactions as indicated in eq. (21) are maximal. Thus, eq. (22) indirectly expresses a hydrophobic effect by an electronic parameter. Had eq. (21) not been found eq. (22) might well have led to incorrect conclusions.

2. Inhibition of the Hill reaction by piperidinoacetanilides (ref. 70):

$$\log BR = -49.52\, q_N + 6.92 \qquad (23)$$
$$r = 0.859 \qquad s = 0.197$$

$$\log BR = 20.69\, E_{HOMO} - 10.57 \qquad (24)$$
$$r = 0.992 \qquad s = 0.047$$

Eq. (23) seems to support the classical hypothesis that the formation of a hydrogen bridge with the NH-group as donor is important for Hill reaction inhibition ($q_N$ = electronic charge at the amide nitrogen). However, $q_N$ is highly correlated with $E_{HOMO}$, the energy of the highest occupied molecular orbital within the training series, and substituting $E_{HOMO}$ for $q_N$ yields a distinctly better equation. This result indicates charge-transfer interactions rather than hydrogen bonding as has also been suggested by Hansch (ref. 71). If so, the amide hydrogen is not essential, and this has been clearly demonstrated by, for example, the high Hill reaction inhibitory potency of triazinones (ref. 72). This example also re-emphasizes the importance of a sufficient spread of all molecular properties influencing biological potency: although it is well known that hydrophobic effects operate in Hill reaction inhibition, a $\pi$-term is missing in eqs.(23) and (24) simply because the substituents considered did not differ enough in their hydrophobicity.

The take-home lesson from these examples is that the exploration of a data space may be incomplete, even when an acceptable QSAR has been found, when not all physically meaningful hypotheses on possible drug-biosystem interactions are considered.

Congeners which do not fit a QSAR or theoretical predictions are of special interest. Such congeners which show a peculiar behaviour as compared with the other compounds can only be detected with the help of QSARs. A great deal of information can be gained from them (Hansch called them "a blessing in disguise" (ref. 66)) and it is not surprising that such outliers have led to information about mechanisms of action or even to potential new drugs (see e.g. refs. 26, 73, 74, 139).

Within SSS reliable predictions are usually possible; some examples are summarized in Table 8. However, QSARs and predictions derived thereby should never be taken as dogma and always considered and used critically. In this sense, and if applied strictly within their limits, QSARs certainly have developed into an important and powerful tool in modern drug research.

TABLE 8

Examples of correct predictions from QSARs

| Types of compounds | Biological activity | Ref. |
|---|---|---|
| Benzothiadiazines | Antihypertensive | 75-77 |
| Clonidine analogs | Antihypertensive | 78 |
| Propynylamines | Inhibition of monoamino oxidase | 79 |
| N-(phenoxyethyl)cyclopropylamines | Inhibition of monoamino oxidase | 80 |
| β-Carbolines | Inhibition of monoamino oxidase | 81 |
| Fusaric acids | Inhibition of dopamine-β-hydroxylase | 82 |
| Sulfonamides | Inhibition of carboanhydrase | 83 |
| Carbamoylpiperidines | Inhibition of cholinesterase | 84,85 |
| Ketones | Inhibition of chymotrypsin | 86 |
| Thiazole β-blockers | Inhibition of adenylate cyclase | 3, 4 |
| Benzylpyridinium ions | Inhibition of complement | 87 |
| Miscellaneous | Binding to BSA | 87 |
| Steroids | Binding to the progesterone receptor | 88<br>88 |
| Esters | Hydrolysis by papain | 66 |
| Dopamine amides | Hydrolysis by arylamidases | 82 |
| Peptidyl-p-nitroanilides | Hydrolysis by subtilisin | 89 |
| Polycyclic aromatic hydrocarbons | Hydroxylation by microsomal oxidase<br>Carcinogenicity | 90 |
| Isatin-β-isothiosemicarbazones | Antiviral | 91 |
| Pyrazoles | Antiviral | 9 |
| Miscellaneous | Cytostatic | 46,92 |
| Aza-cytidine derivatives | Cytostatic<br>Immunosuppressive | 93 |
| Nitrosoureas | Cytostatic | 94 |
| Mitomycins | Cytostatic | 95 |
| Hydantoin derivatives | Cytostatic | 96 |
| Rifamycin-β-amides | Antibacterial | 97 |
| Sulfonamides | Antibacterial<br>Pharmacokinetics | 98,99 |
| Erythromycins | Antibacterial | 92 |
| Quinoxaline 1,4-dioxides | Antibacterial | 100 |
| Phenanthrenes | Antimalarial | 101 |
| Naphthoquinones | Antimalarial | 102 |
| Phenylamidinureas | Antimalarial | 103,104 |
| Tuberins | Antimycoplasma | 4 |
| Methoxychlors | Insecticidal | 22 |
| N-Hydroxypyridones | Antifungal | 105 |
| Pyridine derivatives | Antifungal | 106 |
| Trifluormethanesulfonamides | Herbicidal | 107,108 |
| Aryl-alkyl-carbonyl compounds | Herbicidal | 109 |
| Arylethers | Herbicidal | 110 |
| Piperidinoacetanilides | Phytoactive | 111 |
| Pyrimidones | Inhibition of Hill reaction | 112 |
| Ureas | Herbicidal | 113 |
| Phenylacetamide derivatives | Hypnotic | 114 |
| Pyridylmethanes | Spasmolytic | 115 |
| Promazines | Neuroleptic | 116 |

TABLE 8 - continued -

| Types of compounds | Biological activity | Ref. |
|---|---|---|
| Miscellaneous | Cholinergic | 117,118 |
| Aromatic and aliphatic acids | Antiphlogistic | 73,119 |
| Benzothiepine derivatives | Neuroleptic | 120 |
| Clonidines | α-Adrenergic | 66,122 |
| Carboxylate esters | Clot lysis | 121 |
| Thyroxin analogs | Thyroxin | 123 |
| Acrylates | Toxic | 124 |
| Miscellaneous | Toxic | 125 |
| Copper chelates | Cytotoxic | 126 |
| Pyraneamines | Immunosuppressive | 127 |
| Azapurine-6-ones | Immunosuppressive | 128 |
| Phenyloxazolidines | Radioprotective | 129 |
| Carbamoylethylamines | Cholinolytic | 130 |
| Miscellaneous | Affinity for the muscarinic receptor | 131 |
| Mescaline analogs | Hallucinogenic | 132 |
| Triazines | Inhibition of dihydrofolate reductase | 133 |
| Benzodiazepines | Antipentilene-tetrazole activity | 134 |
| Cyanocyclohexylamines | Antifungal | 134 |
| Cycloalkanol ethers | Several | 134 |
| Piperidinoacetanilides | Antiserotonin | 135 |
| Miscellaneous | $H_2$-Antagonistic | 136 |
| Analogs of somatostatin | Antidiabetic | 137 |
| Steroids | Progestational | 5-7 |
| Azacycloalkanes | Narcotic | 138 |
| Organosilicon amines | Antifungal | 46,139 |
| Indandione-1,3 derivatives | Toxic<br>Anticonvulsive | 46 |

REFERENCES


1 G. Lambrecht, U. Moser and E. Mutschler, Eur. J. Med. Chem., 15(1980)305.
2 E.J. Lien, E.J. Ariens and A.J. Beld, Eur. J. Pharmacol., 35(1976)245.
3 S.H. Unger, K. Untch, B. Lewis, B. Berkoz, J. Edwards, A. Strosberg, R. Weissberg and R. Alvarez, in J. Knoll and F. Darvas (Eds.), Chemical Structure - Biological Activity Relationships, Akadémiai Kiadó, Budapest, 1980, p.3.
4 S.H. Unger, in E.J. Ariens (Ed.), Drug Design, Vol. IX, Academic Press, New York etc., 1980, p.48.
5 A.J. v.d. Broek, A.I.A. Broess, M.J. v.d. Heuvel, H.P. de Jongh, J. Leemhuis, K.H. Schönemann, J. Smits, J. de Visser, N.P. van Vliet and F.J. Zeelen, Steroids, 30(1977)481.
6 F.J. Zeelen,in J.A. Keverling Buisman (Ed.), Biological Activity and Chemical Structure, Elsevier, Amsterdam, 1977, p.147.
7 F.J. Zeelen, in J. Knoll and F. Darvas (Eds.), Chemical Structure - Biological Activity Relationships, Adadémiai Kiadó, Budapest, 1980, p.43.
8 R.D. Cramer III, K.M. Snader, C.R. Willis, L.W. Chakrin, J. Thomas and B.M. Sutton, J. Med. Chem., 22(1979)714
9 H.-J. Michel, R. Franke and H.Willitzer, in R. Franke and P. Oehme (Eds.), Quantitative Structure - Activity Analysis, Akademie-Verlag, Berlin, 1978, p.89.
10 W.Laass, G. Eichler, S. Dove, W.-E. Vogt, R. Franke and H. Vahle, in R. Franke and P. Oehme (Eds.), Quantitative Structure - Activity Analysis, Akademie-Verlag, Berlin, 1978, p.267.
11 R. Franke, Il Farmaco,34(1979)545.

12 R. Franke, Optimierungsmethoden in der Wirkstofforschung, Akademie-Verlag, Berlin, 1980.
13 R. Franke, Theory and Practice in Quantitative Structure-Activity Relationships, Elsevier, Amsterdam, in preparation.
14 Y.C. Martin and H.N. Panas, J. Med. Chem., 22(1979)784.
15 W.-J. Streich, S. Dove and R. Franke, J. Med. Chem., 23(1980)1452.
16 M.J. Box and N.R. Draper, Technometrics, 13(1971)682.
17 N.R. Draper and H.Smith, Applied Regression Analysis, Wiley, New York, 1966.
18 T.J. Mitchell, Technometrics, 16(1974)203.
19 C. Hansch, S.H. Unger and A.B. Forsythe, J. Med. Chem., 16(1973)1217.
20 R. Wootton, R. Cranfield, G.C. Sheppey and P.J. Goodford, J. Med. Chem., 18 (1975)607.
21 P.J. Goodford, A.T. Hudson, G.C. Sheppey, R. Wootton, M.M. Blank, G.J. Sutherland and J.C. Wickham, J. Med. Chem., 19(1976)1239.
22 W.J. Dunn, M.G. Greenberg and S.S. Callojas, J. Med. Chem., 19(1976)1299.
23 K.J. Shah and E.A. Coats, J. Med. Chem., 20(1977)1001.
24 R.Cranfield, P.J. Goodford, F.E. Norrington and W.H.G. Richards, Brit. J. Pharmac., 52(1974)87.
25 Y.C. Martin, J. Med. Chem., 24(1981)229.
26 R. Franke, W.-J. Streich and S. Dove,in E. Knoll and F. Darvas (Eds.), Chemical Structure - Biological Activity Relationships, Akadémia Kiadó, Budapest, 1980, p.153.
27 R. Franke, in A. Simkins (Ed.), Medicinal Chemistry VI, Cotswold Press, Oxford, 1979, p.237.
28 S.Dove, W.-J. Streich and R. Franke, J. Med. Chem., 23(1980)1456.
29 C. Hansch, in J.A. Keverling Buisman (Ed.), Biological Activity and Chemical Structure, Elsevier, Amsterdam, 1977, pp.47 and 287.
30.S.H. Unger, cited in Y.C. Martin, Drug Design Methods: A Critical Introduction, Marcell Dekker, New York, 1978.
31 H.H. Harman, Modern Factor Analysis, 2nd edition, Univ. of Chicago Press, Chicago, 1967.
32 P.A.J. Janssen, in J.A. Keverling Buisman (Ed.), Biological Activity and Chemical Structure, Elsevier, Amsterdam, 1977, p.37.
33 A. Barth and R. Franke, in F. Coulston and I. Korte (Eds.), Pesticides, EQS Suppl. Vol. III, Georg-Thieme-Verlag, Stuttgart, 1975, p.467.
34 A. Barth, R. Franke and D. Börnert, Pharmazie, 31(1976)100.
35 A. Barth, R. Franke and M. Orlick, in R. Franke and P. Oehme (Eds.), Quantitative Structure-Activity Analysis, Akademie-Verlag, Berlin, 1978, p.395.
36 A. Barth and R. Franke, in P. Oehme (Ed.), Theoretische Aspekte der Wirkstofforschung, VEB Verlag Volk und Gesundheit, Berlin, 1978.
37 R. Hagemann, R. Franke and A. Barth, paper presented at the 17th Congress of the Society of Pharmacology and Toxicology of the GDR, Berlin, 1975.
38 R. Franke and A. Barth, Proceedings of the second Conference on Plant Growth Regulators, Akademie-Verlag, Sofia, 1977, p.314.
39 K. Schmidt, H.-J. Michel, R. Franke and A. Barth, in R. Franke and P. Oehme (Eds.), Quantitative Structure-Activity Analysis, Akademie-Verlag, Berlin, 1978, p.417.
40 A.J. Stuper, W.E. Brügger and P.C. Jurs, Computer Assisted Studies of Chemical Structure and Biological Function, Wiley, New York etc., 1979.
41 C. Albano, W. Dunn, U. Edlund, E. Johansson, B. Nordén, M. Sjöström and S. Wold, Anal. Chim. Acta Comp. Tech. und Optim., 2(1978)429.
42 S. Dove, R. Franke, O.L. Mndshojan, W.A. Schkuljev and and L.W. Chashakian, J. Med. Chem., 22(1979)90.
43 H. Ruschig, G. Korger, H. Aumüller, H. Wagner and R. Weyer, Arzneim.-Forsch., 8(1958)448.
44 H. Ruschig, G. Korger, W. Aumüller, H. Wagner and R. Weyer, Medizin u. Chemie, 6(1958)61.
45 S. Richman, J. Med. Chem., 20(1977)469.
46 V.E. Golender and A.B. Rozenblit, in E.J. Ariens (Ed.), Drug Design, Vol. IX, Academic Press, New York etc., 1980, p.300.
47 S. Hübel, T. Rösner and R. Franke, Pharmazie, 35(1980)424.

48 R. Franke, Tables Rondes Roussel Uclaf, 38(1980)20.
49 K. Enslein and P.N. Craig, J. Environ. Pathol. Toxicol., 2(1978)115.
50 M. Waldrop, Chem. Eng. News, 57(1979)29.
51 J. Tinker, J. Chem. Inf. Comput. Sci., 21(1981)3.
52 R.F. Rekker, TIPS, 2(1980)1.
53 P.P. Mager, in E.J. Ariens (Ed.), Drug Design, Vol. IX, Academic Press, New York, 1980, p.187.
54 P.J. Lewi, in E.J. Ariens (Ed.), Drug Design, Vol. VII, Academic Press, New York, 1976, p.209.
55 R. Franke, A. Barth, S. Dove and W. Laass, Pharmazie,35(1980)181.
56 I. Lukovits and A. Lopata, J. Med. Chem., 23(1980)449.
57 P.J. Lewi, W.F.M. van Berger and P.A.J. Janssen, Eur. J. Pharmacol.,35(1976)403.
58 A. Cammarata and G.K. Menon, J. Med. Chem., 19(1976)739.
59 G.K. Menon and A. Cammarata, J. Pharm. Sci., 66(1977)304.
60 W. Laass, D. Modersohn and E. Scheer, in J. Knoll and F. Darvas (Eds.), Chemical Structure - Biological Activity Relationships, Akadémiai Kiadó, Budapest, 1980, p.165.
61 E.J. Ariens and R. De Miranda, in F. Gualtieri, M. Gianella and C. Melchiorre (Eds.), Recent Advances in Receptor Chemistry, Elsevier, Amsterdam, 1979.
62 L. Terenius, J. Pharm. Pharmac.,26(1974)146.
63 G. Krause, W.-J. Streich and R. Franke, Pharmazie, 35(1980)488.
64 G. Krause, W.-J. Streich and R. Franke, in J. Knoll and F. Darvas (Eds.), Chemical Structure - Biological Activity Relationships, Akadémiai Kiadó, Budapest, 1980, p.145.
65 G. Krause, R. Franke and G.N. Vassilev, Biochem. Physiol. Pflanzen, 174(1979)128.
66 C. Hansch, in J.A. Keverling Buisman (Ed.), Biological Activity and Chemical Structure, Elsevier, Amsterdam, 1977, p.47.
67 C. Hansch and D. F. Calef, J. Org. Chem., 41(1976)1240.
68 C. Hansch, R.N. Smith, A. Rockoff, D.F. Calef, P.Y.C. Jow and J.Y. Fukunaga, Arch. Biochem. Biophys., 183(1977)383.
69 C.L. Johnson and J.P. Green, Int. J. Quantum. Chem., QBS, 1(1974)159.
70 R. Franke, in J.A. Keverling Buisman (Ed.), Biological Activity and Chemical Structure, Elsevier, Amsterdam, 1977, p.251.
71 C.Hansch, Progr. Photosynthesis Res., 3(1969)1685.
72 A. Trebst and E. Harth, Naturforsch., 29c(1974)232.
73 M. Kuchař, in R. Franke and P. Oehme (Eds.), Quantitative Structure-Activity Analysis, Akademie-Verlag, Berlin, 1978, contribution to general discussion, p.449.
74 F.J. Zeelen, in R. Franke and P. Oehme (Eds.), Quantitative Structure-Activity Analysis, Akademie-Verlag, Berlin, 1978, contribution to general discussion, p.440.
75 J.A. Wohl, in L.B. Kier (Ed.), Molecular Orbital Studies in Chemical Pharmacology, Springer, New York, 1970, p.262.
76 A. Aranda, C.R. Acad.Sci., 276(1973)1301.
77 J.G. Topliss and M.D. Yudis, J. Med. Chem., 15(1972)394
78 B. Rouot, G. Leclerc, C.G. Wermuth and F. Miesch, J. Pharmac.,8(1977)95
79 Y.C. Martin, W.B. Martin and J.D. Taylor, J. Med. Chem., 18(1975)883.
80 R.W. Fuller, M.M. Marsh and J.J. Mills, J. Med. Chem., 11(1968)397.
81 Y.C. Martin and J.H. Biel, in E. Usdin (Ed.), Neuropsychopharmacology of Monoamines and their Regulatory Enzymes, Raven Press, New York, 1974, p.37.
82 Y.C. Martin, Quantitative Drug Design, Marcell Dekker, New York, 1978.
83 N.Kakeya, M. Aoki, A. Kamada and N. Yata, Chem. Pharm. Bull., 17(1969)1010.
84 W.P. Purcell, Biochim. Biophys. Acta, 105(1965)201.
85 J.C. Beasley and W.P. Purcell, Biochim. Biophys. Acta, 178(1969)175.
86 G. Grieco, C. Silipo, A. Vittorio and C. Hansch, J. Med. Chem.,20(1977)586.
87 C. Hansch, M. Yoshimoto and M.H. Doll, J. Med. Chem., 19(1976)1068.
88 D.L.Lee, P.A. Kollman, F.J. Marsh and M.E. Wolff, J. Med. Chem., 20(1977)1139.
89 M. Pozsgay, R. Gaspar, J. Beejusz and P. Elodi, Eur. J. Biochem., 95(1979)115.
90 T. Rösner, K. Türschman, R. Franke, D. Schönfelder and S. Unger, paper presented at the 17th Congress of the Pharmacological Society of the GDR, Berlin, 1975.
91 R. Franke, D. Labes, M. Tonew, W. Zschiesche and L. Heinisch, Acta Biol. Med. Germ., 34(1975)491.

92 K.C. Chu, R.J. Feldmann, M.B. Shapiro, G.F. Hazard and R.I. Geran, J. Med. Chem., 18(1975)539.
93 W.J. Wechter, M.A. Johnson, C.M. Hall, D.T. Warner, A.E. Berger, H.A. Wenzel, D.T. Gish and G.L. Neil, J. Med. Chem., 18(1975)339.
94 J.L. Montero and J.L. Imbach, C.R. Acad. Sci. Ser. C279(1974)809.
95 W.A. Remers and C.S. Schepman, J. Med. Chem., 17(1974)729.
96 G.W. Peng, V.E. Marquez and J.S. Driscoll, J. Med. Chem., 18(1975)846.
97 F.R. Quinn, J.S. Driscoll and C. Hansch, J. Med. Chem., 18(1975)332.
98 J.K. Seydel and E. Wempe, Arzneimittel-Forsch., 21(1971)187.
99 J.K. Seydel and K.-J. Schaper, Chemische Struktur und biologische Aktivität von Wirkstoffen, Verlag Chemie, Weinheim, 1979.
100 J.P.Dirmla, L.J. Czuba, B.W. Doming, R.B. James, R.M. Pezullo, J.E. Presslitz and R.M. Windisch, J. Med. Chem., 22(1979)1118.
101 C. Hansch and J. Fukunaga, Chem. Technol., 7(1977)120.
102 Y.C. Martin, T.M. Bustard and K.R. Lynn, J. Med. Chem., 16(1973)1089.
103 P.J. Goodford and F.E. Norrington, in M. Tichý (Ed.), Quantitative Structure-Activity Relationships, Akadémia Kiadó, Budapest, 1976, p.79.
104 P.J. Goodford, F.E. Norrington, W. Richards and L.P. Walls, Br. J. Pharmac., 48(1973)650.
105 W. Dittmar, E. Druckrey and H. Urbach, J. Med. Chem., 17(1974)753.
106 E. Druckrey and W. Dittmar, in M. Tichý (Ed.), Quantitative Structure-Activity relationships, Akadémiai Kiadó, Budapest, 1976, p.59.
107 A.F. Yapel Jr., Adv. in Chemistry Series, 114(1972)183.
108 F.F. Yapel Jr., Adv. in Chemistry Series, 114(1972)252.
109 R. Franke and E. Gäbler, unpublished results.
110 D. Schönfelder and R. Franke, unpublished results.
111 S. Scholz, H. Sprinz, R. Hagemann, R. Franke, G. Hübner and A. Barth, Pharmazie, 31(1976)162.
112 L.K.Gibbons, E.F. Koldenboven, A.A. Nethery, R.E. Montgomery and W.P. Purcell, J. Agr. Food Chem., 24(1976)203.
113 P.S. Magee, ACS Symposium Series, 112(1979)319.
114 E. Druckrey, H. Schwarz and H. Leditschke,Chim. Ther., 7(1972)188.
115 H.Cousse, C. Mouzin and L.D. d'Hinterland, Chim. Ther., 4(1973)466.
116 J.J.Kaufman and W.S. Koski, Int. J. Quantum Chem.: QBS 2(1975)35.
117 H. Weinstein, S. Maayani, S. Srebenik, J. Cohen and M. Sokolovsky, Mol. Pharmacol 9(1973)820.
118 H. Weinstein, Int. J. Quantum Chem.: QBS 2(1975)59.
119 M. Kuchař, in J. Knoll and F. Darvas (Eds.), Chemical Structure-Biological Activity Relationships Akadémia Kiadó, Budapest, 1980, p.15.
120 J.P. Tollenaere, H. Moereels and M. Protiva, Eur. J. Med. Chem., 11(1976)298.
121 R. Rouot, G. Leclerc, C.G. Wermuth, F. Miersch and J. Schwatz, J. Med. Chem., 19(1976)1049.
122 E.C. Jorgensen and J.A. Reid, J. Med. Chem., 8(1965)533.
123 G.E. Bass, W.H. Lawrence, W.P. Purcell and U. Autrian, J. Dent. Res., 53(1974) 756.
124 K. Enslein, Genesee Statistik Newsletter, 6(1978)714.
125 E.A. Coats, S.R. Milstein, G. Holbein, J. McDonald, R. Reed and H.G. Petering J. Med. Chem., 19(1976)131.
126 R.D. Cramer, K.M. Snader, C.R. Willis, L.W. Chakrin, J. Thomas and B.M. Sutton, J. Med. Chem., 22(1979)714.
127 B.J. Broughton, P. Chaplin, P. Knowles, E. Lunt, S.M. Marshall, D.L. Pain and K.R.H. Woolridge, J. Med. Chem., 18(1975)1117.
128 J. Fernandez, G. Grassy, A. Terol, Y. Robbe, P. Chapar, R. Granger and H. Sentena Roumanou, Eur. J. Med. Chem., 13(1978)245.
129 K. Bowden and R.C. Young, J. Med. Chem., 13(1970)225.
130 L.B Kier and L.H. Hall, J. Pharm. Sci., 67(1978)1408.
131 R.A. Glennon, L.B. Kier and A.T. Shulgin, J. Pharm. Sci., 68(1979)906.
132 A.J. Hopfinger, J. Am. Chem. Soc., 102(1980)7196.
133 F. Darvas, in J. Knoll and F. Darvas (Eds.), Chemical Structure-Biological Activity Relationships, Adadémia Kiadó, Budapest, 1980, p.25.

134 H.J. Henkel, V. Hagen, A. Hagen, I. Schimke and A. Barth, in J. Knoll and F. Darvas (Eds.), Chemical Structure-Biological Activity Relationships, Akademia Kiadó, Budapest, 1980, p.25.
135 J.P. Green, H. Weinstein and S. Maayani, NIDA Res. Monograph, 25(1978)38.
136 P. Gund, Science, 208(1980)1425.
137 C. Humblet and G. Marshall, Tables Rondes Roussel Uclaf, 38(1980)38.
138 S.A. Hiller, V.E. Golender, A.B. Rosenblit, R.S. Sturkovich and E.Ya. Lukevic, Kim.-Farm. Zh., 10(1976)29.
139 J.K. Seydel and K.-J. Schaper, in J.A. Keverling Buisman (Ed.), Strategy in Drug Design, Elsevier, Amsterdam, 1981.

J.A. Keverling Buisman (Editor), *Strategy in Drug Research*



# SOME ASPECTS OF A QSAR ANALYSIS OF TRIMETHOPRIM ANALOGUES

R.M. HYDE
Wellcome Research Laboratories, Beckenham, Kent, England, and
B. ROTH
Burroughs Wellcome Co., Research Triangle Park, North Carolina, U.S.A.

## INTRODUCTION

It has long been established that the anti-bacterial action of Trimethoprim (TMP); 2,4-diamino-5-(3,4,5-trimethoxybenzyl)-pyrimidine, is attributable to its inhibitory activity on the enzyme dihydrofolate reductase (DHFR) (1,2,3). Specific inhibition of bacterial rather than mammalian DHFR is an important characteristic of TMP. A QSAR study has been undertaken using data available for a series of analogues of TMP in which substitution in the benzene ring is varied. The objective of this study was to identify those substituents associated with high inhibition which are specific for bacterial DHFR and to interpret this association in terms of the physico-chemical properties of the substituents. Attention has been focussed on data for just one bacterial enzyme, E.coli DHFR, and one mammalian enzyme, DHFR from rat liver. Similar studies have been described by Hansch et al., who have compared inhibition of E.coli DHFR with inhibition of bovine liver DHFR(4-12). In those, and the present studies, QSAR appears in the role of a technique for probing the nature of the interactions between enzyme and inhibitors.

The techniques of QSAR were originally most often applied to biological data obtained at the level of complexity of the cell or above. The concept of a series of compounds, equiactive on the ultimate biological target, but differing in their ease of access to the target represents the classical view of QSAR. Processes such as membrane transport are, it seems, often interpretable in terms of substituent hydrophobicity, and the optimum compound - having the best transport properties -can often be predicted. Thus there is an understandable tendency to regard the QSAR approach as a method which is restricted to improving the distributive properties of a set of compounds. In the context of anti-bacterial design, QSAR would naturally be considered as an approach to the interpretation of data relating to the inhibition of growth of whole cells. However, the present discussion has been confined to a consideration of the application of QSAR in the design of compounds at the enzyme level, using $I_{50}$ values as an expression of inhibitory activity.

*References p. 409*

An important pre-requisite to any QSAR study is that the range of substituents as exemplified in the data set is associated with an acceptable level of variation in biological activity. It is obvious that a QSAR study of an enzyme-inhibitor system would be of potential value, but only if the nature of the substituents affected receptor binding as well as transport. In the case of TMP analogues, the effect of substituents on the $I_{50}$ values is considerable, as shown by the examples in Table I.

TABLE I

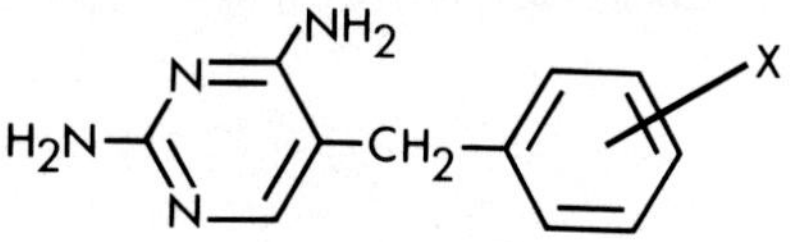

| SUBSTITUENT | E.COLI DHFR $I_{50} \times 10^8$, M | RAT LIVER DHFR $I_{50} \times 10^8$, M | REFERENCES |
|---|---|---|---|
| H | 340 | 15000 | (3,13,14) |
| 3-$OC_6H_5$ | 48 | 450 | (15) |
| 3,4,5-$OMe_3$ | 0.56 | 34560 | (1,16,17) |

These three compounds alone cover a range of between two and three orders of magnitude for bacterial $I_{50}$, nearly two orders of magnitude for the mammalian $I_{50}$ and more than three orders of magnitude for relative potency. The direct involvement of benzene ring substituents is therefore clearly indicated and the case for a physico-chemical interpretation is strong. If such an interpretation proves possible, then the "probing" of a receptor by QSAR becomes an important complement to approaches to drug design based on a knowledge of the crystalline structure of the enzyme.

Perhaps the most important conceptual difference between QSAR of this type and QSAR involving transport processes lies in the extent to which the substituents have their effect directly. "Classically", QSAR theory accounts for the effects of substituents in terms of their indirect contribution to a whole molecule property such as bulk, partition coefficient, or degree of ionisation. In the context of enzyme inhibition data, a direct interaction between substituent and biological macromolecule would also be considered. The effects would be essentially localised. In the following, we have limited our study to the effects of changing the substitution pattern in the benzene nucleus only.

## The Analysis-Preliminary Considerations

The $I_{50}$ data available for both E.coli and Rat Liver DHFR encompassed more than 200 compounds. At the time of analysis the series was already highly developed - a fact which posed some special problems in QSAR analysis. Firstly, the development of the series had naturally been accompanied by an increasing representation of the "successful" substituent groups. However, the objective of the analysis was not merely to identify the active compounds but to interpret their activity in physico-chemical terms so as to give relationships which could be used predictively. In order, therefore, to understand what it was that made substituent patterns such as 3,4,5 trimethoxy so effective, it was necessary to compare them with the less successful compounds, which were not so well represented in the data set as a whole. In general, the approach to well-conditioned data sets was made with the help of a programme known as SELECT. The purpose of this programme was (1) to provide the analyst with a representation of the distribution of individual compounds in each of a chosen set of physico-chemical parameters and (2) to provide interparameter correlations. The form of the programme allowed the effect of each new compound on the "condition" of the existing set to be scrutinised prior to making a decision about its inclusion. Thus compounds chosen by the analyst (by whatever criteria) could be conveniently assessed in terms of effect on spread and orthogonality.(18)

A second major problem arose from the fact that compounds having good specific activity for E.coli DHFR were generally tri-substituted. Successful QSAR depends on the confident prediction of physicochemical properties. However, for compounds such as TMP, which have three adjacent substituents, an estimate of, for example, hydrophobicity from positional $\pi$ constants is subject to error through intersubstituent interactions. Thus, measured values of log P would be desirable for such compounds.

Within the data set as a whole, therefore, the singly-substituted compounds were particularly suitable for a first approach to analysis, since parameter values could be more confidently assigned. The representation of substituent types was also better than for the totality of compounds. The use of compounds with relatively lower inhibitory activity also carried the advantage that differences in activity were more accurately reflected by the $I_{50}$ values. However, the concern was that since they were, as a group, so much less active than the tri-substituted analogues, they may not even provide a model for substituent effects in the more active series. Indeed it was ultimately found that those respects in which the mono-substituted failed to model trends observed for trisubstituted compounds gave an important clue to the interpretation of the bacterial enzyme data.

Examination of the total data set had consistently shown the importance of the 3-substituent position in determining activity against both mammalian and bacterial DHFR. These findings are consistent with the work of Hansch et al. The present treatment is specifically concerned with an examination of effects at the 3-position and the analysis begins with a series of compounds (TABLE II) having a single substituent in this position. Compounds having long and flexible substituents were not included in Table II, since their conformations would be subject to ambiguity. Parameter values were taken from refs. (19-21).

TABLE II

Mono substituted meta compounds (2,4-diamino-5-(3-substituted-benzyl)pyrimidines).

| Substituent | E.coli $I_{50} \times 10^8$,M | Rat Liver $I_{50} \times 10^8$,M | References |
|---|---|---|---|
| H | 340 | 15000 | (3,13,14) |
| I | 13.7 | 1950 | (22) |
| OEt | 45 | 2800 | (23) |
| OPh | 48 | 450 | (15) |
| OMe | 49 | 4300 | (1) |
| Br | 50 | 2300 | (24) |
| CN | 71 | 18000 | (25) |
| Cl | 93 | 2600 | (24) |
| Me | 160 | 18000 | (25) |
| $NMe_2$ | 37 | 14200 | (25) |
| F | 385 | 8800 | (24) |
| OnPr | 34 | 1730 | (25) |

## Analysis

The compounds in Table II are substituted at the 3-position only. Their inhibitory activities against E.coli DHFR and rat liver DHFR are expressed as $I_{50}$ values. In Table III an indication is given of the distribution of compounds in each of the physico-chemical dimensions; $\pi$,F,R and MR. The interparameter correlation matrix shows a potential problem in the correlation between $\pi$ and MR (r = 0.706). However, the compound set exemplifies an acceptable range of chemical types and the results of a preliminary analysis are shown in Table IV.

TABLE III

Spread and orthogonality of all compounds in Table II.

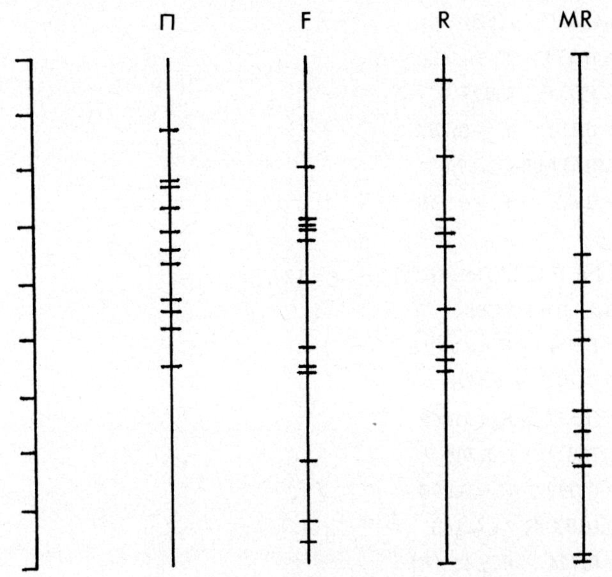


| | π | F | R | MR |
|---|---|---|---|---|
| π | 1.000 | 0.194 | -0.127 | 0.706 |
| F | | 1.000 | 0.291 | 0.062 |
| R | | | 1.000 | -0.439 |
| MR | | | | 1.000 |

TABLE IV

Single Term Regression Equations for mono meta substituted compounds of Table II (numbers in parentheses are 95% confidence limits, F (below each equation) is variance ratio).

a) $Log_{10}\ 1/I_{50}$ E.coli ENZYME (Ece) n = 12

$$Ece = 0.438\ (\pm\ 0.191)\pi - 2.132$$

$$r = 0.586 \quad F = 5.237$$

$$Ece = 0.530\ (\pm\ 0.416)\ F - 2.120$$

$$r = 0.373 \quad F = 1.620$$

$$Ece = -0.434\ (\pm 1.357)\ R - 1.927$$

$$r = 0.101 \quad F = 0.102$$

$$Ece = 0.034\ (\pm\ 0.014)\ MR - 2.194$$

$$r = 0.623 \quad F = 6.338$$

b) $Log_{10}\ I_{50}$ RAT LIVER ENZYME (Rle) n = 12

$$Rle = -0.875\ (\pm\ 0.108)\pi + 4.188$$

$$r = 0.931 \quad F = 65.052$$

$$Rle = -0.709\ (\pm\ 0.518)\ F + 4.008$$

$$r = 0.397 \quad F = 1.869$$

$$Rle = 0.535\ (\pm\ 1.708)\ R + 3.746$$

$$r = 0.099 \quad F = 0.098$$

$$Rle = -0.050\ (\pm\ 0.015)MR + 4.148$$

$$r = 0.726 \quad F = 11.141$$

The equation of highest significance is that which relates rat liver enzyme activity to $\pi_3$. For the E.coli enzyme data the correlation with $MR_3$, although nominally the best, is unconvincing. It is clear, however, that for both enzymes, the bulk/steric (MR) and hydrophobic ( $\pi$ ) properties of a single 3-substituent are more important than the electronic properties as expressed by F and R. It is particularly important to distinguish between the effects described by $\pi$ and those described by MR since there is a suggestion that this distinction may be associated with specificity. On the basis of this preliminary analysis it might be inferred that the substitution of a hydrophilic group in the 3-position would minimise the mammalian enzyme activity without necessarily affecting the bacterial enzyme activity. In order to determine whether physicochemical criteria for specificity can be identified two questions must be answered. The first of these concerns the significance which can be attached to the apparent superiority of the $\pi_3$ equation, for rat liver enzyme activity, over the equation in $MR_3$. The second concerns the interpretation of the E.Coli enzyme data - specifically whether the $MR_3$ equation provides even a basis for further interpretation.

The tendency for $\pi$ and MR to be correlated is an often-encountered problem in QSAR studies. A discussion of the physical significance of the close relationship between these descriptors is not appropriate at this stage although they should perhaps always be seen as two ends of an overlapping scale. For the data set in Table II the correlation between MR and $\pi$ ($r = 0.706$), although acceptable under some circumstances, is higher than desirable when separation of the two effects is sought. An attempt was made, using the programme SELECT, to reduce this correlation while retaining acceptable spread in physicochemical properties. A subset of compounds has been derived in which the correlation has been reduced to 0.474 and the relevant data are shown in Table V. Regression analysis on this data set, chosen specifically to separate $\pi$ and MR reinforces the previous conclusions and the results are shown in Table VI.

TABLE V

Spread and orthogonality of SELECT subset of monosubstituted compounds of Table II (omitting H, OEt, Br and OPh).

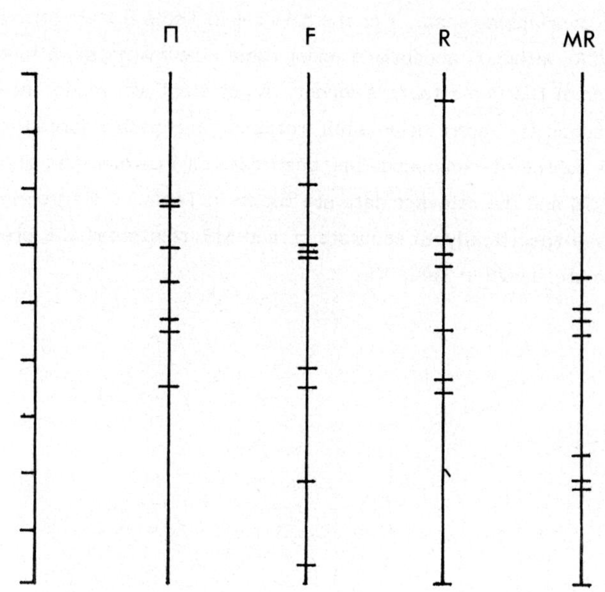


| | Π | F | R | MR |
|---|---|---|---|---|
| Π | 1.000 | -0.086 | -0.050 | 0.474 |
| F | | 1.000 | 0.522 | -0.311 |
| R | | | 1.000 | -0.496 |
| MR | | | | 1.000 |

TABLE VI

Single Term Regression Equations for "SELECT" Set.

a) $Log_{10}$ $1/I_{50}$ E.coli ENZYME (Ece) n = 8

$Ece = 0.453\ (\pm\ 0.294)\pi - 2.089$

$r = 0.533 \quad F = 2.375$

$Ece = 0.245\ (\pm\ 0.580)\,F - 1.994$

$r = 0.170 \quad F = 0.179$

$Ece = 0.338\ (\pm 1.608)\,R - 1.842$

$r = 0.085 \quad F = 0.044$

$Ece = 0.053\ (\pm\ 0.023)\,MR - 2.300$

$r = 0.682 \quad F = 5.215$

b) $Log_{10}$ $I_{50}$ RAT LIVER ENZYME (Rle) n = 8

$Rle = -0.760\ (\pm\ 0.160)\pi + 4.183$

$r = 0.888 \quad F = 22.463$

$Rle = -0.445\ (\pm\ 0.563)\,F + 4.040$

$r = 0.307 \quad F = 0.625$

$Rle = -0.0089\ (\pm\ 1.623)\,R + 3.832$

$r = 0.002 \quad F = 0.000$

$Rle = -0.034(\pm\ 0.028)\,MR + 4.108$

$r = 0.444 \quad F = 1.472$

A formal analysis, in which linear correlations were assessed between the two enzyme activities and each of the parameters, $\pi$ ,F, R and MR, has led therefore to the following conclusions. Rat liver enzyme activity is best correlated with the hydrophobicity of the 3-substituent. E.coli enzyme activity, like the mammalian activity is independent of F and R, but is not well correlated with $\pi_3$. For E.coli enzyme activity, the equation in $MR_3$ is nominally the best although it is far from convincing. Thus an association between hydrophilicity of the 3-substituent and specificity is evident, but a physicochemical description of criteria for anti-bacterial potency is not clear. The broad conclusions at this stage are consistent with the work of Hansch et al. The correlation equation between E.coli enzyme activity and $MR_3$, although of low significance, was nevertheless taken as a basis for the further development of the QSAR analysis which is described in the following section.

## DISCUSSION

In an attempt to determine whether there was any foundation to the possible relationship between E.coli enzyme and $MR_3$, the following five possibilities were considered.

1) That it is simply not possible to interpret the variation in activity in terms of $\pi$, F, R, MR or any other plausible, physicochemical substituent constant. This would suggest that binding interactions involving the 3-substituent were too specific to each member of the series to be accountable in terms of a systematic relationship. This would be in contrast to the situation for the rat liver enzyme, where the principal variation in binding was seen in terms of substituent hydrophobicity. This would mean that anti-bacterial activity was unpredictable.

2) That there is an overall correlation which, if recognised, would be a useful predictive tool, but which is obscured by "outlier" points. This danger is always present if correlations are assessed merely on the basis of computed correlation coefficients and not graphically. Indeed the identification and interpretation of outliers to a general trend can be most important in this type of analysis.

3) If the "outliers" are numerous and systematic, they may be interpretable in terms of a second physicochemical parameter. The significance of two (and higher-) term equations can be tested by regression analysis. Multiple equations, although harder to rationalise physically, can nevertheless be useful predictively.

4) Mathematical modelling suggests that non-linear relationships can often be expected in QSAR analyses (26,27). Whether a "model-based" equation or a purely empirical one is used, an apparently uncorrelated data set can often be interpreted if the "linear" assumption is abandoned. This reinforces the case for graphical inspection of the data.

5) The last option to be considered is that a suggested "correlation" of low apparent significance may reflect an approach to a true interpretation which is masked by the inadequacy of the physicochemical parameter. By this, it is not intended to suggest artefacts, but merely that the chosen parameter is based on a model system which is only partially relevant to the biological system. This is especially likely for steric/bulk relationships where the term MR, commonly used as a first approximation, must be regarded as no more than a compromise candidate. A correlation with a steric/bulk term could have so many physical meanings that it is inconceivable that a single descriptor could be adequate. Hence, a mere suggestion of a correlation with MR should always be pursued further.

For a biological system in which transport is relevant, it is quite reasonable to expect that biological activity will be less for the bulkier members of a series which are less able to diffuse to the site of action. In such a case, MR or even Molecular Weight may be an adequate descriptor. In the present context, a suggestion of the importance of bulk at a particular position implies a fit to a specific site on the receptor. Such a site is unlikely to be completely tolerant of the shape of the interacting group and hence an expression of steric rather than pure bulk effects will be required for an adequate interpretation of the data. Nevertheless a term such as MR should be of use in alerting the analyst to the true situation.

In Fig. 1 a plot is shown of E.coli enzyme activity against MR.

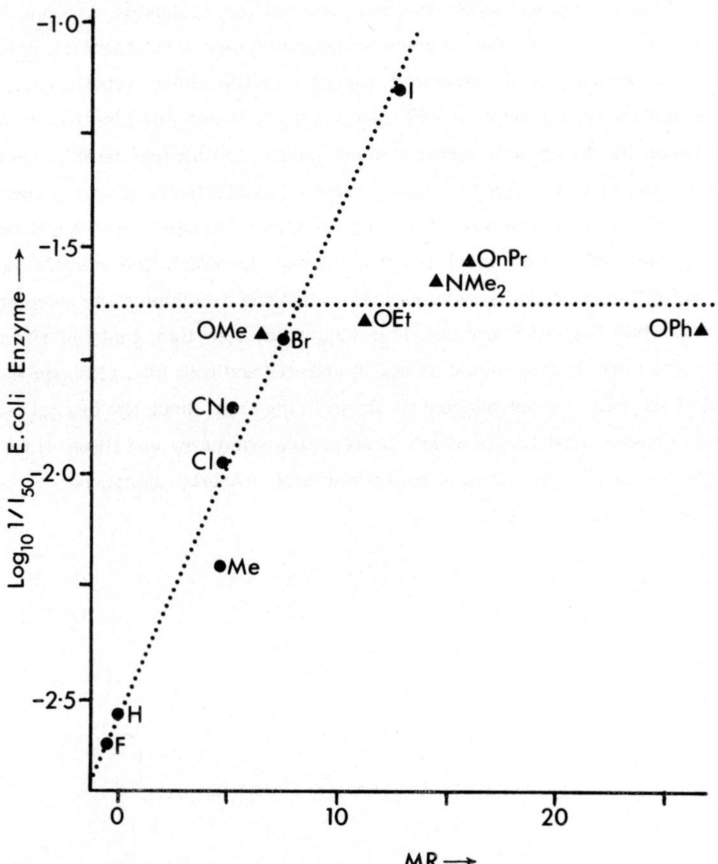


**Figure 1** Plot of $\log_{10}$ $1/I_{50}$ E.coli enzyme versus MR for symmetrical (●) mono meta substituents and asymmetrical (▲) mono meta substituents of Table II (see text).

Firstly, it is clear that hope of finding a systematic relationship should not be abandoned. Secondly, it does not appear that an underlying relationship is being obscured by one or two inexplicable outlier points. The possibility of a nonlinear relationship must be considered. Data in the form log (1/(effective concentration) ) would be expected to correlate with a physicochemical parameter in a non-linear form providing the parameter was in the form of log (equilibrium constant). For a relationship with a descriptor such as MR, which expresses pure size, a non linear relationship is, in the limit, almost inevitable. For a given cavity on the receptor, the binding contribution of a substituent would be expected to increase until its size approached that of the cavity, after which a plateau or a decline would be anticipated. An effect of this kind is suggested by the data although it is not on its own sufficient to interpret the data.

Inspection of the data to see whether systematic outliers suggested a second term was encouraging at first sight. For the electron withdrawing halo-substituents, E.coli enzyme activity and $MR_3$ are very well correlated,whereas for the alkoxy substituents, activity appears to be almost independent of MR. However, it is not just electron-withdrawing substituents which lie in the well-correlated sub series, and indeed there is no evidence from regression analysis to suggest a second term in an electronic property such as F or R. However, there is a fundamental difference in shape between those substituents for which activity and $MR_3$ are correlated and those for which the correlation is not observed. The former are radially symmetrical around the axis joining the benzene ring to the substituent, while the latter are not. It is suggested, therefore, that the effectiveness of a 3-substituent may be determined by steric criteria and that MR, although expressing this for limited sub-sets, cannot adequately do so in general. Since the crucial difference appears to be between substituents which possess this symmetry and those which do not, then a parameter which expresses a conformational property orthogonal to the ring-substituent axis should be relevant.

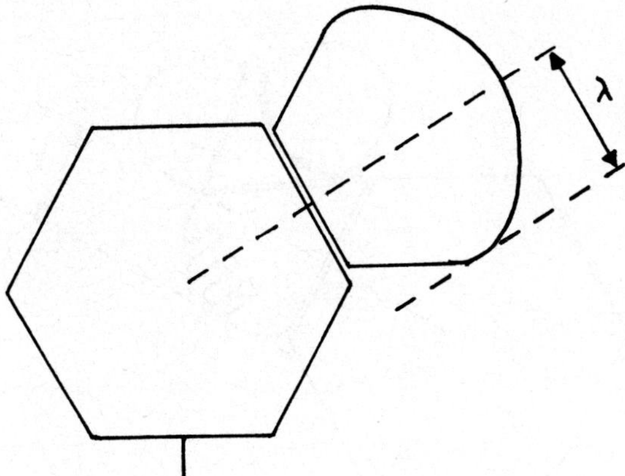


**Figure 2** Projection of CPK-model of 3-bromo compound.

In Fig 2 the distance, λ, represents a projection in the plane of the benzene ring and runs perpendicular to the axis of attachment for the 3-substituents. For a substituent such as this, λ can readily be calculated. However, for an alkoxy group, free to rotate, it is ambiguous (Fig 3). On a dynamic model, a time-averaged distance could be assigned and this would be intermediate between the maximum and minimum values derived on a static model. It is proposed that the effective capacity of a substituent to fill space in the direction indicated by λ is associated with activity against E.coli enzyme. (28) A clear difference exists between symmetrical substituents, such as iodo and those such as the rotating methoxy, whose space filling properties would change as interaction with a cavity in a binding site takes place. Repulsive forces would tend to constrain the methoxy substituent towards that part of its locus of rotation where they were minimised. In the limit, that point would be reached where no further compression could occur - ie. the effective λ-dimension of the group would be equivalent to the minimum as seen on a static model. This minimum does not vary through the alkoxy series - which is consistent with the trend observed for the biological activity.

*References p. 409*

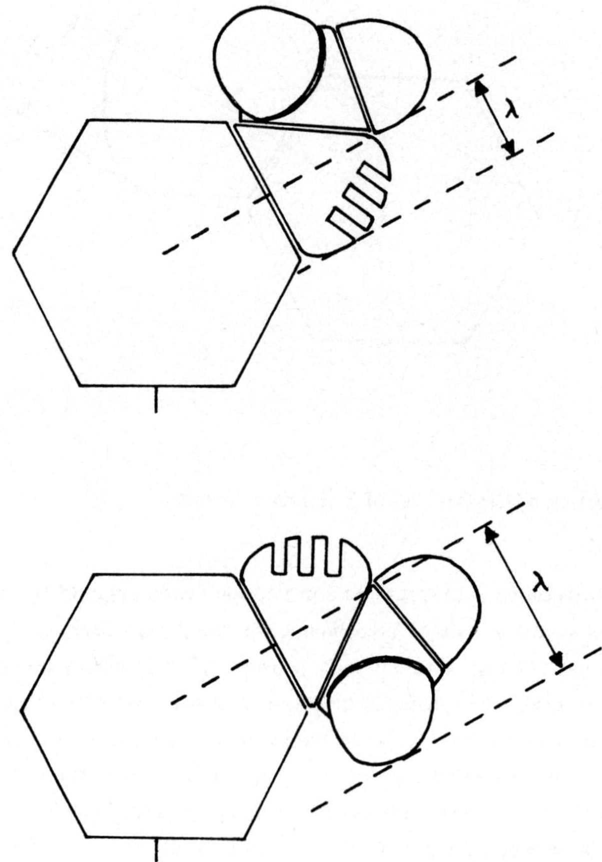


**Figure 3** Projection of CPK model of 3-methoxy compound in two extreme positions (minimum and maximum λ).

At this stage, closer examination of a QSAR relationship has led to the suggestion of a steric property which may be associated with activity. Ideally dynamic molecular mechanical calculations would be made for each substituted TMP analogue and from these, a quantity chosen as expressing the "sense" of $\lambda$ would be correlated with activity. However, such calculations are lengthy, and the essence of the QSAR approach is the ready availability of the physicochemical parameter. If the relevance of $\lambda$ could be established, to a first approximation, in terms of a pre-defined and accessible steric parameter, then the molecular mechanics could be embarked on with confidence. It was decided to attempt an interpretation using the STERIMOL system of Verloop et al.(29). $\lambda$, it was suggested, would be represented by the smallest of the "STERIMOL" "B" parameters. This would express the most pessimistic view of the group's ability to fill the desired space.

An important consequence of this hypothesis is that for 3-substituents such as methoxy, the presence of a 4-substituent would have an effect on $\lambda$. Inhibition of free rotation by an adjacent substituent would clearly increase the capacity of such a group to fill space in the desired direction (Fig 4.). In other words, the limit to which a substituent can be compressed is raised. Thus, a 3-methoxy group adjacent to a 4-substituent would be more effective than if it were on its own. The concept that it is both the environment and the nature of a 3-substituent which are important for activity is consistent with the considerable increase in activity observed when a 4-methoxy group is added to the 3,5-dimethoxy compound.

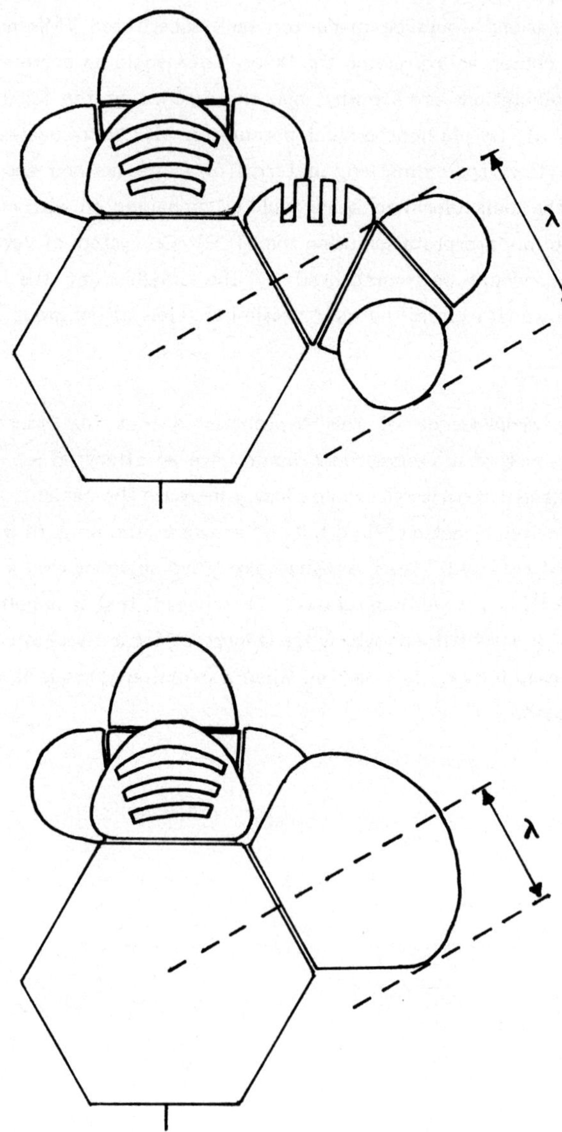


**Figure 4** Projection of CPK models of 3,4-dimethoxy and 3-bromo,4-methoxy compounds.

The 4-methoxy compound itself is relatively inactive and its contribution to the activity of TMP is therefore largely through its effect on the conformations of its neighbours. The case for regarding the entire substituent system as an interacting dynamic entity is strong, (28) but the time involved in calculating dimensions on this basis is considerable. However, for tri-substituted compounds, the STERIMOL system can again provide an appropriate parameter in the absence of rigorous conformational calculations. This has been exemplified for TMP analogues having substituents 3-OMe, 4-OMe, 5-X. For a data set containing compounds some of which have 4-substituents, the following rule is proposed to define the appropriate STERIMOL "B" value:

For a 3-substituent with no neighbour at the 4-position, the smallest STERIMOL "B" expresses $\lambda$. Where a 4-substituent is present, the "B" value opposite the smallest is used. The assumption is made that a non-symmetrical substituent would tend to present its smallest lateral dimension to a neighbouring group at the 4-position. Using this definition, it would be anticipated that the true $\lambda$ was underestimated for mono-substituted compounds, but was better defined for poly-substituted analogues. For the latter, an improvement over MR might be expected in the interpretation of the data.

One more factor must be accounted for in drawing up a list of parameter values. It is that the effect of a neighbouring substituent upon conformation can only extend a short distance from the ring. For example, (see Fig. 5), while a 4-substituent would have a pronounced effect on the methylene group of an ethoxy substituent, forcing it in the direction indicated by $\lambda$, the terminal methyl group would not be directly affected. Since, in the definition of the STERIMOL system, a substituent is assumed to be compressed lengthwise, allowance must be made for this discrepancy. Thus, the adjacent substitutent effect is only allowed for until the second atom. For example, the value of the required steric parameter for a higher alkoxy would be the same as for methoxy (see Table VII).

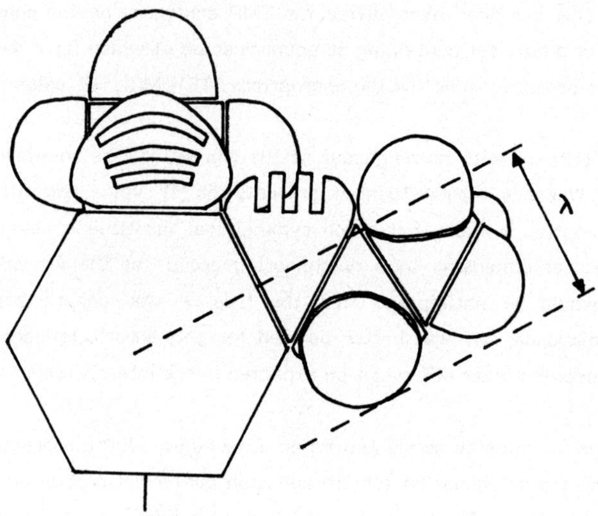


**Figure 5** Projection of CPK models of 3-ethoxy, 4-methoxy compound.

TABLE VII

Steric Parameter λ (based on STERIMOL)

| 3-substituent | Alone | Adjacent to 4-OMe |
|---|---|---|
| H | 1.00 | 1.00 |
| Me | 1.52 | 2.04 |
| Et | 1.52 | 2.97 |
| nPr | 2.04 | 2.76 |
| tBu | 2.59 | 2.97 |
| OH | 1.35 | 1.93 |
| OMe | 1.35 | 2.87 |
| OEt | 1.35 | 2.87 |
| OnPr | 1.35 | 2.87 |
| OiPr | 1.35 | 2.87 |
| OnBu | 1.35 | 2.87 |
| OtBu | 1.35 | 3.12 |
| OnAm | 1.35 | 2.87 |
| $NMe_2$ | 1.50 | 2.80 |
| COMe | 2.36 | 2.93 |
| CN | 1.60 | 1.60 |
| F | 1.35 | 1.35 |
| Cl | 1.80 | 1.80 |
| Br | 1.95 | 1.95 |
| I | 2.15 | 2.15 |

There are clearly limitations to this approach which must be borne in mind. Firstly, an attempt has been made to represent a dynamic and interactive system of substituents in terms of a static model. The distances derived from this model are projections in an arbitrarily chosen plane, that of the benzene ring, and represent only an approximation to the proposed space-filling property. Possibly more serious is the problem of the second meta substituent. Since the benzene ring is free to rotate relative to the pyrimidine, whose binding site is assumed fixed, then a cavity corresponding to a 3-substituent could equally well interact with an identical substituent in the other meta position (30). Thus the probability of binding is increased if both meta positions are substituted. Furthermore, the possibility of more than one cavity has to be considered so that, for two meta substituents, four possible interactions corresponding to two different whole molecule conformations may be important. Mathematical models for treating the general situation are complex, and it is for this reason that the present discussion is restricted to a trisubstituted series in which variation occurs at just one of the meta substituent positions. The assumption that the variable meta position substituent always interacts with the same cavity and that the contribution to binding of the meta methoxy group is constant has therefore been made.

This illustrates the point that in QSAR studies of this kind, the characteristics of the receptor are implicitly probed a piece at a time. The essential requirement is a fixed point of reference whose contribution to binding can be assumed constant and considerable. The evidence for this may be direct, e.g. through crystallographic binding studies or indirect, by virtue of the fact that this part of the molecule is essential for inhibition. When structural variation takes place at a position which is unambiguously known relative to this point of reference, then it is relatively easy to build up a picture of the part of the receptor corresponding to the point of variation.

In the present case, the simplifying assumption is made that there is a constant contribution to binding which is attributable to the 3-methoxy group and that this contribution is missing from the series in which just a single meta-substituent is present. A regression equation in which E.coli enzyme activity is correlated with the steric parameter expressing $\lambda$ , for the tri-substituted series is shown below. The data are taken from Table VIII.

TABLE VIII

| Substituent | E. coli DHFR $I_{50} \times 10^8$, M | References |
|---|---|---|
| I | 1.62 | (31) |
| OEt | 0.19 | (32) |
| OMe | 0.56 | (1, 16, 17) |
| Br | 2.0 | (1) |
| CN | 4.25 | (33) |
| Cl | 4.0 | (1, 14) |
| nPr | 0.39 | (32) |
| OnPr | 0.38 | (32) |
| OiPr | 0.5 | (33) |
| OH | 2.0 | (34) |

$\log 1/I_{50} = 0.859\ (\pm 0.090)\ \lambda - 2.03(\pm 0.217)$
$(r = 0.959 \qquad F = 91.05 \qquad n = 10\ )$

This equation expresses the dependence of $\log 1/I_{50}$ on $\lambda$ for the series 3,4-dimethoxy, 5X. The corresponding equation in MR is shown below:-

$\log 1/I_{50} = 0.063(\pm 0.024)MR - 0.598\ (\pm 0.255)$
$(r = 0.685 \qquad F = 7.07 \qquad n = 10)$

If an indicator variable, I, is used to express the contribution of the 3,4-dimethoxy groups, both series can be treated together (I = 0 for mono meta series, I = 1 for 3,4-dimethoxy, 5-X series).
$\log 1/I_{50} = 0.826\ (\pm 0.149)\lambda + 1.150\ (\pm 0.174)\ I - 3.099\ (\pm 0.241).$
$(r = 0.966 \qquad F = 132.37 \qquad n = 22\ ).$

(The dominant effect of the I term should be borne in mind (Fig. 6).

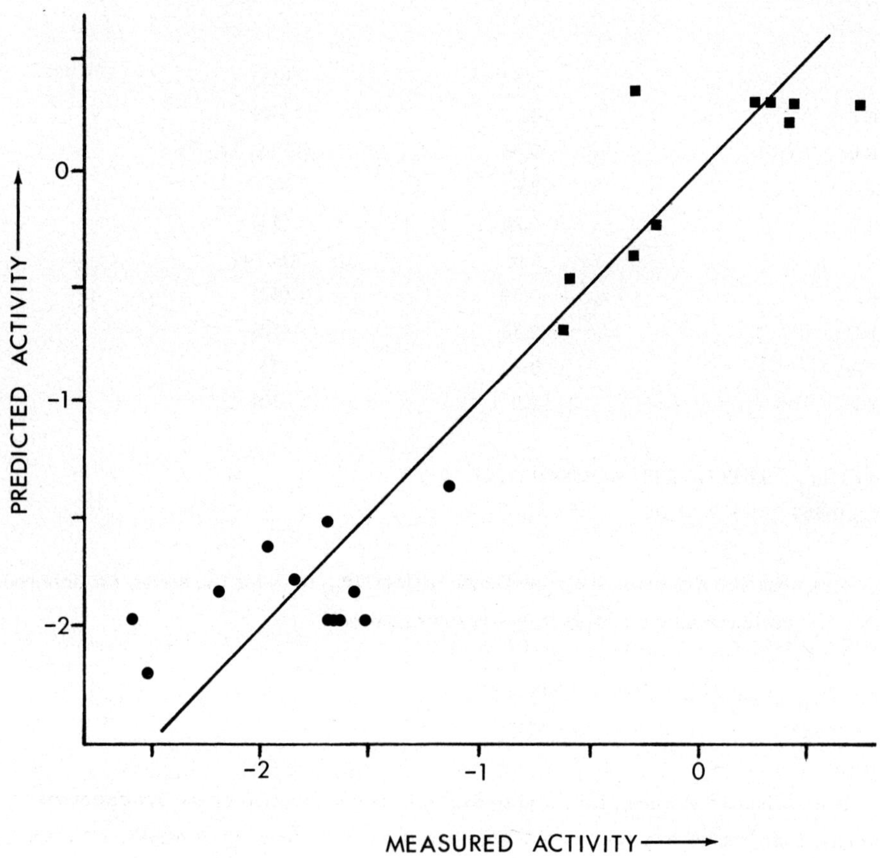


**Figure 6** Predicted versus measured E.coli enzyme activity for 3-X compounds (●) and 3,4-dimethoxy, 5-X (■) compounds (log $1/I_{50}$) .

As larger 3-substituents are considered, the difficulties of predicting conformation, or any property dependent on conformation, become considerable. The possibilities for a substituent to make specific interactions elsewhere on the receptor multiply with increasing length and a corresponding increase in the locus of the end of the chain. To probe these "outer space" effects, further points of reference would be necessary.

CONCLUSIONS

Some facets have been described of an attempt to identify 3-substituent properties associated with high potency as an inhibitor of E.coli DHFR accompanied by relatively little effect on Rat Liver DHFR within the series:-

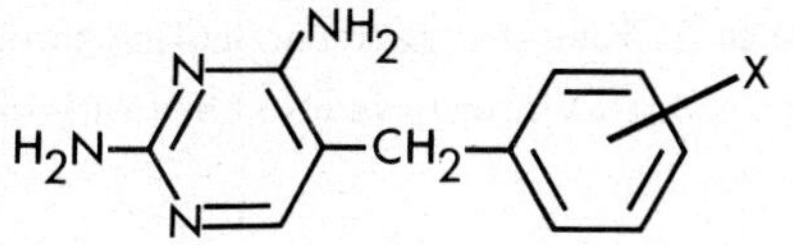

$NH_2$ / N / $H_2N$ / N / $CH_2$ / X

Activity against rat liver DHFR was associated with hydrophobicity at the 3-position. For E.coli DHFR, a tentative relationship with $MR_3$ has been refined, using a steric parameter based on the Verloop STERIMOL approach. An important feature of this treatment is that activity is associated with a specific conformational property of the 3-position and that the 4-substituent consequently contributes to binding, it is suggested, largely through its effect on the conformation of neighbouring substituents.

This "association" was tested using an approach based on Verloop's STERIMOL. Although a static approximation to a dynamic situation, the data were sufficiently well explained to confirm the potential value of undertaking comprehensive calculations of substituent conformation.

An approach which is based on actual biological measurements and careful physicochemical description of a series of compounds, is an attractive and rewarding way of understanding the properties of drug-receptor interactions. Unlike the structurally based molecular modelling approach to which it is complementary, QSAR provides an extremely detailed view of the properties of fractions of the receptor. However, since variation in biological activity associated with changes involving these fractions is the basis of QSAR, then they must by definition be of high relevance.

Finally, a general point must be made, which is equally applicable to QSAR whether it is applied to transport or receptor binding: The approach is, in the limit, simply a formalisation and quantification of the fundamental intuitive approach of the Medicinal Chemist. Perhaps the most immediately relevant example of this, is trimethoprim itself, which was developed along classical lines and yet in itself holds so much of the essential key to physicochemical criteria for the series. The concept of the hydrophilic meta methoxy groups, their conformations inextricably bound up with the para methoxy substituent, represents an extraordinarily effective fulfilment of the criteria for selective potency which have been subsequently identified.

## ACKNOWLEDGEMENTS

The authors are indebted to Miss E. Rahr for her contribution throughout this work. Discussions with Dr. S. Daluge and Dr. J. G. Vinter have also been very much appreciated.

REFERENCES


1. B. Roth, E. A. Falco, G. H. Hitchings and S. R. M. Bushby, J. Med. Pharm. Chem. 5 (1962) 1103-1123.
2. G. H. Hitchings and S. R. M. Bushby, in 5th Internat. Congress of Biochem, Moscow (1961) 165.
3. J. J. Burchall and G. H. Hitchings, Mol. Pharmacol. 1 (1965) 126-136.
4. C. Silipo and C. Hansch, J. Am. Chem. Soc. 97 (1975) 6849-6861.
5. C. Hansch, C. Silipo and E. E. Steller, J. Pharm. Sci. 64 (1975) 1186-1191.
6. J. Y. Fukunaga, C. Hansch and E. E. Steller, J. Med. Chem. 19 (1976) 605-611.
7. C. Hansch, J. Y. Fukunaga, P.Y.C. Jow and J. B. Hynes, J. Med. Chem. 20 (1977) 96-102.
8. S. W. Dietrich, R. N. Smith, J. Y. Fukunaga, M. Olney and C. Hansch, Arch. Biochem. Biophys. 194 (1979) 600-611.
9. S. W. Dietrich, R. N. Smith, S. Brendler and C. Hansch, Arch. Biochem. Biophys. 194 (1979) 612-619.
10. J. M. Blaney, S. W. Dietrich, M. A. Reynolds and C. Hansch, J. Med. Chem. 22 (1979) 614-617.
11. S. W. Dietrich, J. M. Blaney, M. A. Reynolds, P.Y.C. Jow and C. Hansch, J. Med. Chem. 23 (1980) 1205-1212.
12. R-L. Li, S. W. Dietrich and C. Hansch, J. Med. Chem. 24 (1981) 538-544.
13. E. A. Falco, S. DuBreuil and G. H. Hitchings, J. Am. Chem. Soc. 73 (1951) 3758-3762.
14. G. H. Hitchings, J. J. Burchall and R. Ferone, Proc. Int. Pharmacol. Meeting, 3rd, 5 (1966) 3-18.
15. D. Maytum, unpublished.
16. B. Roth, J. Z. Strelitz and B. S. Rauckman, J. Med. Chem. 23 (1980) 379-384.
17. D. P. Baccanari, A. Phillips, S. Smith, D. Sinski and J. J. Burchall, Biochemistry 14 (1975) 5267.
18. R. Wootton, R. Cranfield, G. C. Sheppey and P. J. Goodford, J. Med. Chem. 18 (1975) 607-613.
19. F. E. Norrington, R. M. Hyde. S. G. Williams and R. Wootton, J. Med. Chem. 18 (1975) 604-607.
20. C. G. Swain and E. C. Lupton Jnr. J. Am. Chem. Soc. 90 (1968) 4328.
21. T. Fujita, J. Iwasa and C. Hansch, J. Am. Chem. Soc. 86 (1964) 5175.
22. J. Burscu, unpublished
23. P. Stenbuck, R. Baltzly and M. Hood, J. Org. Chem. 28 (1963) 1983.
24. P. Stenbuck, unpublished.
25. B. Roth and B. S. Rauckman, to be published.
26. R. M. Hyde, J. Med. Chem. 18 (1975) 231-233.
27. H. Kubinyi, J. Med. Chem. 20 (1977) 625-629.
28. B. Roth, E. Aig, B.S. Rauckman, J.Z. Strelitz, A.P. Phillips, F. Ferone, S.R.M. Bushby and C.W. Sigel, J. Med. Chem. 24 (1981) (In press).
29. A Verloop, W. Hoogenstraaten and J. Tipker, in E. J. Ariens (Ed.), Drug Design, Vol. VII, Academic Press, London, 1976, Ch. 4, pp 165-207.
30. G. C. K. Roberts, in R. Porter and D. W. Fitzsimons (Eds), Molecular Interactions and Activity in Proteins, Ciba Foundation Symposium 60 (1978) pp 89-104.
31. B. Roth, E. Aig and R. Ferone, publication in preparation.
32. B. Roth and M. Y. Tidwell, to be published.
33. S. Daluge and P. Skonezny, to be published.
34. G. Rey-Bellet and R. Reiner, Helv. Chim. Acta 53 (1970) 945-950.

# GENERAL (ROUND TABLE) DISCUSSION: "PERSPECTIVES IN QSAR"

Ample consideration made us decide to abandon a full reporting on the general discussion at the end of the Satellite Symposium QSAR.

We intend, however, to extract from the abundant material a few topics, which are, in our opinion, interesting enough for a rewriting into a paper suited for publication in the Eur. J. Med. Chem.

The four 'satellite' speakers will take full responsibility for this publication.

R.F. REKKER
J.K. SEYDEL
R. FRANKE
R.M. HYDE

# List of symbols used in Q S A R publications

Ar = aromatic ring as chemical substituent

B E = biological effect

B R = biological response

$E_s$ = steric substituent constant (Taft)

f = hydrophobic fragmental constant (Rekker)

F (originally written character) = field effect substituent constant (Swain and Lupton)

$K_m$ = Michaelis - Menten constant

M I C = minimal inhibitory concentration

M R = molecular refractivity

M W = molecular weight

(log) P = (log) partition coefficient (mostly octanol-1 / water)

Q S A R = quantitative structure activity relationship

Q S P R = quantitative structure pharmacokinetic relationship

R (originally written character) = resonance effect substituent constant (Swain and Lupton)

R, $R_1$, $R_2$ ... = various chemical substituents

$R_M$ = chromatographic value, calculated from paper chromatographic procedures

S = electronic substituent constant for inductive effect

S S S = spanned substituent space

$V_W$ = van der Waals' volume

$\pi$ (pi) = hydrophobic substituent constant

$\sigma$ = electronic substituent constant (Hammett)

$\sigma^-$ = electronic substituent constant accounting for intramolecular "through resonance effects"

$\sigma_D$ = electronic substituent constand of the resonance type (D = delocalization, Charton)

$\sigma^*$ = polar electronic substituent constant for substituent on aliphatic carbon atom (Taft)

$\sigma'_R$ = electronic substituent constant corrected for inductive effects (Taft)

## Statistical symbols

F = variance ratio

n = number of data points

r, R = correlation coefficient

s = standard deviation

t = Student's test value

SUBJECT INDEX